Assessment made Incredibly Easy!®

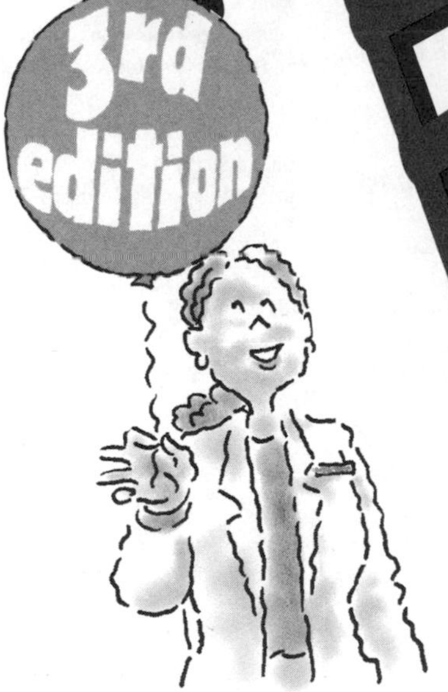

3rd edition

LIPPINCOTT WILLIAMS & WILKINS
A **Wolters Kluwer** Company
Philadelphia • Baltimore • New York • London
Buenos Aires • Hong Kong • Sydney • Tokyo

Staff

Executive Publisher
Judith A. Schilling McCann, RN, MSN

Editorial Director
David Moreau

Clinical Director
Joan M. Robinson, RN, MSN

Senior Art Director
Arlene Putterman

Art Director
Mary Ludwicki

Editorial Project Manager
Jaime Stockslager Buss

Clinical Project Managers
Beverly Ann Tscheschlog, RN, BS; Jana L. Sciarra, RN, MSN, CRNP

Editors
Dave Beverage, Brenna H. Mayer, Liz Schaeffer, Gale Thompson

Copy Editors
Kimberly Bilotta (supervisor), Scotti Cohn, Shana Harrington, Lisa Stockslager, Pamela Wingrod

Designer
Lynn Foulk

Illustrator
Bot Roda

Digital Composition Services
Diane Paluba (manager), Joyce Rossi Biletz

Manufacturing
Patricia K. Dorshaw (director), Beth J. Welsh

Editorial Assistants
Megan L. Aldinger, Karen J. Kirk, Linda K. Ruhf

Indexer
Barbara Hodgson

Photo credits
Squamous cell carcinoma, Psoriasis: Reprinted with permission from Bickley, L.S. *Bates' Guide to Physical Examination and History Taking,* 8th ed. Philadelphia: Lippincott Williams & Wilkins, 2003.
Malignant melanoma: Courtesy of The American Cancer Society; American Academy of Dermatology.
Kaposi's sarcoma: From Sanders, C.V. & Nesbitt, L.T., Jr. *The Skin and Infection: A Color Atlas and Text.* Baltimore: Williams and Wilkins, 1995.
Telangiectasia: From Willis, M.C., CMA-AC. *Medical Terminology: A Programmed Learning Approach to the Language of Health Care.* Baltimore: Lippincott Williams & Wilkins. 2002.
Basal cell carcinoma, Candidiasis, Contact dermatitis, Eczema, Herpes zoster, Impetigo, Systemic lupus erythematosus, Tinea corporis, Urticaria: Goodheart, H.P., M.D. *Goodheart's Photoguide of Common Skin Disorders,* 2nd ed. Philadelphia: Lippincott Williams & Wilkins, 2003.
Scabies, Vitiligo: Stedman's Medical Dictionary, 27th ed. Philadelphia: Lippincott Williams & Wilkins, 2000.

The clinical treatments described and recommended in this publication are based on research and consultation with nursing, medical, and legal authorities. To the best of our knowledge, these procedures reflect currently accepted practice. Nevertheless, they can't be considered absolute and universal recommendations. For individual applications, all recommendations must be considered in light of the patient's clinical condition and, before administration of new or infrequently used drugs, in light of the latest package-insert information. The authors and publisher disclaim any responsibility for any adverse effects resulting from the suggested procedures, from any undetected errors, or from the reader's misunderstanding of the text.

ASMTMIE3—D N O S A J J M A M F J
07 06 05 10 9 8 7 6 5 4 3 2 1

Library of Congress Cataloging-in-Publication Data

Assessment made incredibly easy.— 3rd ed.
p. ; cm.
Includes bibliographical references and index.
1. Nursing assessment—Handbooks, manuals, etc. I. Lippincott Williams & Wilkins.
[DNLM: 1. Nursing Assessment—methods—Handbooks. 2. Physical Examination—methods—Handbooks. WY 49 A846 2005]

RT48.A876 2005
616.07'54—dc22
ISBN 1-58255-391-2 (alk. paper) 2004023256

Contents

Contributors and consultants

Deborah A. Andris, RN,CS, MSN, APNP
Nurse Practitioner
Bariatric Surgery Program
Medical College of Wisconsin
Milwaukee

Jemma Bailey-Kunte, APRN-BC, MS, FNP
Clinical Lecturer
Binghamton (N.Y.) University
Nurse Practitioner
Lourdes Hospital
Binghamton

Cheryl A. Bean, APRN,BC, DSN, ANP, AOCN
Associate Professor
Indiana University School of Nursing
Indianapolis

Natalie Burkhalter, RN, MSN, ACNP, CS, FNP
Associate Professor
Texas A&M International University
Laredo

Shelba Durston, RN, MSN, CCRN
Nursing Instructor
San Joaquin Delta College
Stockton, Calif.
Staff Nurse
San Joaquin General Hospital
French Camp, Calif.

Tamara D. Espejo, RN, MS
Registered Nurse and Clinical Educator
Aurora Behavioral Healthcare-Charter Oak
Covina, Calif.

Michelle L. Foley, RN,C, MA
Director of Nursing Education
Charles E. Gregory School of Nursing
Raritan Bay Medical Center
Perth Amboy, N.J.

Catherine B. Holland, RN, PhD, ANP, APRN,BC, CNS
Associate Professor
Southeastern Louisiana University
Baton Rouge

Julia Anne Isen, RN, MS, FNP-C
Nurse Practitioner—Internal Medicine
Veterans Administration Medical Center
San Francisco
Assistant Clinical Professor
School of Nursing
University of California at San Francisco

Nancy Banfield Johnson, RN, MSN, ANP (INACTIVE)
Nurse-Manager
Kendal at Ithaca (N.Y.)

Gary R. Jones, MSN, CNS, FNP
ARNP, Disease Management Program
Mercy Health Center
Fort Scott, Kans.

Vanessa C. Kramasz, RN, MSN, FNP-C
Nursing Faculty & Family Nurse Practitioner
Gateway Technical College
Kenosha, Wis.

Priscilla A. Lee, MN, FNP
Instructor in Nursing
Moorpark (Calif.) College

Susan Luck, RN, MS, CCN
Director of Nutrition
Biodoron Immunology Center
Hollywood, Fla.

Ann S. McQueen, RNC, MSN, CRNP
Family Nurse Practitioner
Healthlink Medical Center
Southampton, Pa.

Dale O'Donnell, RN, BSN
Administrator Community Surgery Center
Community Hospital
Munster, Ind.

William J. Pawlyshyn, RN, MS, MN, APRN,BC
Nurse Practitioner Consultant
New England Geriatrics
West Springfield, Mass.

Catherine Pence, RN, MSN, CCRN
Assistant Professor
Good Samaritan College of Nursing
Cincinnati

Abby Plambeck, RN, BSN
Freelance Writer
Milwaukee, Wis.

Theresa Pulvano, RN, BSN
Nursing Educator
Ocean County Vocational Technical School
Lakehurst, N.J.

Monica Narvaez Ramirez, RN, MSN
Faculty
University of the Incarnate Word
San Antonio, Tex.

Regina Reed, MSN, FNP
Associate Professor
Washington State Community College
Marrietta, Ohio

Foreword

For several years, I've taught health assessment courses to prelicensure registered nursing students and experienced registered nurses in graduate nursing studies or continuing education courses. It has always been a challenge to select a text that provides a strong introduction to health assessment for the prelicensure nursing student yet also offers a solid reference for seasoned clinicians to use for refreshing or updating their assessment techniques. To be frank, I did not think that any one text could help these varied learners meet their educational needs without being several hundred pages in length, excessively detailed, and extraordinarily monotonous. I am pleased to report, however, that *Assessment Made Incredibly Easy*, Third Edition, offers such opportunities for new and seasoned nurse clinicians alike.

The third edition of *Assessment Made Incredibly Easy* builds on the unique user-friendly format found in previous editions. The book is divided into two main sections. Part I emphasizes the assessment elements that are often completed at the beginning of a comprehensive health assessment or that warrant understanding prior to conducting a head-to-toe physical examination: the health history; fundamental physical assessment techniques, which includes a definition of the generic physical examination techniques; nutritional assessment; and mental health assessment. Part II guides the reader through an objective assessment of the body systems. Each chapter contains learning objectives, a quick-review summary of essential concepts, and a quiz to gauge understanding. Finally, the book includes a section called *Practice makes perfect* with comprehensive NCLEX-style question-and-answer exercises, including alternate-format questions, that put your assessment knowledge to the test.

Throughout the book, hundreds of illustrations and photographs help you to hone your clinical assessment skills. What's more, text-specific logos highlight critical information:

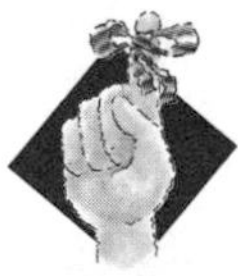

Memory jogger helps the reader remember important points.

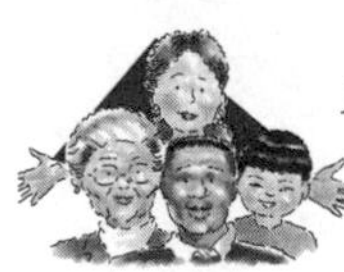

Bridging the gap explains cultural variables that may influence the health assessment.

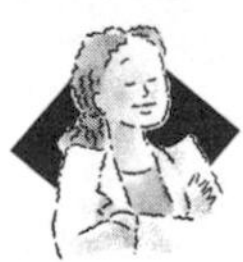

Peak technique illustrates and describes the best ways to perform specific physical examination techniques.

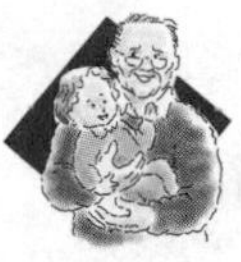

Ages and stages pinpoints age-related variations in assessment findings.

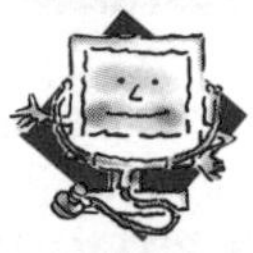

Interpretation station provides surefire guidelines for interpreting assessment findings quickly and easily.

With a dash of strategically placed levity, *Assessment Made Incredibly Easy,* Third Edition, makes the challenge of understanding such a sizable amount of information less daunting. This one-of-a-kind health assessment text is sure to be invaluable to a wide audience of nurses studying or working in a variety of health settings.

JoAnne M. Saxe, RN, MS, ANP,BC
Clinical Professor
Director, Adult Nurse Practitioner Program
University of California, San Francisco
School of Nursing, Department of Community Health Systems

Part I Beginning the assessment

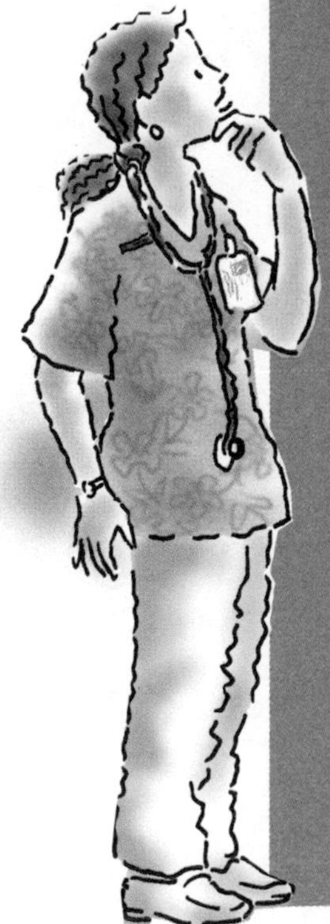

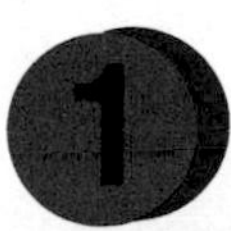

Health history

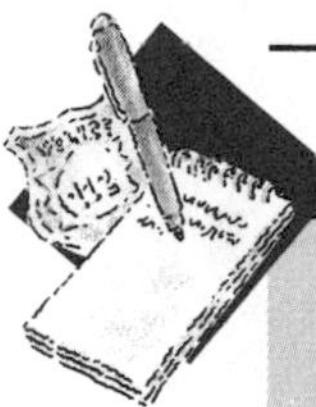

Just the facts

In this chapter, you'll learn:

- reasons for performing a health history
- techniques for communicating effectively during a health history assessment
- essential steps in a complete health history
- questions specific to each step of a health history.

A look at the health history

Knowing how to complete an accurate assessment — from taking the health history to performing the physical examination — can help you uncover significant problems and make an appropriate care plan.

Any assessment involves collecting two kinds of data: objective and subjective. *Objective data* are obtained through observation and are verifiable. For instance, a red, swollen arm in a patient who's complaining of arm pain is an example of data that can be seen and verified by someone other than the patient. *Subjective data* can't be verified by anyone other than the patient; they're gathered solely from the patient's own account — for example, "My head hurts" or "I have trouble sleeping at night."

Here's a way to remember the two types of data: you "observe" objective data, whereas only the "subject" provides subjective data.

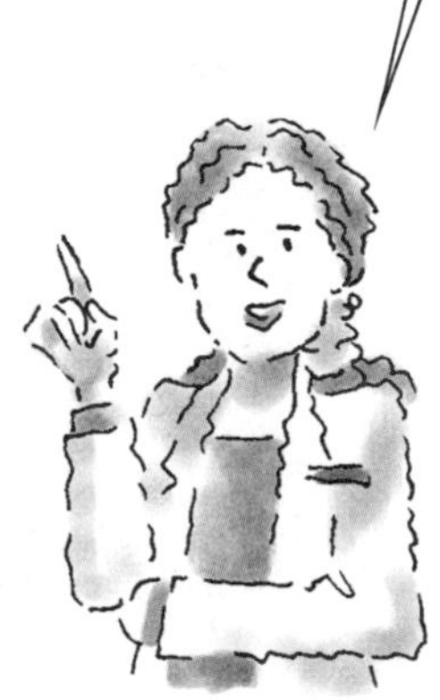

Exploring past and present

You'll use a health history to gather subjective data about the patient and explore past and present problems. To begin, ask the patient about his general physical and emotional health; then ask him about specific body systems and structures.

Skills for getting the scoop

Keep in mind that the accuracy and completeness of your patient's answers largely depend on your skill as an interviewer. Therefore, before you start asking questions, review the following communication guidelines.

Beginning the interview

To make the most of your patient interview, before you begin, you'll need to create an environment in which the patient feels comfortable. During the interview, you'll want to use various communication strategies to make sure you communicate effectively.

Create the proper environment

Before asking your first question, try to establish a rapport with the patient and explain what you'll cover during the interview. Consider the following guidelines when selecting a location for the interview.

Settling in

- Choose a quiet, private, well-lit interview setting. Such a setting makes it easier for you and your patient to interact and helps the patient feel more at ease.
- Make sure that the patient is comfortable. Sit facing him, 3′ to 4′ (1 to 1.5 m) away.
- Introduce yourself and explain that the purpose of the health history and assessment is to identify key problems and gather information to aid in planning care.
- Reassure the patient that everything he says will be kept confidential.
- Tell the patient how long the interview will last and ask him what he expects from the interview.
- Use touch sparingly. Many people aren't comfortable with strangers hugging, patting, or touching them.

Take a moment to set the stage. A supportive, encouraging approach will make your patient much more forthcoming and will enable you to provide optimal care.

Watch what you say

- Assess the patient to see if language barriers exist. For example, does he speak and understand English? Can he hear you? (See *Overcoming interview obstacles.*)
- Speak slowly and clearly, using easy-to-understand language. Avoid using medical terms and jargon.
- Address the patient by a formal name such as "Mr. Jones." Don't call him by his first name unless he asks you to. Avoid using terms of endearment, such as "honey" or "sweetie." Treating the patient with respect encourages him to trust you and provide more accurate and complete information.

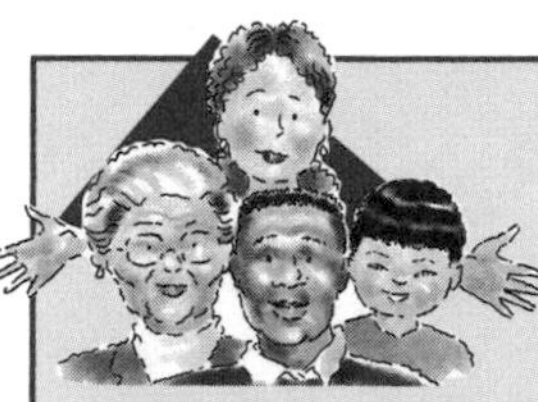

Bridging the gap

Overcoming interview obstacles

With a little creativity, you can overcome barriers to interviewing. For example, if a patient doesn't speak English, your facility may have a bank of interpreters you can call on for help. A trained medical interpreter—one who is familiar with medical terminology, knows interpreting techniques, and understands the patient's rights—would be ideal. Be sure to tell the interpreter to translate the patient's speech verbatim.

Avoid using one of the patient's family members or friends as an interpreter. Doing so violates the patient's right to confidentiality.

Breaking the sound barrier

Is your patient hearing impaired? You can overcome this barrier, too. First, make sure the light is bright enough for him to see your lips move. Then face him and speak slowly and clearly. If necessary, have the patient use an assistive device, such as a hearing aid or an amplifier. If the patient uses sign language, see if your facility has a sign-language interpreter.

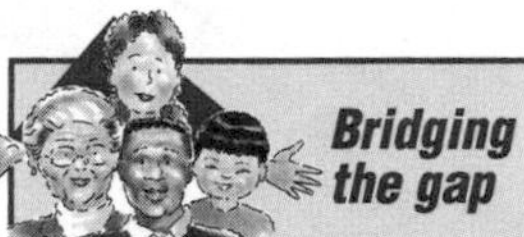

Bridging the gap

Overcoming cultural barriers

To maintain a good relationship with your patient, remember that his cultural behaviors and beliefs may differ from your own. For example, most people in the United States make eye contact when talking with others. However, people with different cultural backgrounds—including Native Americans, Asians, and people from Arabic-speaking countries—may find eye contact disrespectful or aggressive. Be aware of these differences and respond appropriately.

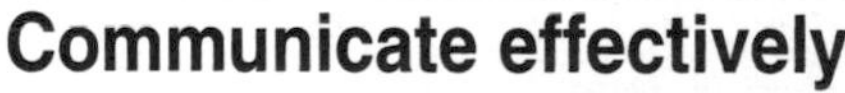

Communicate effectively

Realize that you and the patient communicate nonverbally as well as verbally. Being aware of these forms of communication will aid you in the interview process.

Nonverbal communication strategies

To make the most of nonverbal communication, follow these guidelines:

- Listen attentively and make eye contact frequently. (See *Overcoming cultural barriers.*)
- Use reassuring gestures, such as nodding your head, to encourage the patient to keep talking.
- Watch for nonverbal clues that indicate the patient is uncomfortable or unsure about how to answer a question. For example, he might lower his voice or glance around uneasily.
- Be aware of your own nonverbal behaviors that might cause the patient to stop talking or become defensive. For example, if you cross your arms, you might appear closed off from him. If you stand while he's sitting, you might appear superior. If you glance at your watch, you might appear to be bored or rushed, which could keep the patient from answering questions completely.
- Observe the patient closely to see if he understands each question. If he doesn't appear to understand, repeat the question using different words or familiar examples. For instance, instead of ask-

ing, "Do you have respiratory difficulty after exercising?" ask, "Do you have to sit down after walking around the block?"

Verbal communication strategies

Verbal communication strategies range from alternating between open-ended and closed questions to employing such techniques as silence, facilitation, confirmation, reflection, clarification, summary, and conclusion.

An open...

Asking open-ended questions such as "How did you fall?" lets the patient respond more freely. His response may provide answers to many other questions. For instance, from the patient's answer, you might learn that he has previously fallen, that he was unsteady on his feet before he fell, and that he fell just before eating dinner. Armed with this information, you might deduce that the patient had a syncopal episode caused by hypoglycemia.

...and shut case

You may also choose to ask closed questions. Although these questions are unlikely to provide extra information, they may encourage the patient to give clear, concise feedback. (See *Two ways to ask.*)

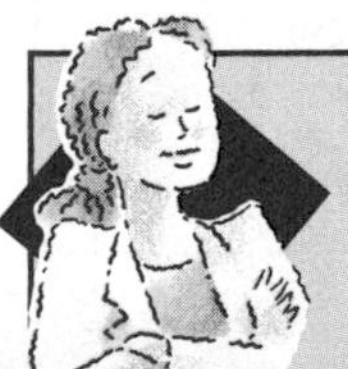

Peak technique

Two ways to ask

You can ask your patient two types of questions: open-ended and closed.

Open-ended questions

Open-ended questions require the patient to express feelings, opinions, and ideas. They also help you gather more information than closed questions. Open-ended questions facilitate nurse-patient rapport because they show that you're interested in what the patient has to say. Examples of such questions include:

- What caused you to come to the hospital tonight?
- How would you describe the problems you're having with your breathing?
- What lung problems, if any, do other members of your family have?

Closed questions

Closed questions elicit yes-or-no answers or one- to two-word responses. They limit the development of nurse-patient rapport. Closed questions can help you "zoom in" on specific points, but they don't provide the patient the opportunity to elaborate. Examples of closed questions include:

- Do you ever get short of breath?
- Are you the only one in your family with lung problems?

Silence is golden

Another technique is to allow moments of *silence* during the interview. Besides encouraging the patient to continue talking, silence also gives you a chance to assess his ability to organize thoughts. You may find this technique difficult (most people are uncomfortable with silence), but the more often you use it, the more comfortable you'll become.

Give 'em a boost

Using such phrases as "please continue," "go on," and even "uh-huh" encourages the patient to continue with his story. Known as *facilitation*, this technique shows him that you're interested in what he's saying.

Confirmation conversation

Confirmation helps ensure that you and the patient are on the same track. For example, you might say, "If I understand you correctly, you said..." and then repeat the information the patient gave. This technique helps to clear misconceptions that you or the patient might have.

Check and reflect

Try using *reflection* (repeating something the patient has just said) to help you obtain more-specific information. For example, a patient with a stomachache might say, "I know I have an ulcer." If so, you can repeat the statement as a question, "You know you have an ulcer?" Then the patient might say, "Yes. I had one before and the pain is the same."

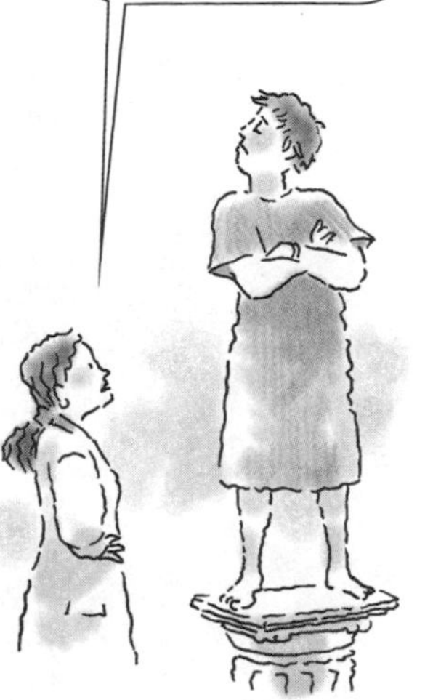

Clear skies

When information is vague or confusing, use the technique of *clarification*. For example, if your patient says, "I can't stand this," you might respond, "What can't you stand?" or "What do you mean by 'I can't stand this?'" Doing so gives the patient an opportunity to explain his statement.

Put the landing gear down...

Get in the habit of restating the information the patient gave you. Known as *summarization*, this technique ensures that the data you've collected are accurate and complete. Summarization also signals that the interview is about to end.

...and come in for a safe landing

Signal the patient when you're ready to conclude the interview. Known as *conclusion*, this signal gives him the opportunity to gather his thoughts and make any pertinent final statements. You can do this by saying, "I think I have all the information I need now. Is there anything you would like to add?"

Reviewing general health

You've just learned how to ask questions. Now it's time to learn the right questions to ask when reviewing the patient's general physical and emotional health. Also, remember to maintain a professional attitude throughout this process.

Asking the right questions

A complete health history requires information from each of the following categories, obtained in this order:

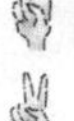 biographic data

 chief complaint

 medical history

 family history

 psychosocial history

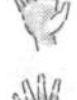 activities of daily living.

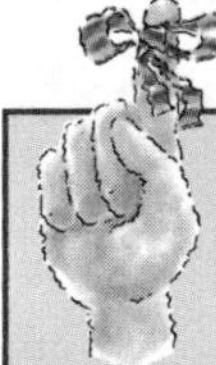

Memory jogger

To remember the categories you should cover in your health history, think: **B**eing **C**omplete **M**akes **F**or **P**roper **A**ssessment:

Biographic data

Chief complaint

Medical history

Family history

Psychosocial history

Activities of daily living.

Biographic data

Start the health history by obtaining biographic information from the patient. Do this first so you don't forget about this information after you become involved in details of the patient's health. Ask the patient for his name, address, telephone number, birth date, age, marital status, religion, and nationality. Find out with whom he lives and get the name and telephone number of a person to contact in case of an emergency.

Also, ask the patient about his health care, including who his primary doctor is and how he gets to the doctor's office. Ask if he has ever been treated for his present problem. Finally, ask if he has advance directives in place. (See *Advance directives*.)

Take a hint

Your patient's answers to basic questions can provide important clues about his personality, medical problems, and reliability. If he can't furnish accurate information, ask him for the name of a friend or relative who can. Document the source of the information as well as whether an interpreter was necessary.

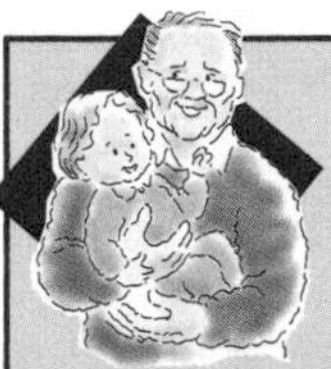

Ages and stages

Advance directives

The Patient Self-Determination Act allows patients to prepare advance directives—written documents that state their wishes regarding health care in the event they become incapacitated or unable to make decisions. Elderly patients in particular may have interest in advance directives because they tend to be concerned with end-of-life issues.

Direction for directives

If a patient doesn't have an advance directive in place, the health care facility must provide him with information about it, including how to establish one.

An advance directive may include:
• name of the person authorized by the patient to make medical decisions if the patient can no longer do so
• specific medical treatment the patient wants or doesn't want
• instructions regarding pain medication and comfort—specifically, whether the patient wishes to receive certain treatment even if the treatment may hasten his death
• information the patient wants to relay to his loved ones
• name of the patient's primary health care provider
• any other wishes.

Chief complaint

Try to pinpoint why the patient is seeking health care, or his *chief complaint.* Document this information in the patient's exact words to avoid misinterpretation. Ask how and when the symptoms developed, what led the patient to seek medical attention, and how the problem has affected his life and ability to function.

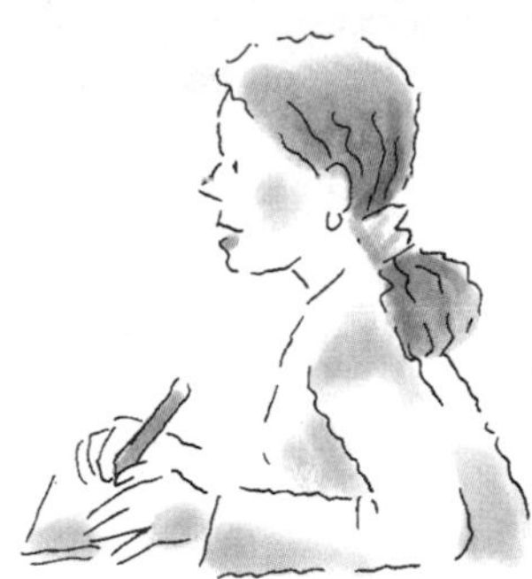

Alphabet soup

To ensure that you don't omit pertinent data, use the PQRSTU mnemonic device, which provides a systematic approach to obtaining information. (See *PQRSTU: What's the story?* page 10.)

Medical history

Ask the patient about past and current medical problems, such as hypertension, diabetes, and back pain. Typical questions include:
• Have you ever been hospitalized? If so, when and why?
• What childhood illnesses did you have?
• Are you being treated for any problem? If so, for what reason and who's your doctor?
• Have you ever had surgery? If so, when and why?
• Are you allergic to anything in the environment or to any drugs or foods? If so, what kind of allergic reaction do you have?
• Are you taking medications, including over-the-counter preparations, such as aspirin, vitamins, and cough syrup? If so, how much do you take and how often do you take it? Do you use home remedies such as homemade ointments? Do you use herbal prepara-

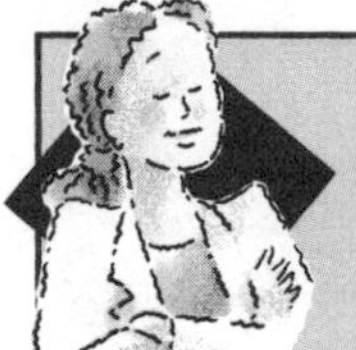

Peak technique

PQRSTU: What's the story?

Use the PQRSTU mnemonic device to fully explore your patient's chief complaint. When you ask the questions below, you'll encourage him to describe his symptoms in greater detail.

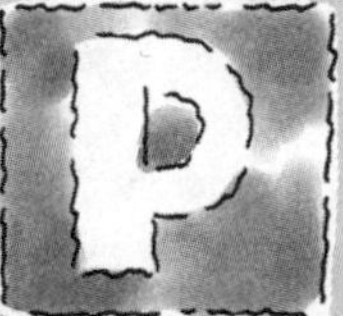

Provocative or palliative
Ask the patient:
- What provokes or relieves the symptom?
- Do stress, anger, certain physical positions, or other factors trigger the symptom?
- What makes the symptom worsen or subside?

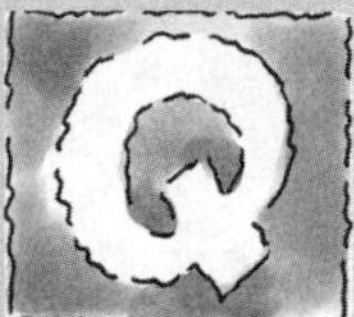

Quality or quantity
Ask the patient:
- What does the symptom feel like, look like, or sound like?
- Are you having the symptom right now? If so, is it more or less severe than usual?
- To what degree does the symptom affect your normal activities?

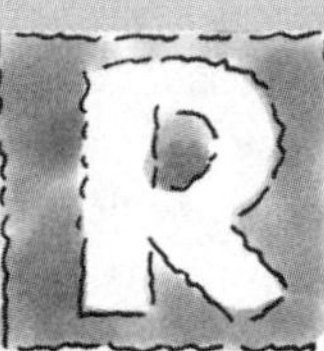

Region or radiation
Ask the patient:
- Where in the body does the symptom occur?
- Does the symptom appear in other regions? If so, where?

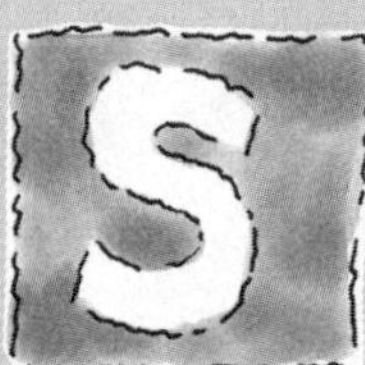

Severity
Ask the patient:
- How severe is the symptom? How would you rate it on a scale of 1 to 10, with 10 being the most severe?
- Does the symptom seem to be diminishing, intensifying, or staying the same?

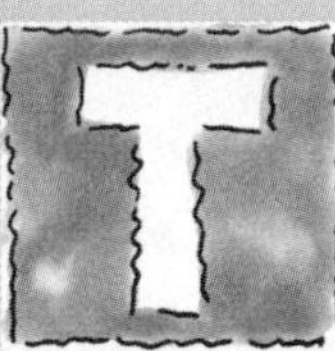

Timing
Ask the patient:
- When did the symptom begin?
- Was the onset sudden or gradual?
- How often does the symptom occur?
- How long does the symptom last?

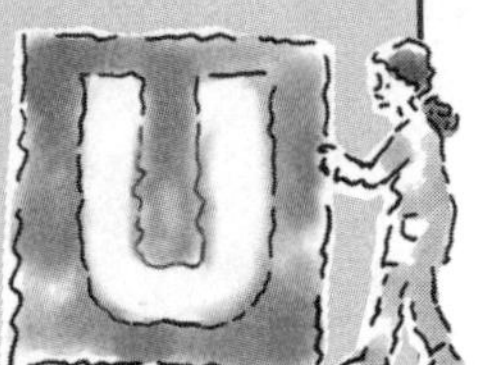

Understanding
Ask the patient:
- What do you think caused the symptom?
- How do you feel about the symptom? Do you have fears associated with it?
- How is the symptom affecting your life?
- What are your expectations of the health care team?

tions or take dietary supplements? Do you use other alternative or complementary therapies, such as acupuncture, therapeutic massage, or chiropractic?

Family history

Questioning the patient about his family's health is a good way to uncover his risk of having certain illnesses. Typical questions include:

- Are your mother, father, and siblings living? If not, how old were they when they died? What were the causes of their deaths?

• If they're alive, do they have diabetes, high blood pressure, heart disease, asthma, cancer, sickle cell anemia, hemophilia, cataracts, glaucoma, or other illnesses?

Want to know if a patient is at risk for certain illnesses? Ask about his family's health history.

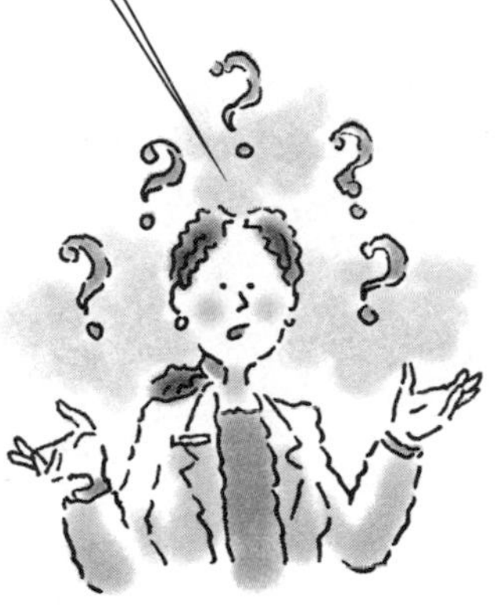

Psychosocial history

Find out how the patient feels about himself, his place in society, and his relationships with others. Ask about his occupation (past and present), education, economic status, and responsibilities. Typical questions include:

• How have you coped with medical or emotional crises in the past? (See *Asking about abuse.*)

• Has your life changed recently? What changes in your personality or behavior have you noticed?

The ties that bind

• How adequate is the emotional support you receive from family and friends?

• How close do you live to health care facilities? Can you get to them easily?

• Do you have health insurance?

• Are you on a fixed income with no extra money for health care?

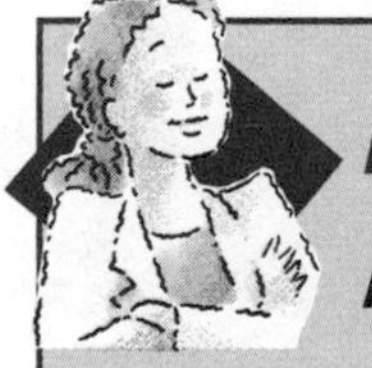

Peak technique

Asking about abuse

Abuse is a tricky subject. Anyone can be a victim of abuse: a boyfriend or girlfriend, a spouse, an elderly patient, a child, or a parent. Also, abuse can come in many forms: physical, psychological, emotional, and sexual. So, when taking a health history, ask two open-ended questions to explore abuse: When do you feel safe at home? When don't you feel safe?

Watch the reaction

Even when you don't immediately suspect an abusive situation, be aware of how your patient reacts to open-ended questions. Is the patient defensive, hostile, confused, or frightened? Assess how he interacts with you and others. Does he seem withdrawn or frightened or show other inappropriate behavior? Keep his reactions in mind when you perform your physical assessment.

Remember, if the patient tells you about any type of abuse, you're obligated to report it. Inform the patient that you must report the incident to local authorities.

Activities of daily living

Find out what's normal for the patient by asking him to describe his typical day. Make sure you ask about the following areas in your assessment.

Diet and elimination

Ask the patient about his appetite, special diets, and food allergies. Can he afford to buy enough food? Who cooks and shops at his house? Ask about the frequency of bowel movements and laxative use.

Exercise and sleep

Ask the patient if he has a special exercise program and, if so, why. Ask him to describe it. Ask how many hours he sleeps at night, what his sleep pattern is like, and whether he feels rested after sleep. Ask him if he has any difficulties with sleep.

You seem a little tired. Are you having any difficulty sleeping?

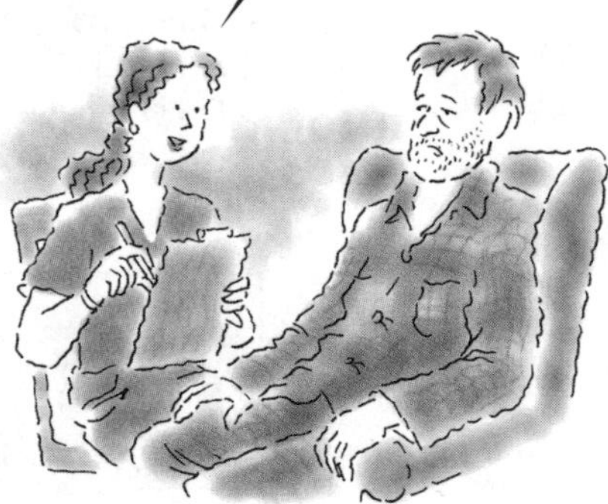

Work and leisure

Ask the patient what he does for a living and what he does during his leisure time. Does he have hobbies?

Use of tobacco, alcohol, and other drugs

Ask the patient if he smokes cigarettes. If so, how many does he smoke each day? Does he drink alcohol? If so, how much each day? Ask if he uses illicit drugs, such as marijuana and cocaine. If so, how often?

Fudging the facts

Patients may understate the amount they drink because of embarrassment. If you're having trouble getting what you believe are honest answers to such questions, you might try overestimating the amount. For example, you might say, "You told me you drink beer. Do you drink about a six-pack per day?" The patient's response might be, "No, I drink about half that."

Religious observances

Ask the patient if he has religious beliefs that affect diet, dress, or health practices. Patients will feel reassured when you make it clear that you understand these points.

Maintaining a professional attitude

Don't let your personal opinions interfere with this part of the assessment. Maintain a professional, neutral approach and don't offer advice. For example, don't suggest that the patient enter a drug rehabilitation program. That type of response puts him on the defensive and he might not answer subsequent questions honestly.

Also, avoid making paternalistic statements, such as, "The doctor knows what's best for you." Such statements make the patient feel inferior and break down communication. Finally, don't use leading questions such as "You don't do drugs, do you?" to get the answer you're hoping for. This type of question, based on your own value system, can make the patient feel guilty and might prevent him from responding honestly.

Reviewing structures and systems

The last part of the health history is a systematic assessment of the patient's body structures and systems. A thorough assessment requires that you follow a process while asking specific questions.

Follow a process

Always start at the top of the head and work your way down the body. This helps keep you from skipping any areas. When questioning an elderly patient, remember that he may have difficulty hearing or communicating. (See *Overcoming communication problems in elderly patients*.)

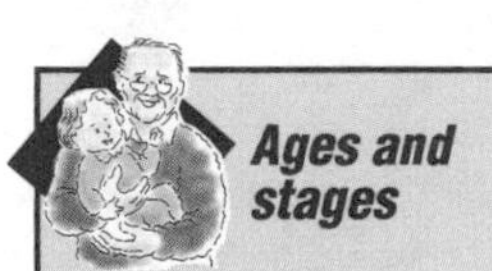

Ages and stages

Overcoming communication problems in elderly patients

An elderly patient might have sensory or memory impairment or a decreased attention span. If your patient is confused or has trouble communicating, you may need to rely on a family member for some or all of the health history.

Ask specific questions

Information gained from a health history forms the basis for your care plan and enables you to distinguish physical changes and devise a holistic approach to treatment. As with other nursing skills, the only way you can improve your interviewing technique is with practice, practice, and more practice. (See *Evaluating a symptom*, page 14.)

Here are some key questions to ask your patient about each body structure and system.

Head first

Do you get headaches? If so, where are they and how painful are they? How often do they occur, and how long do they last? Does anything trigger them, and how do you relieve them? Have you ever had a head injury? Do you have lumps or bumps on your head?

Evaluating a symptom

Your patient is vague in describing his chief complaint. Using your interviewing skills, you discover his problem is related to abdominal distention. Now what? This flowchart will help you decide what to do next, using abdominal distention as the patient's chief complaint.

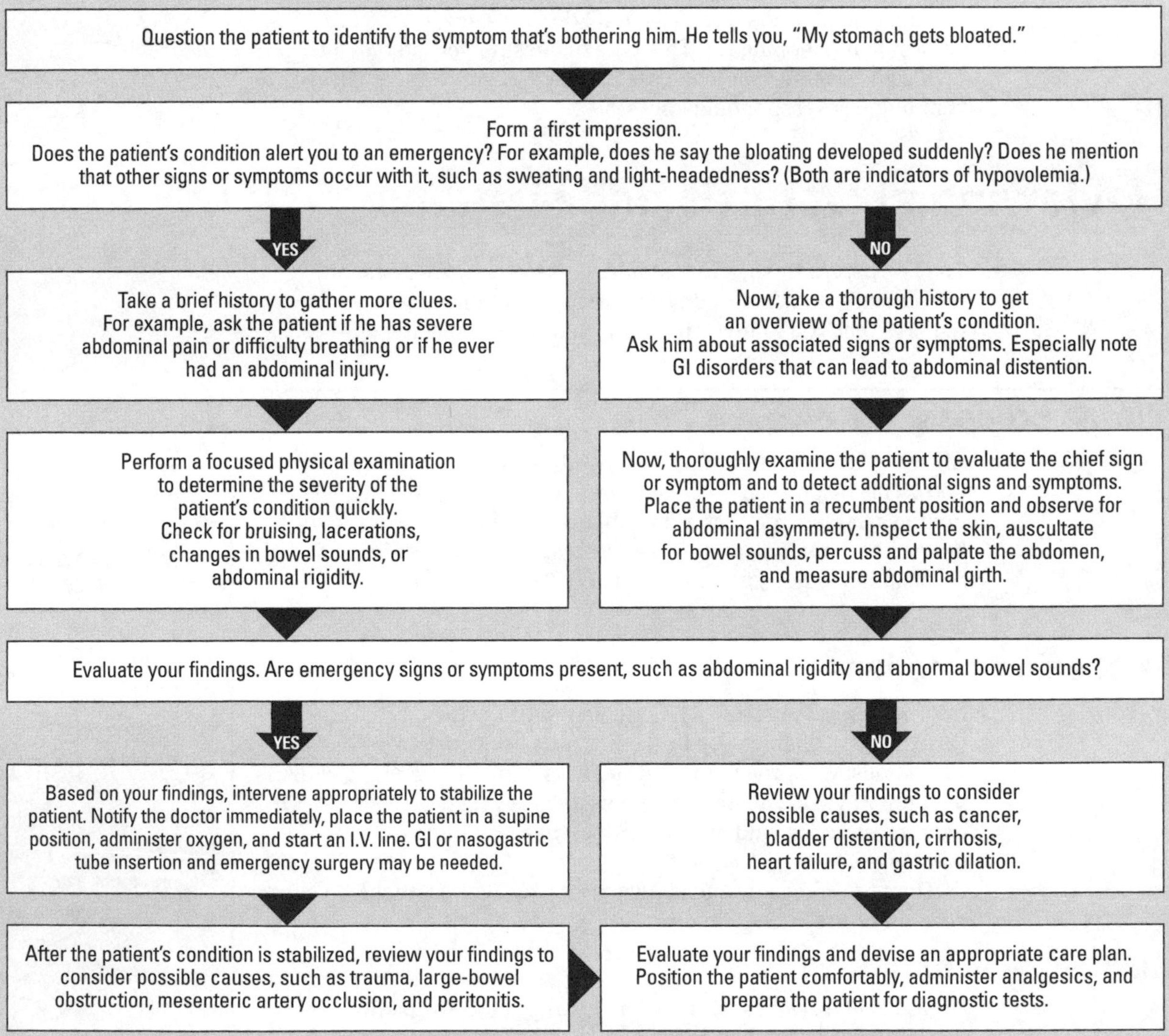

Question the patient to identify the symptom that's bothering him. He tells you, "My stomach gets bloated."

Form a first impression.
Does the patient's condition alert you to an emergency? For example, does he say the bloating developed suddenly? Does he mention that other signs or symptoms occur with it, such as sweating and light-headedness? (Both are indicators of hypovolemia.)

YES

Take a brief history to gather more clues.
For example, ask the patient if he has severe abdominal pain or difficulty breathing or if he ever had an abdominal injury.

Perform a focused physical examination to determine the severity of the patient's condition quickly.
Check for bruising, lacerations, changes in bowel sounds, or abdominal rigidity.

NO

Now, take a thorough history to get an overview of the patient's condition.
Ask him about associated signs or symptoms. Especially note GI disorders that can lead to abdominal distention.

Now, thoroughly examine the patient to evaluate the chief sign or symptom and to detect additional signs and symptoms. Place the patient in a recumbent position and observe for abdominal asymmetry. Inspect the skin, auscultate for bowel sounds, percuss and palpate the abdomen, and measure abdominal girth.

Evaluate your findings. Are emergency signs or symptoms present, such as abdominal rigidity and abnormal bowel sounds?

YES

Based on your findings, intervene appropriately to stabilize the patient. Notify the doctor immediately, place the patient in a supine position, administer oxygen, and start an I.V. line. GI or nasogastric tube insertion and emergency surgery may be needed.

After the patient's condition is stabilized, review your findings to consider possible causes, such as trauma, large-bowel obstruction, mesenteric artery occlusion, and peritonitis.

NO

Review your findings to consider possible causes, such as cancer, bladder distention, cirrhosis, heart failure, and gastric dilation.

Evaluate your findings and devise an appropriate care plan. Position the patient comfortably, administer analgesics, and prepare the patient for diagnostic tests.

Vision quest

When was your last eye examination? Do you wear glasses? Do you have glaucoma, cataracts, or color blindness? Does light bother your eyes? Do you have excessive tearing; blurred vision; double vision; or dry, itchy, burning, inflamed, or swollen eyes?

An earful

Do you have loss of balance, ringing in your ears, deafness, or poor hearing? Have you ever had ear surgery? If so, why and when? Do you wear a hearing aid? Are you having pain, swelling, or discharge from your ears? If so, has this problem occurred before and how frequently?

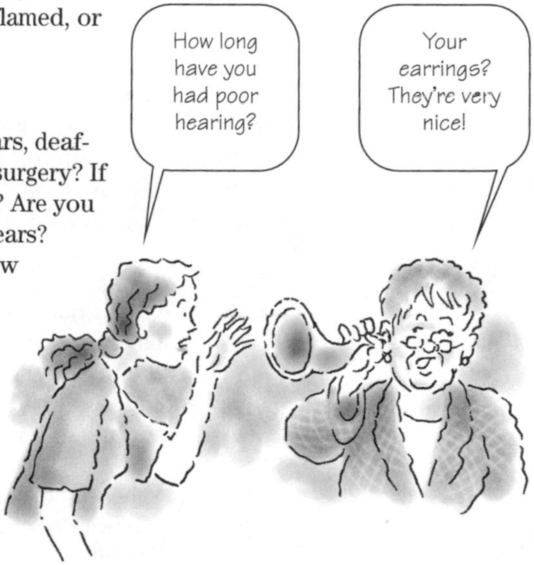

Nose knows

Have you ever had nasal surgery? If so, why and when? Have you ever had sinusitis or nosebleeds? Do you have nasal problems that impair your ability to smell or that cause breathing difficulties, frequent sneezing, or discharge?

Mouth and throat run-through

Do you have mouth sores, a dry mouth, loss of taste, a toothache, or bleeding gums? Do you wear dentures and, if so, do they fit? Do you have a sore throat, fever, or chills? How often do you get a sore throat, and have you seen a doctor for this?

Do you have difficulty swallowing? If so, is the problem with solids or liquids? Is it a constant problem or does it accompany a sore throat or another problem? What, if anything, makes it go away?

Neck check

Do you have swelling, soreness, lack of movement, stiffness, or pain in your neck? If so, did something specific cause it to happen such as too much exercise? How long have you had this symptom? Does anything relieve it or aggravate it?

Respiratory research

Do you have shortness of breath on exertion or while lying in bed? How many pillows do you use at night? Does breathing cause pain or wheezing? Do you have a productive cough? If so, do you cough up blood-tinged sputum? Do you have night sweats?

Have you ever been treated for pneumonia, asthma, emphysema, or frequent respiratory tract infections? Have you ever had a chest X-ray or tuberculin skin test? If so, when and what were the results?

Asking these questions will help you get to the root of the patient's problem.

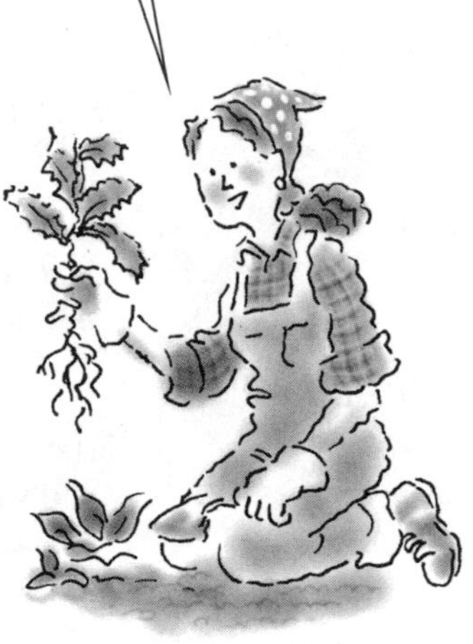

Heart health hunt

Do you have chest pain, palpitations, irregular heartbeat, fast heartbeat, shortness of breath, or a persistent cough? Have you ever had an electrocardiogram? If so, when?

Do you have high blood pressure, peripheral vascular disease, swelling of the ankles and hands, varicose veins, cold extremities, or intermittent pain in your legs?

Breast test

Ask women these questions: Do you perform monthly breast self-examinations? Have you noticed a lump, a change in breast contour, breast pain, or discharge from your nipples? Have you ever had breast cancer? If not, has anyone else in your family had it? Have you ever had a mammogram? When and what were the results?

Ask men these questions: Do you have pain in your breast tissue? Have you noticed lumps or a change in contour?

Stomach symptom search

Have you had nausea, vomiting, loss of appetite, heartburn, abdominal pain, frequent belching, or passing of gas? Have you lost or gained weight recently? How often do you have a bowel movement, and what color, odor, and consistency are your stools? Have you noticed a change in your regular elimination pattern? Do you use laxatives frequently?

Have you had hemorrhoids, rectal bleeding, hernias, gallbladder disease, or liver disease?

GU interview

Do you have urinary problems, such as burning during urination, incontinence, urgency, retention, reduced urinary flow, and dribbling? Do you get up during the night to urinate? If so, how many times? What color is your urine? Have you ever noticed blood in it? Have you ever been treated for kidney stones?

Reproduction review

Ask women these questions: How old were you when you started menstruating? How often do you get your period, and how long does it usually last? Do you have pain or pass clots? If you're postmenopausal, at what age did you stop menstruating? If you're in the transitional stage, what perimenopausal symptoms are you experiencing? Have you ever been pregnant? If so, how many times? What was the method of delivery? How many pregnancies resulted in live births? How many resulted in miscarriages? Have you had an abortion?

What's your method of birth control? Are you involved in a long-term, monogamous relationship? Have you had frequent vaginal infections or a sexually transmitted disease (STD)? When was your last gynecologic examination and Papanicolaou test? What were the results?

Ask men these questions: Do you perform monthly testicular self-examinations? Have you ever had a prostate examination and, if so, when? Have you noticed penile pain, discharge, or lesions or testicular lumps? Which form of birth control do you use? Have you had a vasectomy? Are you involved in a long-term, monogamous relationship? Have you ever had an STD?

Don't forget to ask male patients about testicular self-examinations.

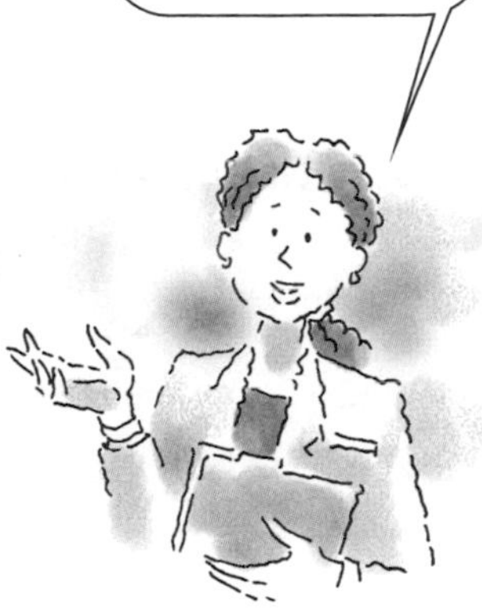

Monitoring muscle

Do you have difficulty walking, sitting, or standing? Are you steady on your feet or do you lose your balance easily? Do you have arthritis, gout, a back injury, muscle weakness, or paralysis?

CNS scrutiny

Have you ever had seizures? Do you ever experience tremors, twitching, numbness, tingling, or loss of sensation in a part of your body? Are you less able to get around than you think you should be? (See *Tips for assessing a severely ill patient.*)

Peak technique

Tips for assessing a severely ill patient

When the patient's condition doesn't allow a full assessment—for instance, if the patient is in severe pain—get as much information as possible from other sources. With a severely ill patient, keep these key points in mind:

- Identify yourself to the patient and his family.
- Stay calm to gain his confidence and allay anxiety.
- Stay on the lookout for important information. For example, if a patient seeks help for a ringing in his ears, don't overlook his casual mention of a periodic "racing heartbeat."
- Avoid jumping to conclusions. Don't assume that the patient's complaint is related to his admitting diagnosis. Use a systematic approach and collect the appropriate information; then draw conclusions.

Endocrine inquiry

Have you been unusually tired lately? Do you feel hungry or thirsty more often than usual? Have you lost weight for unexplained reasons? How well can you tolerate heat or cold? Have you noticed changes in your hair texture or color? Have you been losing hair? Do you take hormone medications?

Circulatory study

Have you ever been diagnosed with anemia or blood abnormalities? Do you bruise easily or become fatigued quickly? Have you ever had a blood transfusion? If so, did you have any type of adverse reaction?

Psychological survey

Do you ever experience mood swings or memory loss? Do you ever feel anxious, depressed, or unable to concentrate? Are you feeling unusually stressed? Do you ever feel unable to cope?

Throughout your initial assessment, be aware of the patient's emotional status. Keep in mind that stress levels and emotional well-being can affect every body system.

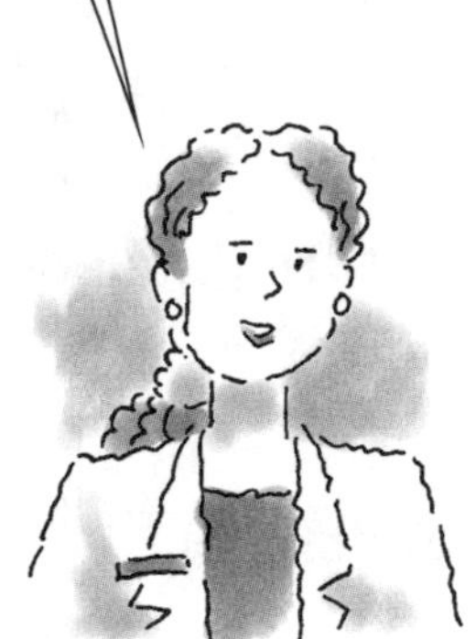

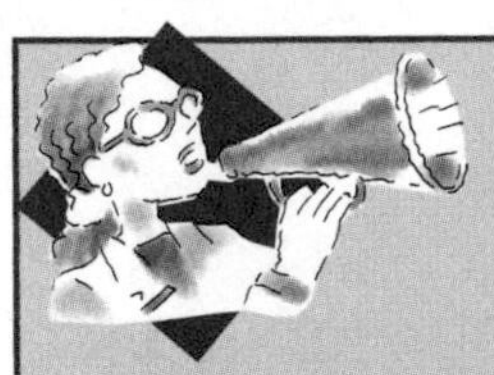

That's a wrap!

Health history review

Obtaining assessment data
- Collect objective data (data that's obtained through observation and is verifiable).
- Collect subjective data (data that can be verified only by the patient).

Patient interview
- Select a quiet, private setting.
- Choose terms carefully and avoid using medical jargon.
- Use appropriate body language.
- Confirm patient statements to avoid misunderstanding.
- Use open-ended questions.

Effective communication
- Use silence effectively.
- Encourage responses.
- Use repetition and reflection to help clarify meaning.
- Use clarification to eliminate misunderstandings.
- Summarize and conclude with "Is there anything else?"

Components of a complete health history
- Biographic data, such as the patient's name, address, birth date, and emergency contact information
- Chief complaint
- Past and current health care
- Health of the patient's family
- Psychosocial history (feelings about self, place in society, and relationships with others)
- Activities of daily living

Review of structures and systems

Head
- Headaches
- Past or present head injury

Health history review *(continued)*

Eyes
- Vision
- Use of glasses or contact lenses
- History of glaucoma, cataracts, color blindness
- Tearing; blurred vision; double vision; dry, itchy, burning, or inflamed eyes

Ears
- Hearing and balance
- History of ear surgery
- Use of hearing aids
- Ear pain or swelling
- Discharge from ears

Nose
- History of nasal surgery
- Breathing or smelling difficulties
- History of sinusitis or nosebleeds

Mouth and throat
- Dentures
- Mouth sores or dryness
- Loss of taste
- Toothache or bleeding gums
- Throat soreness or difficulty swallowing

Neck
- Swelling
- Soreness
- Lack of movement, stiffness, or pain

Respiratory
- Shortness of breath
- Pain or wheezing with breathing
- Cough (productive or nonproductive)
- History of pneumonia, asthma, emphysema, or frequent respiratory tract infections
- Tuberculin skin test or chest X-ray results

Cardiovascular
- Chest pain, palpitations, irregular or fast heartbeat, shortness of breath, persistent cough
- Results of electrocardiogram
- History of high blood pressure, peripheral vascular disease, swelling of the extremities, varicose veins, or intermittent pain in the legs

Breasts
- Women
  - Monthly breast self-examination
  - Lumps, changes in breast contour, pain, discharge from nipples
  - History of breast cancer
  - Results of mammograms
- Men
  - Pain
  - Lumps
  - Change in contour

Gastrointestinal
- Recent weight changes
- Frequency and characteristics of bowel movements
- Laxative use
- Nausea, vomiting, loss of appetite, heartburn, abdominal pain, frequent belching, passing of gas
- Hemorrhoids, rectal bleeding, hernias, gallbladder disease, liver disease

Urinary
- Color of urine
- Nighttime urination
- Burning, incontinence, urgency, retention, reduced urinary flow, or dribbling

(continued)

Health history review *(continued)*

Reproductive
- Women
  - Menstruation and menopause
  - Pregnancies
  - Birth control
  - Papanicolaou test results
  - Vaginal infections
  - STDs
- Men
  - Monthly testicular self-examinations
  - Results of prostate examinations
  - STDs
  - Birth control
  - Penile pain, discharge, or lesions
  - Testicular lumps

Musculoskeletal
- Balance
- Difficulty walking, sitting, or standing
- History of arthritis, gout, back injury, muscle weakness, or paralysis

Neurologic
- Tremors, twitching, numbness, tingling, or loss of sensation
- History of seizures

Endocrine
- Unusual fatigue or tiredness
- Hunger and thirst
- Unexplained weight loss or gain
- Tolerance of heat and cold
- Hair loss or changes in color or texture
- Hormone medications

Hematologic
- History of anemia, blood abnormalities, or blood transfusions
- Fatigue or bruising

Psychological
- Mood swings or memory loss
- Anxiety, depression, or difficulty concentrating
- Stress and coping mechanisms

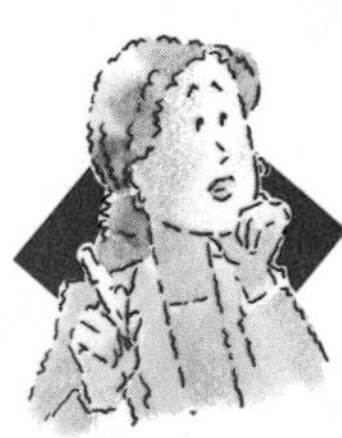

Quick quiz

1. Leading questions may initiate untrue or inaccurate responses because such questions:

A. encourage short or vague answers.
B. require an educational level the patient may not possess.
C. prompt the patient to try to give a particular answer.
D. confuse the patient.

Answer: C. Because of how they're phrased, leading questions may prompt the patient to give the answer you're looking for.

2. When obtaining a health history from a patient, ask first about:

A. family history.
B. his chief complaint.
C. health insurance coverage.
D. biographic data.

Answer: D. Take care of the biographic data first; otherwise, you might get involved in the patient history and forget to ask basic questions.

3. Silence is a communication technique used during an interview to:

A. show respect.
B. change the topic.
C. encourage the patient to continue talking.
D. clarify information.

Answer: C. Silence allows the patient to collect his thoughts and continue to answer your questions.

4. Data are considered subjective if you obtain them from:

A. the patient's verbal account.
B. your observations of the patient's actions.
C. the patient's records.
D. X-ray reports.

Answer: A. Data from the patient's own words are subjective.

5. "If I understand you correctly, you said..." is an example of the interviewing technique:

A. clarification.
B. confirmation.
C. reflection.
D. facilitation.

Answer: B. The phrase is an example of confirmation, a technique that can help clear up misconceptions you or the patient might have.

6. Which of the following questions is considered open-ended?

A. Does your pain last through the night?
B. Have you ever had heart surgery?
C. Do you frequently get headaches?
D. How would you describe your pain?

Answer: D. Open-ended questions require the patient to express feelings, opinions, or ideas. They elicit more than just a simple yes-or-no response.

Scoring

☆☆☆ If you answered all six questions correctly, bravo! You're an intrepid interviewer.

☆☆ If you answered four or five questions correctly, that's cool! You're a hip historian.

☆ If you answered fewer than four questions correctly, that's okay! This is only the first chapter. We have many more questions for you.

2

Fundamental physical assessment techniques

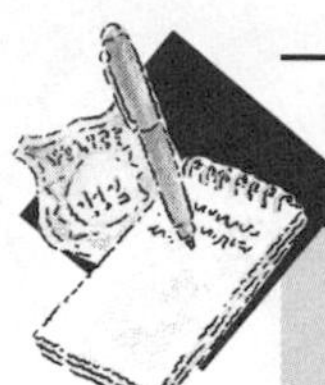

Just the facts

In this chapter, you'll learn:

- types of equipment used in an assessment and the proper ways to use them
- skills for performing an initial observation of the patient
- ways to prepare your patient for an assessment
- techniques for performing inspection, palpation, percussion, and auscultation.

A look at physical assessment

During the physical assessment you'll use all of your senses and a systematic approach to collect information about your patient's health. As you proceed through the physical examination, you can also teach your patient about his body. For instance, you can explain how to perform a testicular self-examination or why the patient should monitor the appearance of a mole. More than anything else, successful assessment requires critical thinking. How does one finding fit in the big picture? An initial assessment guides your whole care plan.

Performing a physical assessment gives me the opportunity to use critical thinking.

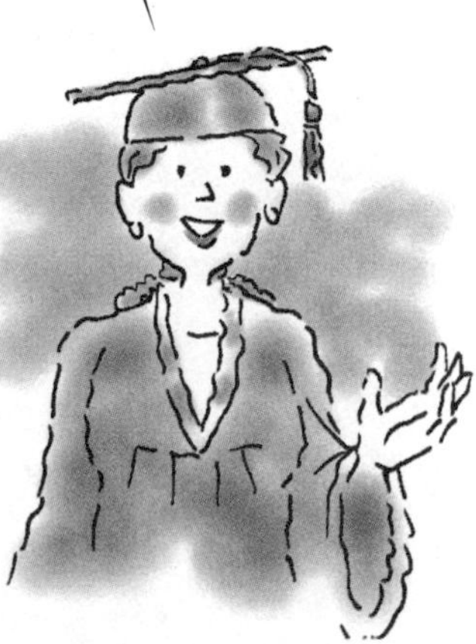

Collecting the tools

Before starting a physical assessment, assemble the necessary tools, which may include cotton balls, gloves, an ophthalmoscope, an otoscope, a penlight, a percussion hammer, safety

Assessment tools

Tools used for assessment include:

- blood pressure cuff
- cotton balls
- gloves
- metric ruler (clear)
- near-vision and visual acuity charts
- ophthalmoscope
- otoscope
- penlight
- percussion hammer
- safety pins
- scale with height measurement
- skin calipers
- specula (nasal and vaginal)
- stethoscope
- tape measure (cloth or paper)
- thermometer
- tuning fork
- wooden tongue blade.

pins, and a stethoscope. (For a more complete list, see *Assessment tools.*)

Two heads are better than one

Use a stethoscope with a diaphragm and a bell. The diaphragm has a flat, thin, plastic surface that picks up high-pitched sounds such as breath sounds. The bell has a smaller, open end that picks up low-pitched sounds, such as third and fourth heart sounds.

All the better to see you with...

You'll need a penlight to illuminate the inside of the patient's nose and mouth, cast tangential light on lesions, and evaluate pupillary reactions. An ophthalmoscope enables you to examine the internal structures of the eye; an otoscope, the external auditory canal and tympanic membrane.

Other tools include cotton balls and safety pins to test sensation and pain differentiation, a percussion hammer to evaluate deep tendon reflexes, and gloves to protect the patient and you.

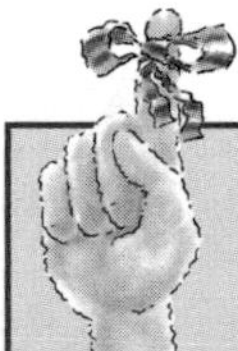

Memory jogger

Remembering that the bell of a stethoscope is used to hear low-pitched sounds and the diaphragm is used to hear high-pitched sounds is easy: *Bell and low both contain the letter l.*

Performing a general survey

After assembling the necessary tools, move on to the first part of the physical assessment: forming your initial impressions of the patient and obtaining his baseline data, including height, weight, and vital signs. This information will direct the rest of your assessment.

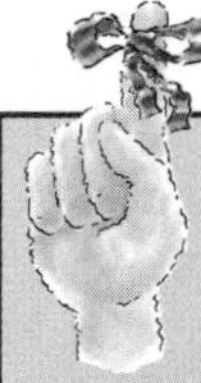

Memory jogger

Use the mnemonic **SOME TEAMS** as a checklist to help you remember what to look for when observing a patient.

Symmetry — Are his face and body symmetrical?

Old — Does he look his age?

Mental acuity — Is he alert, confused, agitated, or inattentive?

Expression — Does he appear ill, in pain, or anxious?

Trunk — Is he lean, stocky, obese, or barrel-chested?

Extremities — Are his fingers clubbed? Does he have joint abnormalities or edema?

Appearance — Is he clean and appropriately dressed?

Movement — Are his posture, gait, and coordination normal?

Speech — Is his speech relaxed, clear, strong, understandable, and appropriate? Does it sound stressed?

Observing the patient

A patient's behavior and appearance can offer subtle clues about his health. Carefully observe him for unusual behavior or signs of illness.

Preparing the patient

If possible, introduce yourself to the patient before the assessment, preferably when he's dressed. Meeting you under less-threatening circumstances might decrease his anxiety when you perform the assessment. (See *Tips for assessment success*.)

Keep in mind that the patient may be worried that you'll find a problem. He may also consider the assessment an invasion of his privacy because you're observing and touching sensitive, private, and perhaps painful body areas.

No surprises

Before you start, briefly explain what you're planning to do, why you're doing it, how long it will take, what position changes it will require, and what equipment you'll use. As you perform the assessment, explain each step in detail. A well-prepared patient won't be surprised or feel unexpected discomfort, so he'll trust you more and cooperate better.

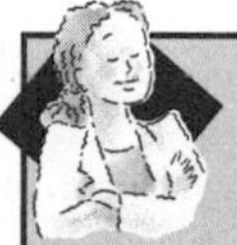

Peak technique

Tips for assessment success

Before starting the physical assessment, follow these guidelines:

- Eliminate as many distractions and disruptions as possible.
- Ask your patient to void before beginning the physical assessment.
- Wash your hands before and after the assessment—preferably in the patient's presence.
- Have all the necessary equipment on hand and in working order.
- Make sure the examination room is well lit and warm.
- Warm your hands and equipment before touching the patient.
- Be aware of your nonverbal communication and possible negative reactions from the patient.

Put your patient at ease but know where to draw the line. Maintain professionalism during the examination. Humor can help put the patient at ease but avoid sarcasm and keep jokes in good taste.

Explaining everything in advance will help the patient relax and ensure his cooperation.

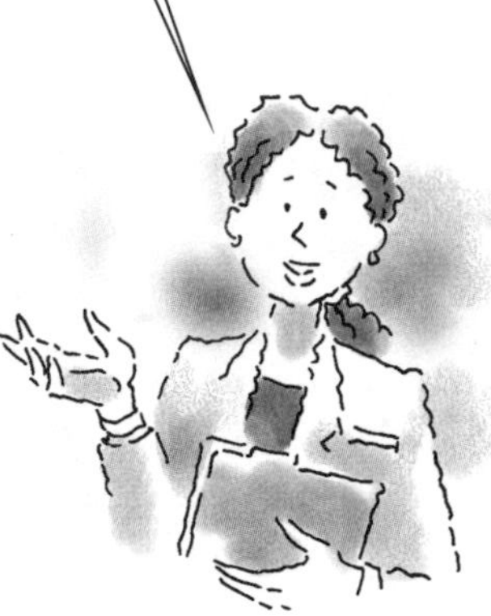

Get it down on paper

Document your findings up to this point in a concise paragraph. Include only essential information that communicates your overall impression of the patient. For example, if your patient has a lesion, simply note it now. You'll describe the lesion in detail when you complete the physical assessment.

Recording vital signs and statistics

Accurate measurements of your patient's height, weight, and vital signs provide critical information about body functions. The first time you assess a patient, record his baseline vital signs and statistics. Afterward, take measurements at regular intervals, depending on the patient's condition and your facility's policy. A series of readings usually provides more valuable information than a single set. (See *Tips for interpreting vital signs.*)

Height and weight

Height and weight are important parameters for evaluating nutritional status, calculating medication dosages, and assessing fluid loss or gain. Take the patient's baseline height and weight so you can gauge future weight changes or calculate medication dosages in an emergency. (See *Measuring height and weight.*) Keep this information handy so you can refer to it quickly, if needed. Note that these measurements differ for pediatric patients. (See *Obtaining pediatric measurements*, page 28.)

Tips for interpreting vital signs

Always analyze vital signs at the same time because two or more abnormal values provide important clues to your patient's problem. For example, a rapid, thready pulse along with low blood pressure may signal shock.

Accuracy

If you obtain an abnormal value, take the vital sign again to make sure it's accurate. Remember that normal readings vary with the patient's age. For example, temperature decreases with age, and respiratory rate may increase with age or with an underlying disease.

Individuality

Also remember that an abnormal value for one patient may be a normal value for another. Each patient has his own baseline values, which is what makes recording vital signs during the initial assessment so important.

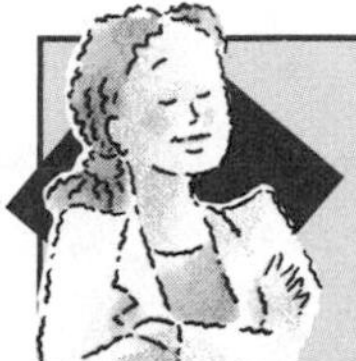

Peak technique

Measuring height and weight

Ask the patient to remove his shoes and to dress in a hospital gown. Then use these techniques to measure his height and weight.

Balancing the scale

Slide both weight bars on the scale to zero. The balancing arrow should stop in the center of the open box. If the scale has wheels, lock them before the patient gets on.

Measuring height

Ask the patient to step on the scale and turn his back to it. Move the height bar over his head and lift the horizontal arm. Then lower the bar until the horizontal arm touches the top of his head. Now read the height measurement from the height bar.

Measuring weight

Slide the lower weight into the groove representing the largest increment below the patient's estimated weight. For example, if you think the patient weighs 145 lb (65.8 kg), slide the weight into the groove for 100 lb (45.4 kg).

Slide the upper weight across until the arrow on the right stops in the middle of the open box. If the arrow hits the bottom, slide the weight to a lower number. If the arrow hits the top, slide the weight to a higher number.

The patient's weight is the sum of these numbers. For example, if the lower weight is on 150 lb (68 kg) and the upper weight is on 12 lb (5.4 kg), the patient weighs 162 lb (73.5 kg).

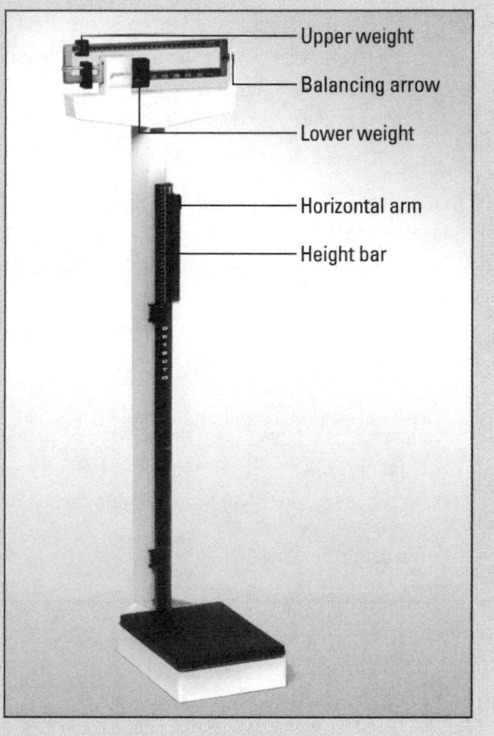

Body temperature

Body temperature is measured in degrees Fahrenheit (F) or degrees Celsius (C). Normal body temperature ranges from 96.7° to 100.5° F (35.9° to 38.1° C), depending on the route used for measurement. Hyperthermia describes an oral temperature above 106° F (41.1° C); hypothermia, a rectal temperature below 95° F (35° C).

From F to C and back again

To convert a Celsius measurement to a Fahrenheit measurement, multiply the Celsius temperature by 1.8 and add 32. To convert Fahrenheit to Celsius, subtract 32 from the Fahrenheit temperature and divide by 1.8. (See *How temperature readings compare*, page 29.)

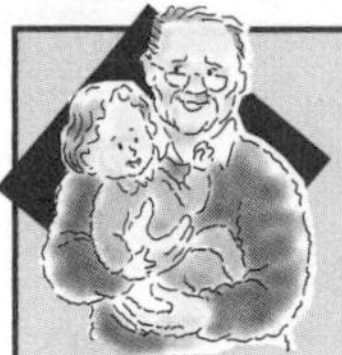

Ages and stages

Obtaining pediatric measurements

The height and weight of an infant or young child are measured differently from those of an adult. In addition to obtaining height and weight, you'll include the patient's head circumference in your measurements.

Height

Until a child is 2 to 3 years old, measure his height from the top of his head to the bottom of his heel while he's lying down. When measured in this fashion, height is commonly referred to as length.

Because infants tend to flex and curl, here are three steps to make measuring length easy and accurate:

1. Hold the infant's head in the midline position.
2. Hold his knees together with your other hand, gently pressing them down toward the table until fully extended.
3. Measure the length.

Weight

If a child is young enough to have his length measured while he's lying down, you'll most likely weigh him on an infant scale. Infant scales may be digital or use a balancing arrow. To obtain the weight, the infant or child either sits or lies down in a "bucket" or other enclosed area.

To prevent injury, never turn away from a child on a scale or leave him unattended. You can usually use an adult scale to weigh children older than age 2 or 3.

Head circumference

You should measure a child's head circumference until he's 36 months old. This measurement reflects the growth of the cranium and its contents.

To measure a child's head circumference, place a flexible measuring tape around the child's head at the widest point, from the frontal bone of the forehead and around the occipital prominence at the back of the head.

Pulse

The patient's pulse reflects the amount of blood ejected with each heartbeat. To assess the pulse, palpate one of the patient's arterial pulse points and note the rate, rhythm, and amplitude of the pulse. A normal pulse for an adult is between 60 and 100 beats/minute.

The radial pulse is the most accessible. However, in cardiovascular emergencies, you may palpate for the femoral or carotid pulses. These vessels are larger and closer to the heart and more accurately reflect the heart's activity. (See *Pinpointing pulse sites*.)

If the patient has an irregular heartbeat, or if he has a pacemaker, be sure to count his pulse for a full minute.

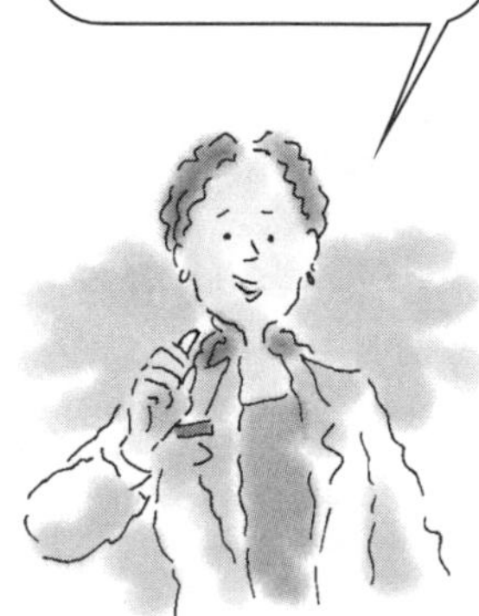

Feeling the beat

To palpate for a pulse, use the pads of your index and middle fingers. Press the area over the artery until you feel pulsations. If the rhythm is regular, count the beats for 30 seconds and then multiply by 2 to get the number of beats per minute. If the rhythm is irregular or your patient has a pacemaker, count the beats for 1 minute.

How temperature readings compare

You can take your patient's temperature in four ways. The chart below describes each method.

Method	Normal temperature	Used with
Oral	97.7° to 99.5° F (36.5° to 37.5° C)	Adults and older children who are awake, alert, oriented, and cooperative
Axillary (armpit)	96.7° to 98.5° F (35.9° to 36.9° C)	Infants, young children, and patients with impaired immune systems when infection is a concern
Rectal	98.7° to 100.5° F (37.1° to 38.1° C)	Infants, young children, and confused or unconscious patients
Tympanic (ear)	98.2° to 100° F (36.8° to 37.8° C)	Adults and children, conscious and cooperative patients, and confused or unconscious patients

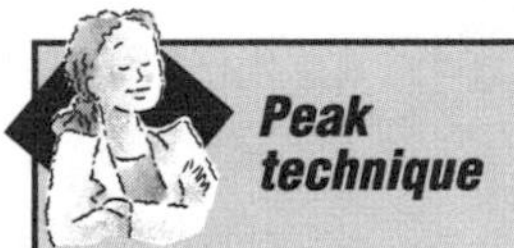

Peak technique

Pinpointing pulse sites

You can assess your patient's pulse rate at several sites, including those shown in the illustration below.

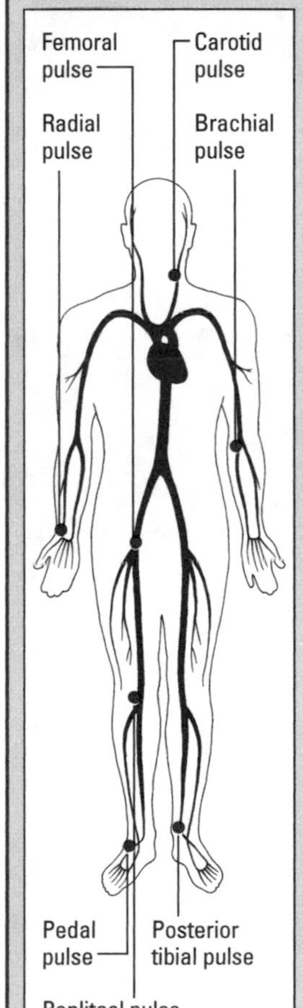

When taking the patient's pulse for the first time (or when obtaining baseline data) count the beats for 1 minute.

Palpation pointers

Avoid using your thumb to count a patient's pulse because the thumb has a strong pulse of its own. If you need to palpate the carotid arteries, avoid exerting a lot of pressure, which can stimulate the vagus nerve and cause reflex bradycardia. Also, don't palpate both carotid pulses at the same time. Putting pressure on both sides of the patient's neck can impair cerebral blood flow and function.

Off beat

When you note an irregular pulse:

- Evaluate whether the irregularity follows a pattern.
- Auscultate the apical pulse while palpating the radial pulse. You should feel the pulse every time you hear a heartbeat.
- Measure the difference between the apical pulse rate and radial pulse rate, a measurement called the *pulse deficit.* Measuring the pulse deficit allows you to evaluate indirectly the ability of each cardiac contraction to eject sufficient blood into the peripheral circulation.

Leaps and bounds

You also need to assess the pulse amplitude. To do this, use a numerical scale or descriptive term to rate or characterize the strength. Numerical scales differ slightly among facilities but the following scale is commonly used:

- *absent pulse*—not palpable, measured as 0
- *weak or thready pulse*—hard to feel, easily obliterated by slight finger pressure, measured as +1
- *normal pulse*—easily palpable, obliterated by strong finger pressure, measured as +2
- *bounding pulse*—readily palpable, forceful, not easily obliterated by pressure from the fingers, measured as +3.

Respirations

As you count respirations, be aware of the depth and rhythm of each breath. To determine the respiratory rate, count the number of respirations for 60 seconds. A rate of 16 to 20 breaths/minute is normal for an adult. If the patient knows you're counting how often he breathes, he may subconsciously alter the rate. To avoid this, take his respirations while you take his pulse.

Pay attention as well to the depth of the patient's respirations by watching his chest rise and fall. Is his breathing shallow, moderate, or deep? Observe the rhythm and symmetry of his chest wall as it expands during inspiration and relaxes during expiration. Be aware that skeletal deformity, fractured ribs, and collapsed lung tissue can cause unequal chest expansion.

Accessory to the act...of breathing

Use of accessory muscles can enhance lung expansion when oxygenation drops. Patients with chronic obstructive pulmonary disease (COPD) or respiratory distress may use neck muscles, including the sternocleidomastoid muscles, and abdominal muscles for breathing. Patient position during normal breathing may also suggest problems such as COPD. Normal respirations are quiet and easy, so note any abnormal sounds, such as wheezing and stridor.

Blood pressure

Blood pressure measurements are helpful in evaluating cardiac output, fluid and circulatory status, and arterial resistance. Blood pressure measurements consist of systolic and diastolic readings. The systolic reading reflects the maximum pressure exerted on the arterial wall at the peak of left ventricular contraction. Normal systolic pressure ranges from 100 to 140 mm Hg.

The diastolic reading reflects the minimum pressure exerted on the arterial wall during left ventricular relaxation. This reading is generally more significant than the systolic reading because it evaluates arterial pressure when the heart is at rest. Normal diastolic pressure ranges from 60 to 90 mm Hg. (See *Blood pressure variations.*)

Unpronounceable and indispensable

The sphygmomanometer, a device used to measure blood pressure, consists of an inflatable cuff, a pressure manometer, and a bulb with a valve. To record a blood pressure, the cuff is centered over an artery, inflated, and deflated. (See *Using a sphygmomanometer.*)

As the cuff deflates, listen with a stethoscope for Korotkoff sounds, which indicate the systolic and diastolic pressures. Blood pressure can be measured from most extremity pulse points. The

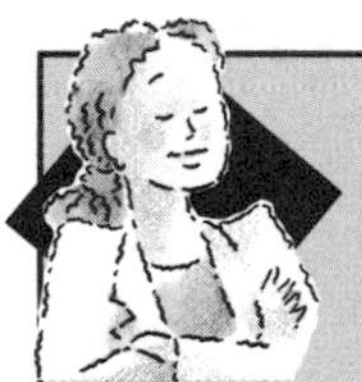

Peak technique

Using a sphygmomanometer

Here's how to use a sphygmomanometer properly:

- For accuracy and consistency, position your patient with his upper arm at heart level and his palm turned up.
- Apply the cuff snugly, 1″ (2.5 cm) above the brachial pulse, as shown in the top photo.
- Position the manometer in line with your eye level.
- Palpate the brachial or radial pulse with your fingertips while inflating the cuff.
- Inflate the cuff to 30 mm Hg above the point where the pulse disappears.
- Place the bell of your stethoscope over the point where you felt the pulse, as shown in the bottom photo. Using the bell helps you better hear Korotkoff sounds, which indicate pulse.
- Release the valve slowly and note the point at which Korotkoff sounds reappear. The start of the pulse sound indicates the systolic pressure.
- The sounds will become muffled and then disappear. The last Korotkoff sound you hear is the diastolic pressure.

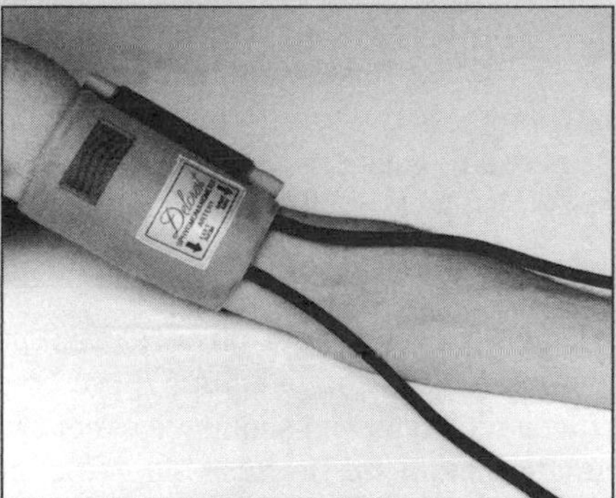

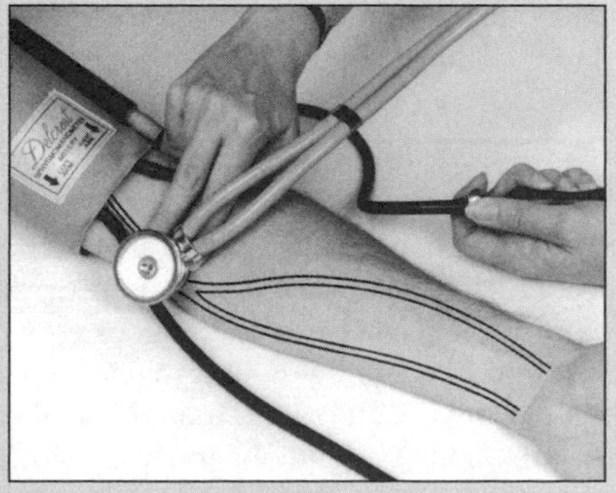

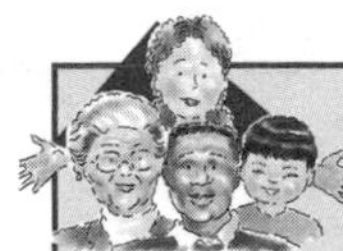

Bridging the gap

Blood pressure variations

Blood pressure may vary depending on the patient's race or sex. For example, black women tend to have higher systolic blood pressures than white women, regardless of age. Furthermore, after age 45, the average blood pressure of black women is almost 16 mm Hg higher than that of white women in the same age-group.

With this in mind, carefully monitor the blood pressures of your black female patients, being alert for signs of hypertension. Early detection and treatment—combined with lifestyle changes—can help prevent such complications as stroke and kidney disease.

Tips for hearing Korotkoff sounds

If you have difficulty hearing Korotkoff sounds, try to intensify them by increasing vascular pressure below the cuff. Here are two techniques.

Have the patient raise his arm
Palpate the brachial pulse and mark its location with a pen to avoid losing the pulse spot. Apply the cuff and have the patient raise his arm above his head. Then inflate the cuff about 30 mm Hg above the patient's systolic pressure. Have him lower his arm until the cuff reaches heart level, deflate the cuff, and take a reading.

Have the patient make a fist
Position the patient's arm at heart level. Inflate the cuff to 30 mm Hg above the patient's systolic pressure and ask him to make a fist. Have him rapidly open and close his hand approximately 10 times; then deflate the cuff and take the reading.

brachial artery is used for most patients because of its accessibility. (See *Tips for hearing Korotkoff sounds.*)

Performing a physical assessment

During the physical assessment, use drapes so only the area being examined is exposed. Develop a pattern for your assessments, starting with the same body system and proceeding in the same sequence. Organize your steps to minimize the number of times the patient needs to change position. By using a systematic approach, you'll also be less likely to forget an area.

A tetrad of techniques

No matter where you start your physical assessment, you'll use four techniques: inspection, palpation, percussion, and auscultation. Use these techniques in sequence except when you perform an abdominal assessment. Because palpation and percussion can alter bowel sounds, the sequence for assessing the abdomen is inspection, auscultation, percussion, and palpation. Let's look at each step in the sequence, one at a time.

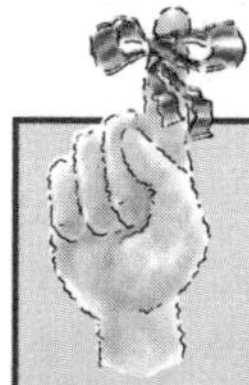

Memory jogger

To remember the order in which you should perform assessment of most systems, just think, "**I**'ll **P**roperly **Per**form **A**ssessment."

Inspection

Palpation

Percussion

Auscultation

Inspection

Inspect the patient using vision, smell, and hearing to observe normal conditions and deviations. Performed correctly, inspection can reveal more than can other techniques.

Inspection begins when you first meet the patient and continues throughout the health history and physical examination. As you assess each body system, observe for color, size, location, movement, texture, symmetry, odors, and sounds.

Palpation

Palpation requires you to touch the patient with different parts of your hands, using varying degrees of pressure. To do this, you need short fingernails and warm hands. Always palpate tender areas last. Tell your patient the purpose of your touch and what you're feeling with your hands. (See *Types of palpation*.)

Don't forget to wear gloves when palpating, especially when palpating mucous membranes or other areas where you might come in contact with body fluids.

Check out these features

As you palpate each body system, evaluate the following features:

- texture — rough or smooth?
- temperature — warm, hot, or cold?
- moisture — dry, wet, or moist?

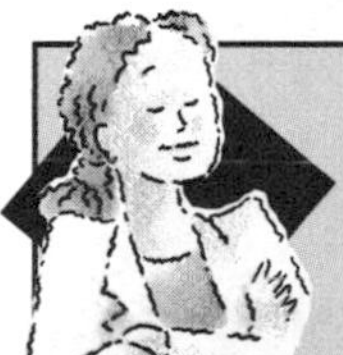

Peak technique

Types of palpation

The two types of palpation, light and deep, provide different types of assessment information.

Light palpation
Perform light palpation to feel for surface abnormalities. Depress the skin ½″ to ¾″ (1 to 2 cm) with your finger pads, using the lightest touch possible. Assess for texture, tenderness, temperature, moisture, elasticity, pulsations, superficial organs, and masses.

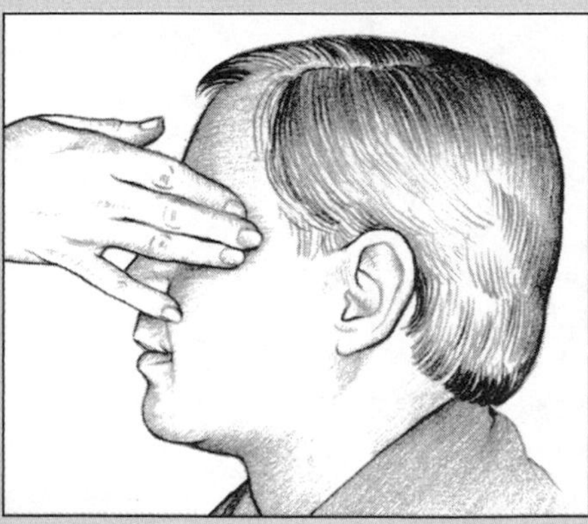

Deep palpation
Deep palpation is used to feel internal organs and masses for size, shape, tenderness, symmetry, and mobility. Depress the skin 1½″ to 2″ (4 to 5 cm) with firm, deep pressure. If necessary, use one hand on top of the other to exert firmer pressure.

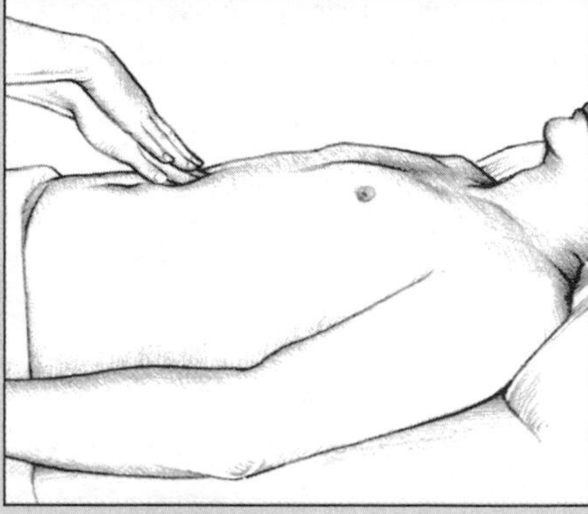

- motion — still or vibrating?
- consistency of structures — solid or fluid-filled?
- patient response — any pain or tenderness?

Percussion

Percussion involves tapping your fingers or hands quickly and sharply against parts of the patient's body, usually the chest or abdomen. The technique helps you locate organ borders, identify organ shape and position, and determine if an organ is solid or filled with fluid or gas. (See *Types of percussion.*)

Subtle sounds

Percussion requires a skilled touch and an ear trained to detect slight variations in sound. Organs and tissues, depending on their

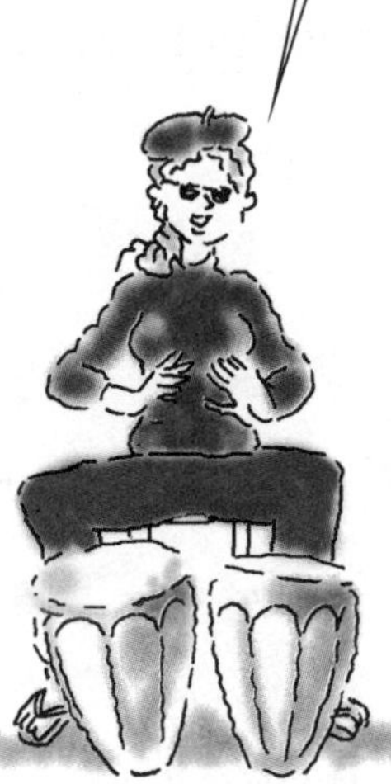

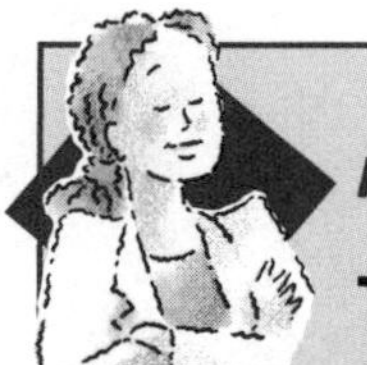

Peak technique

Types of percussion

You can perform percussion using the direct or indirect method.

Direct percussion
Direct percussion reveals tenderness. Using one or two fingers, tap directly on the body part. Ask the patient to tell you which areas are painful and watch his face for signs of discomfort. This technique is commonly used to assess an adult patient's sinuses for tenderness.

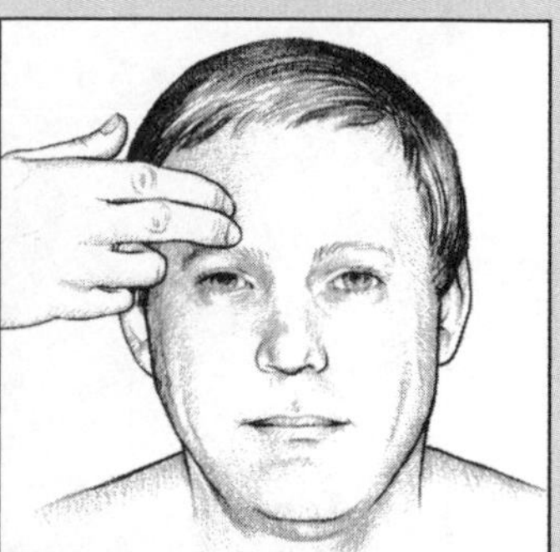

Indirect percussion
Indirect percussion elicits sounds that give clues to the makeup of the underlying tissue. Press the distal part of the middle finger of your nondominant hand firmly on the body part. Keep the rest of your hand off the body surface. Flex the wrist of your dominant hand. Using the middle finger of your dominant hand, tap quickly and directly over the point where your other middle finger touches the patient's skin. Listen to the sounds produced.

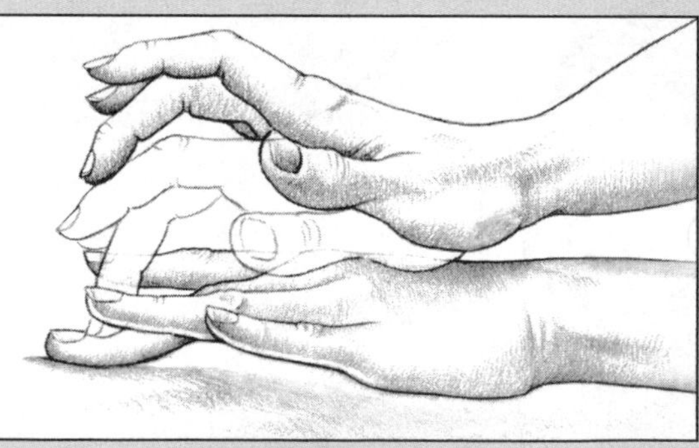

Sounds and their sources

As you practice percussion, you'll recognize different sounds. Each sound is related to the structure underneath. This chart offers a quick guide to percussion sounds and their sources.

Sound	Quality of sound	Where it's heard	Source
Tympany	Drumlike	Over enclosed air	Air in bowel
Resonance	Hollow	Over areas of part air and part solid	Normal lung
Hyperresonance	Booming	Over air	Lung with emphysema
Dullness	Thudlike	Over solid tissue	Liver, spleen, heart
Flatness	Flat	Over dense tissue	Muscle, bone

density, produce sounds of varying loudness, pitch, and duration. For instance, air-filled cavities such as the lungs produce markedly different sounds than the liver and other dense tissues. (See *Sounds and their sources.*)

As you percuss, move gradually from areas of resonance to those of dullness and then compare sounds. Also, compare sounds on one side of the body with those on the other side.

Auscultation

Auscultation, usually the last step, involves listening for various breath, heart, and bowel sounds with a stethoscope. To prevent the spread of infection among patients, clean the heads and end pieces of the stethoscope with alcohol or a disinfectant before each use. (See *Using a stethoscope*, page 36.)

Recording your findings

Begin your documentation with general information, including the patient's age, race, sex, general appearance, height, weight, body mass, vital signs, communication skills, behavior, awareness, orientation, and level of cooperation. Next, precisely record all information you obtained using the four physical assessment techniques. (See *Documenting your findings*, page 37.)

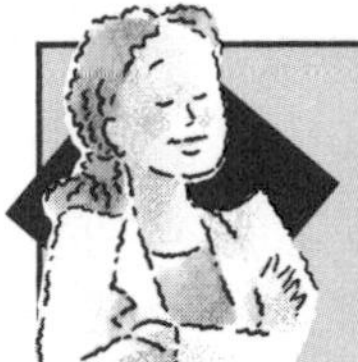

Peak technique

Using a stethoscope

Even if using a stethoscope is second nature to you, it might still be a good idea to brush up on your technique. First, your stethoscope should have these features:

- snug-fitting ear plugs, which you'll position toward your nose
- tubing no longer than 15″ (38.1 cm) with an internal diameter no greater than ⅛″ (0.3 cm)
- diaphragm
- bell.

How to auscultate

Hold the *diaphragm* firmly against the patient's skin, enough to leave a slight ring afterward. Hold the *bell* lightly against the patient's skin, just enough to form a seal. Holding the bell too firmly causes the skin to act as a diaphragm, obliterating low-pitched sounds.

Hair on the patient's chest may cause friction on the end piece, which can mimic abnormal breath sounds such as crackles. You can minimize this problem by lightly wetting the hair before auscultating.

A few more tips

Also keep these points in mind:

- Provide a quiet environment.
- Make sure the area to be auscultated is exposed. Don't try to auscultate over a gown or bed linens because they can interfere with sounds.
- Warm the stethoscope head in your hand.
- Close your eyes to help focus your attention.
- Listen to and try to identify the characteristics of one sound at a time.

Just as you should follow an organized sequence in your examination, you should also follow an organized pattern for recording your findings. Document all information about one body system, for example, before proceeding to another.

Locate landmarks

Use anatomic landmarks in your descriptions so other people caring for the patient can compare their findings with yours. For instance, you might describe a wound as "1½″ × 2½″ located 2½″ below the umbilicus at the midclavicular line."

Documenting your findings

Whether documenting an initial assessment of a patient admitted to your unit or writing a routine assessment note after a home visit, you'll need to use the appropriate form. The illustration below is an example of part of an initial assessment form similar to one you might use.

GENERAL INFORMATION

Age *55* Sex *M* Height *163 cm* Weight *57 kg*
T *37° C* P *76* R *14* B/P(R) *150/90 sitting* (L) ______

Room *328*
Admission time *0800*
Admission date *12-28-04*
Doctor *Manzel*
Admitting diagnosis *Pneumonia*

Patient's stated reason for hospitalization *To get rid of the pneumonia*

Allergies *penicillin, codeine*
Current medications *None*

Name	Dosage	Last taken

GENERAL SURVEY

In no acute distress, slender, appears younger than stated age. Is alert and well-groomed. Communicates well. Makes eye contact and expresses appropriate concern throughout exam. C. Smith, RN

With some structures, such as the tympanic membrane and breast, you can pinpoint a finding by its position on a clock. For instance, you might write "breast mass at 3 o'clock." If you use this method, however, make sure others recognize the same landmark for the 12 o'clock reference point.

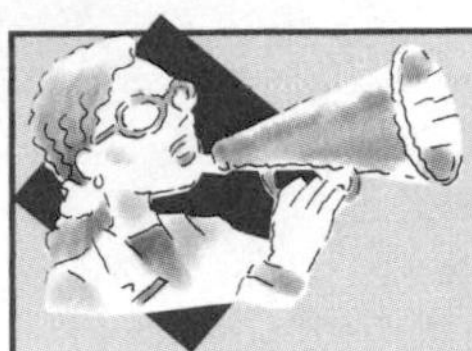

That's a wrap!

Physical assessment review

Performing a physical assessment

- Introduce yourself and help alleviate the patient's anxiety.
- Explain the entire procedure, including expected duration.
- Briefly document essential information.

Body temperature

- Remember that normal body temperature ranges from 96.7° to 100.5° F (35.9° to 38.1° C).
- To convert from Celsius to Farenheit, multiply the Celsius temperature by 1.8 and add 32.
- To convert from Farenheit to Celsius, subtract 32 from the Farenheit temperature and divide by 1.8.

Pulse

- Remember that a normal pulse is between 60 and 100 beats/minute.
- To palpate a pulse, press the area over the artery using the pads of your index and middle fingers until you feel pulsations.
- Avoid using your thumb to assess pulse, and never palpate both carotid arteries at the same time.

Respirations

- Remember that 16 to 20 breaths/minute is normal.
- Assess respiratory rate while taking the pulse.
- Observe the number and rhythm of the breaths and the symmetry of the chest.
- Watch for the use of accessory muscles, wheezing, and stridor.

Blood pressure

- Remember that normal systolic pressure is 100 to 140 mm Hg; normal diastolic pressure, 60 to 90 mm Hg.
- Use the brachial artery under normal circumstances.
- Use techniques to intensify Korotkoff sounds as needed.

Physical assessment techniques

- Use drapes, exposing only the area being examined.
- Organize your approach: Start with the same body system; proceed in the same sequence.
- Perform inspection, palpation, percussion, and auscultation in that order for most body systems. However, when examining the abdomen, use inspection, auscultation, percussion, and palpation in that order.

Inspection

- Use your vision, smell, and hearing to inspect the patient.
- Observe the patient for color, size, location, movement, texture, symmetry, odors, and sounds.

Palpation

- Always tell the patient when and why you're going to touch him.
- Use different parts of your hand to touch the patient. Always palpate tender areas last.
- Use light palpation to assess for surface abnormalities, texture, tenderness, temperature, moisture, pulsations, and masses.
- Use deep palpation to feel internal organs and masses.

Physical assessment review *(continued)*

Percussion

- Tap your fingers or hands quickly and sharply against parts of the patient's body to locate organ borders, identify organ shape and position, and determine consistency.
- Listen to the sounds produced: Observe their loudness, pitch, and duration.
- Use direct percussion to reveal tenderness.
- Use indirect percussion to determine the makeup of the underlying tissue.

Auscultation

- Use a stethoscope to listen for breath, heart, and bowel sounds.
- Hold the diaphragm of the stethoscope firmly against the patient's skin to listen for high-pitched sounds.
- Hold the bell of the stethoscope lightly against the patient's skin to listen for low-pitched sounds.
- Don't auscultate over a gown. Wet excess hair on the patient's chest to eliminate interference.
- Close your eyes to focus during auscultation.

Documenting findings

- Begin by documenting general information.
- Next, document information you obtained from your assessment. Record your findings by body system to organize the information.
- Use anatomic landmarks in your descriptions.

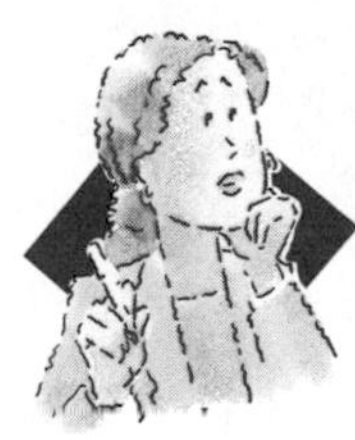

Quick quiz

1. The first technique in your physical assessment sequence is:
A. palpation.
B. auscultation.
C. inspection.
D. percussion.

Answer: C. The assessment of each body system begins with inspection. It's the most commonly used technique, and it can reveal more than can any other technique.

2. When palpating the abdomen, begin by palpating:
A. lightly.
B. firmly.
C. deeply.
D. indirectly.

Answer: A. Light palpation is always done first to detect surface characteristics.

3. If you're auscultating the lungs of a man with chest hair:
A. shave the chest first.
B. auscultate through the patient's gown.
C. use the diaphragm instead of the bell.
D. lightly wet the hair.

Answer: D. Because the friction caused by chest hair can mimic abnormal breath sounds, wet the hair slightly to prevent friction.

4. The pulse deficit measures the difference between the:
A. apical and radial pulse rates.
B. systolic and diastolic blood pressure.
C. systolic blood pressure and atrial pulse rate.
D. systolic blood pressure and radial pulse rate.

Answer: A. The pulse deficit is the difference between the apical and radial pulse rates. It provides an indirect evaluation of the ability of each heart contraction to eject enough blood into the peripheral circulation.

5. During percussion you hear a flat sound. The most likely source of this sound is:
A. normal tissue.
B. lung with emphysema.
C. muscle.
D. air in the bowel.

Answer: C. Flatness is most commonly heard over dense tissue, such as muscle and bone.

Scoring

☆☆☆ If you answered all five questions correctly, hooray! You're a history-takin', physical-assessin', proudly palpatin' assessment whiz.

☆☆ If you answered four questions correctly, terrific! You're a hands-on winner.

☆ If you answered fewer than four questions correctly, it's okay. In our assessment, you have unfulfilled potential.

Nutritional assessment

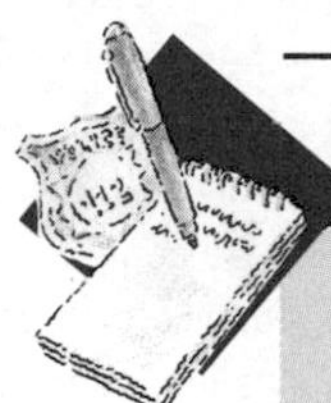

Just the facts

In this chapter, you'll learn:

- ways in which nutrition affects health
- questions to ask your patient during a nutritional health history
- methods for assessing body systems as part of a nutritional assessment
- the proper way to take anthropometric measurements
- specific laboratory tests to help diagnose nutritional problems
- abnormal findings that you may discover during a nutritional assessment.

A look at nutritional assessment

A patient's nutritional health can influence his body's response to illness and treatment. Regardless of your patient's overall condition, an evaluation of his nutritional health should be a critical part of your total assessment. A better understanding of your patient's nutritional status can help you plan his care more effectively. (See *Parts of a nutritional assessment.*)

Parts of a nutritional assessment

Remember the four parts of a nutritional assessment, shown here.

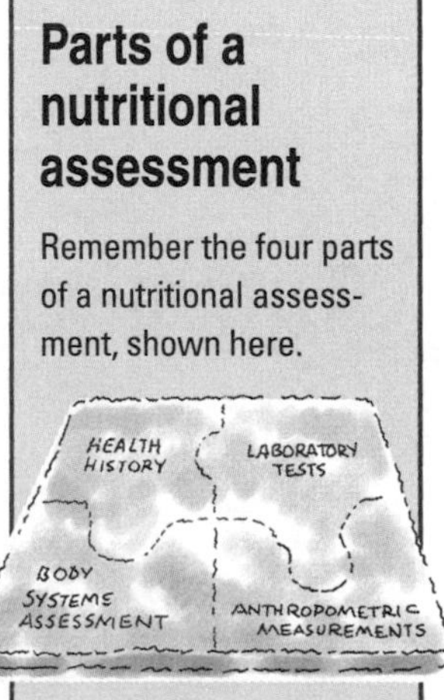

Normal nutrition

Nutrition refers to the sum of the processes by which a living organism ingests, digests, absorbs, transports, uses, and excretes nutrients. For nutrition to be adequate, a person must receive the proper nutrients, including proteins, fats, carbohydrates, water, vitamins, and minerals. Also, his digestive system must function properly for his body to make use of nutrients.

Break it down

The body breaks down nutrients mechanically and chemically into simpler compounds for absorption in the stomach and intestines. The mechanical breakdown of food begins in the mouth with chewing and continues in the stomach and intestine as food is churned in the GI tract. The chemical processes start with the salivary enzymes in the mouth and continue with acid and enzyme action throughout the rest of the GI tract.

Now...or later

Nutrients can be used for the body's immediate needs, or they can be stored for later use. For example, glucose, a carbohydrate, is stored in the muscles and the liver. It can be converted quickly when the body needs energy fast. If glucose is unavailable, the body breaks down stored fat, a source of energy during periods of starvation. (See *Anabolism and catabolism.*)

Protein power

The body needs protein to ensure normal growth and function and to maintain body tissues. Protein is stored in muscle, bone, blood, skin, cartilage, and lymph. Because the body preserves protein to maintain body functions, the body breaks down protein as a source of energy only when the supply of carbohydrates and fat—the primary sources of energy for the body—is inadequate. Carbohydrate and fat are the primary sources of energy for the body, while protein is preserved to maintain body functions. Vitamins, minerals, and water are also essential for normal functioning.

Lipids on the loose

Lipids and other fats are also essential for the body's normal functioning. To be transported throughout the body, they must combine with plasma proteins to form lipoproteins. Likewise, free fatty acids combine with albumin, whereas cholesterol, triglycerides, and phospholipids bind to globulin.

Anabolism and catabolism

Anabolism is a building up process that occurs when simple substances such as nutrients are converted into more complex compounds to be used for tissue growth, maintenance, and repair.

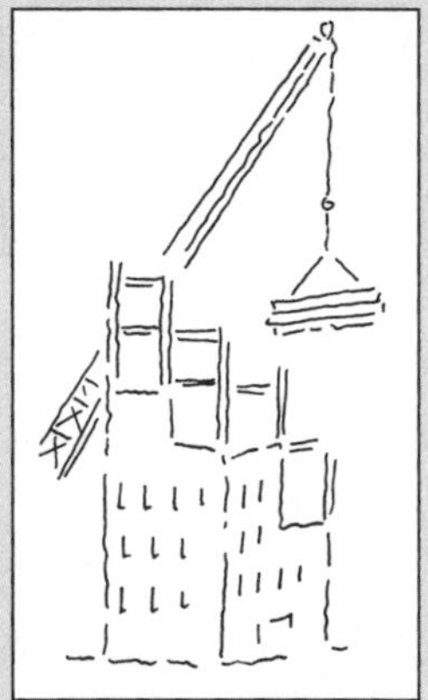

Catabolism is a breaking down process that occurs when complex substances are converted into simple compounds and stored or used for energy.

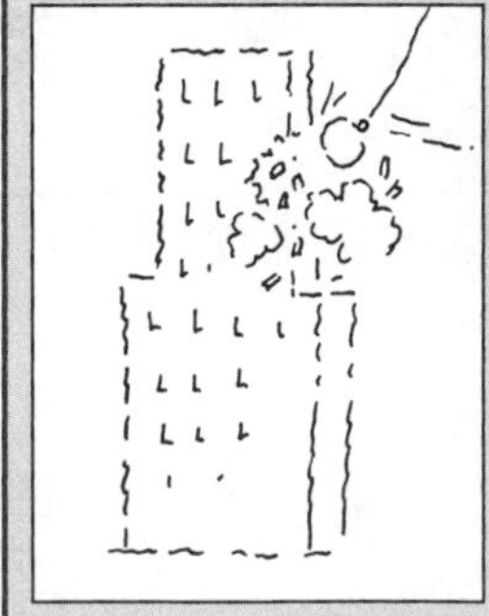

Obtaining a nutritional health history

A patient may come to you with various nutrition-related complaints, such as weight gain or loss; changes in energy level, appetite, or taste; dysphagia; GI tract problems, such as nausea, vomiting, and diarrhea; or other body system changes, such as skin and nail abnormalities. After establishing the patient's chief complaint, start the nutritional assessment by obtaining the patient's nutritional health history.

Blast from the past

During your interview, ask the patient about previous medical problems, surgical history, current medications (including over-the-counter medications, vitamins, and herbal preparations), unusual physical activity, weight loss or gain, allergies, smoking, eating patterns, alcohol or drug use, food choices, and dietary restrictions. Also, ask about a family history of obesity, diabetes, metabolic disorders such as hypercholesterolemia, and stomach and GI disturbances. These problems commonly occur in families.

The patient's description of his typical day can reveal important information about his activity level and eating habits.

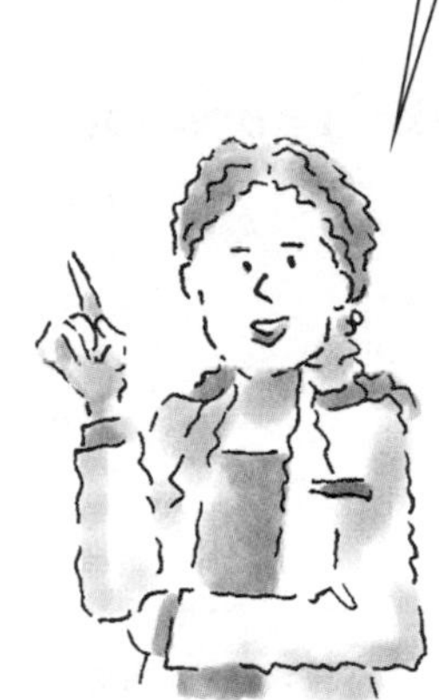

A day in the life

Also, ask the patient to describe his typical day. This will give you important information about his routine activity level and eating habits.

Ask him to recount what and how much he ate yesterday, how the food was cooked, and who cooked it. This information not only tells you about the patient's usual intake but also gives clues about food preferences, eating patterns, and even the patient's memory and mental status. (See *Understanding differences in food intake*.)

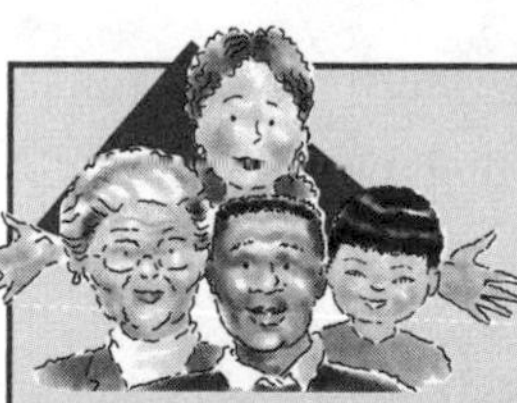

Bridging the gap

Understanding differences in food intake

What your patient eats depends on various cultural and economic influences. Understanding these influences can give you more insight into the patient's nutritional status:

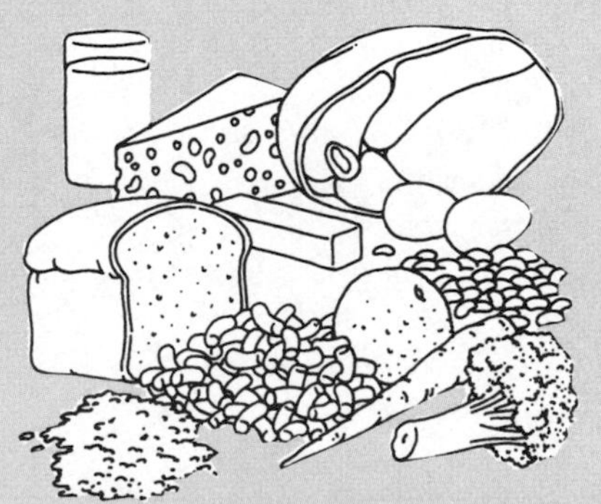

- *Socioeconomic status* may affect a patient's ability to afford healthful foods in the quantities needed to maintain proper health. Low socioeconomic status can lead to nutritional problems, especially for small children and pregnant women, who may give birth to infants with a low birth weights or experience complications during labor.
- *Work schedule* can affect the amount and type of food a patient eats, especially if the patient works full-time at night.
- *Religion* can restrict food choices. For example, some Jews and Muslims don't eat pork products, and many Roman Catholics avoid meat on Ash Wednesday and on Fridays during Lent.
- *Ethnic background* influences food choices. For example, fish and rice are staple foods for many Asians.

Performing the assessment

After completing the health history, you'll perform a two-part nutritional physical assessment. In part one, you'll assess several key body systems. In part two, you'll take anthropometric measurements. You'll also need to evaluate laboratory studies. Remember that nutritional problems may be associated with various disorders or factors. (See *Tips for detecting nutritional problems.*)

Take a good look

Before starting your physical assessment, quickly evaluate the patient's general appearance. Does he look rested? Is his posture good? Is his speech clear? Are his height and weight proportional to his body build? Are his physical movements smooth with no apparent weaknesses? Is he free from skeletal deformities?

Tips for detecting nutritional problems

Nutritional problems may stem from physical conditions, drugs, diet, or lifestyle factors. Listed below are factors that might indicate your patient is particularly susceptible to nutritional problems.

Physical conditions

- Chronic illnesses such as diabetes and neurologic, cardiac, or thyroid problems
- Family history of diabetes or heart disease
- Draining wounds or fistulas
- Obesity or a weight gain of 20% above normal body weight
- Unplanned weight loss of 20% below normal body weight
- Cystic fibrosis
- History of GI disturbances
- Anorexia or bulimia
- Depression or anxiety
- Severe trauma
- Recent chemotherapy, radiation therapy, or bone marrow transplantation
- Physical limitations, such as paresis or paralysis
- Recent major surgery
- Pregnancy, especially teen or multiple-birth pregnancy
- Burns

Drugs and diet

- Fad diets
- Steroid, diuretic, or antacid use
- Mouth, tooth, or denture problems
- Excessive alcohol intake
- Strict vegetarian diet
- Liquid diet or nothing by mouth for more than 3 days

Lifestyle factors

- Lack of support from family or friends
- Financial problems

Assessing each body system

Once you've assessed the patient's general appearance, you're ready to perform a head-to-toe assessment of the patient's major body systems. In addition to observing the patient's body structure, assess the following areas.

Skin, hair, and nails

When assessing the patient's skin, hair, and nails, ask yourself these questions: Is his hair shiny and full? Is his skin free from blemishes and rashes? Is it warm and dry, with normal color for that particular patient? Are his nails firm with pink beds?

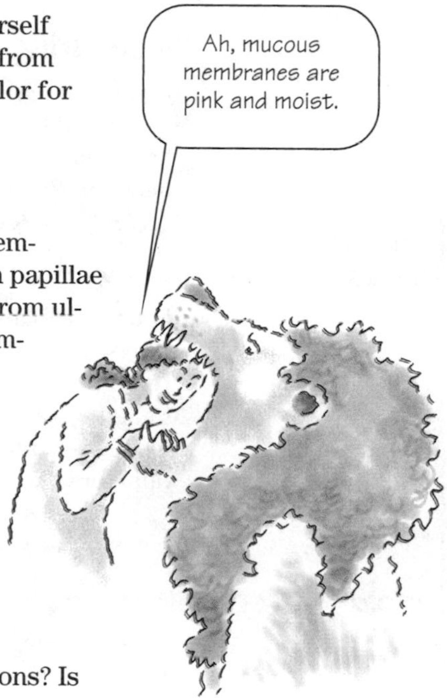

Eyes, nose, throat, and neck

Are the patient's eyes clear and shiny? Are the mucous membranes in his nose moist and pink? Is his tongue pink with papillae present? Are his gums moist and pink? Is his mouth free from ulcers or lesions? Is his neck free from masses that would impede swallowing?

Cardiovascular system

Is the patient's heart rhythm regular? Are his heart rate and blood pressure normal for his age? Are his extremities free from swelling?

Respiratory system

Are the patient's lungs clear? Can he clear his own secretions? Is his chest expansion with breathing normal?

GI system

Is the patient's appetite satisfactory? Is he free from GI problems? Are his elimination patterns regular? Is his abdomen free from abnormal masses on palpation?

Neuromuscular system

Is the patient alert and responsive? Are his reflexes normal? Is his behavior appropriate? Is there any evidence of muscle wasting? Does he have calf pain? Are his legs and feet free from paresthesia?

Anthropometric measurements

The second part of the physical assessment is taking anthropometric measurements. These measurements can help identify nutritional problems, especially in patients who are seriously overweight or underweight. You won't always need to take all measurements but height and weight are usually necessary. Let the results of the patient's health history guide you.

Measuring height and weight

If your patient can stand without assistance, weigh him using a calibrated balance beam scale, and measure his height using the height bar on the scale. If he's weak or bedridden, measure his height with a measuring stick or tape and weigh him using a bed scale. (See *Overcoming problems in measuring height.*)

That elusive ideal weight

You've probably heard the term *ideal body weight,* a term that refers to standard weights associated with various heights on a reference table. Weight as a percentage of ideal body weight is obtained by dividing the patient's true weight by an ideal body weight — a number found on a table — and then multiplying that number by 100. (See *Height and weight table.*)

A body weight of 120% or more of the ideal body weight indicates obesity. Below 90% indicates less-than-adequate weight.

Weighty terms

Here are some weight-related definitions:

- *normal weight* — 10% above or below recommended weight
- *overweight* — 10% to 20% above recommended weight
- *obese* — 20% or more above recommended weight
- *underweight* — 10% to 20% below recommended weight
- *seriously underweight* — 20% or more below recommended weight.

Mass-ive formula

An alternative method of evaluating a patient's weight is by using body mass index (BMI). BMI is a measure of body fat based on height and weight. To determine a patient's BMI, consult a BMI chart or use this formula:

$$\text{BMI} = \left(\frac{\text{weight in pounds}}{(\text{height in inches}) \times (\text{height in inches})}\right) \times 703$$

Overcoming problems in measuring height

Is your patient confined to a wheelchair? Is he unable to stand straight because of scoliosis? Despite such problems, you can still get an approximate measurement of his height using the "wingspan" technique.

Have the patient hold his arms straight out from the sides of his body. Tell children to hold their arms out "like bird wings." Then measure from the tip of one middle finger to the tip of the other. That distance is the patient's approximate height.

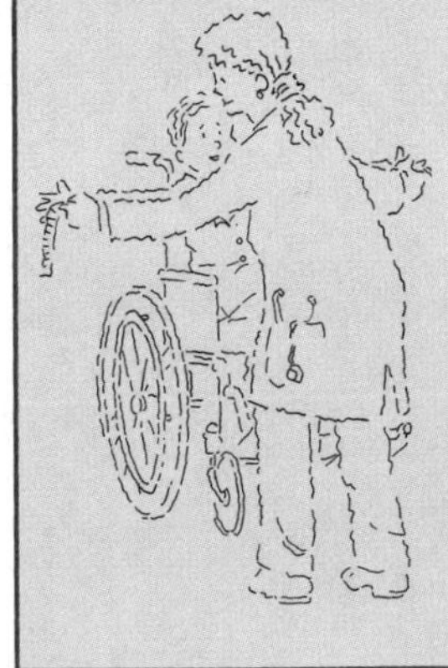

Height and weight table

Because people of the same height may differ in muscle and bone makeup, a range of weights for each height is shown in the table below. The higher weights in each category apply to men, who typically have more muscle and bone than women. Height measurements are for patients not wearing shoes; weight measurements are for patients not wearing clothes.

Height	Weight	
	Ages 19 to 34	***Age 35 and older***
5′0″	97 to 128 lb	108 to 138 lb
5′1″	101 to 132 lb	111 to 143 lb
5′2″	104 to 137 lb	115 to 148 lb
5′3″	107 to 141 lb	119 to 152 lb
5′4″	111 to 146 lb	122 to 157 lb
5′5″	114 to 150 lb	126 to 162 lb
5′6″	118 to 155 lb	130 to 167 lb
5′7″	121 to 160 lb	134 to 172 lb
5′8″	125 to 164 lb	138 to 178 lb
5′9″	129 to 169 lb	142 to 183 lb
5′10″	132 to 174 lb	146 to 188 lb
5′11″	136 to 179 lb	151 to 194 lb
6′0″	140 to 184 lb	155 to 199 lb
6′1″	144 to 189 lb	159 to 205 lb
6′2″	148 to 195 lb	164 to 210 lb
6′3″	152 to 200 lb	168 to 216 lb
6′4″	156 to 205 lb	172 to 222 lb
6′5″	160 to 211 lb	177 to 228 lb
6′6″	164 to 216 lb	182 to 234 lb

Discussing a patient's weight may seem like a heavy topic, but don't be shy. Being significantly overweight or underweight can have serious health consequences.

Here are some weight definitions based on BMI:

- *normal weight*—BMI between 18.5 and 24.9
- *overweight*—BMI between 25 and 29.9
- *obese*—BMI of 30 or greater
- *underweight*—BMI less than 18.5.

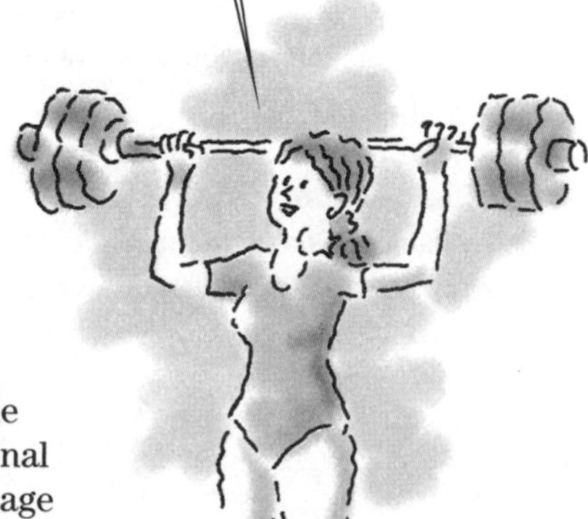

Anthropometric alternatives

Other anthropometric measurements include midarm circumference, midarm muscle circumference, and skin-fold thickness. These measurements are used to evaluate muscle mass and subcutaneous fat, both of which relate to nutritional status. (See *Taking anthropometric arm measurements*, page 48.)

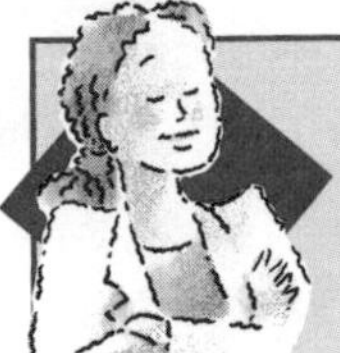

Peak technique

Taking anthropometric arm measurements

Follow these steps to determine the triceps skin-fold thickness, midarm circumference, and midarm muscle circumference.

Triceps skin-fold thickness

1. Find the arm's midpoint circumference by placing the tape measure halfway between the axilla and the elbow. Then grasp the patient's skin with your thumb and forefinger, about ⅜″ (1 cm) above the midpoint, as shown below.
2. Place the calipers at the midpoint and squeeze for 3 seconds.
3. Record the measurement to the nearest millimeter.
4. Take two more readings and use the average.

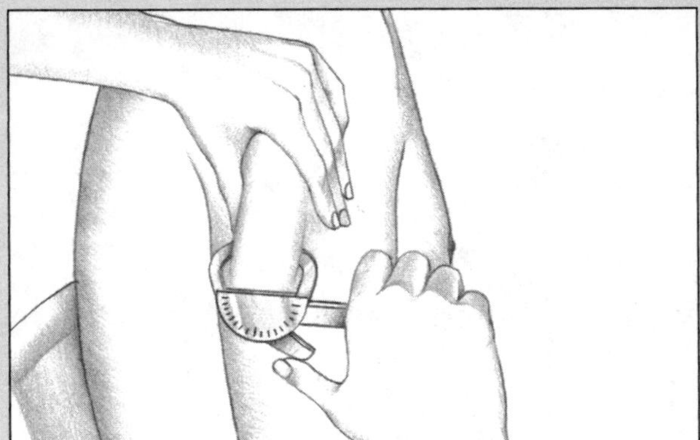

Midarm circumference and midarm muscle circumference

1. At the midpoint, measure the midarm circumference, as shown below. Record the measurement in centimeters.
2. Calculate the midarm muscle circumference by multiplying the triceps skin-fold thickness—measured in millimeters—by 3.14.
3. Subtract this number from the midarm circumference.

Recording the measurements

Record all three measurements as a percentage of the standard measurements (see chart below), using this formula:

$$\frac{\text{Actual measurement}}{\text{Standard measurement}} \times 100 = \%$$

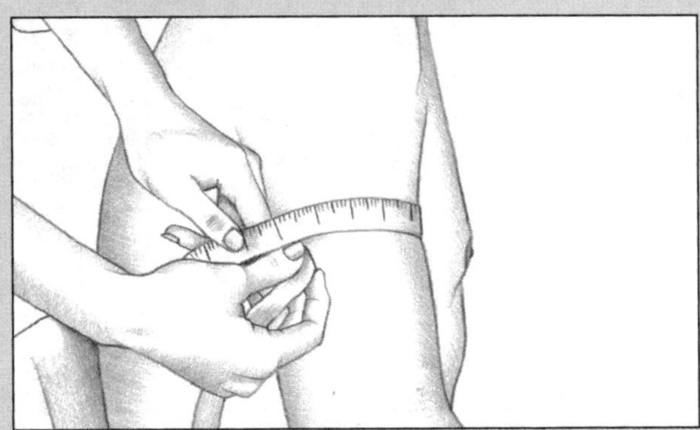

After you've taken all the measurements, apply these rules:

- A measurement less than 90% of the standard indicates caloric deprivation.
- A measurement more than 90% indicates adequate or more than adequate energy reserves.

Measurement	Standard	90%
Triceps skin-fold thickness	Men: 12.5 mm Women: 16.5 mm	Men: 11.3 mm Women: 14.9 mm
Midarm circumference	Men: 29.3 cm Women: 28.5 cm	Men: 26.4 cm Women: 25.7 cm
Midarm muscle circumference	Men: 25.3 cm Women: 23.3 cm	Men: 22.8 cm Women: 20.9 cm

Laboratory studies

The last part of the nutritional assessment is an evaluation of the patient's laboratory test results. Below are some common biochemical tests that may be performed as part of a nutritional assessment as well as possible outcomes and interpretations. Other tests, such as thyroid function tests and serum electrolyte and vitamin levels, may also be ordered.

All about albumin

Serum albumin level is used to assess protein levels in the body. Albumin makes up more than 50% of total proteins in the serum and affects the cardiovascular system because it helps maintain plasma osmotic pressure. It also functions as a carrier protein for various substances important for nutritional health, such as iron. Keep in mind that albumin production requires functioning liver cells and an adequate supply of amino acids, which are the building blocks of proteins.

Serum albumin level is decreased with serious protein deficiency and loss of blood protein resulting from burns, malnutrition, liver or renal disease, heart failure, major surgery, infections, or cancer.

Here's to hemoglobin!

Hemoglobin is the main component of red blood cells (RBCs), which transport oxygen. Its formation requires an adequate supply of protein in the form of amino acids. Hemoglobin values help assess the blood's oxygen-carrying capacity and are useful in diagnosing anemia, protein deficiency, and hydration status.

A decreased hemoglobin level suggests iron deficiency anemia, protein deficiency, excessive blood loss, or overhydration. An increased hemoglobin level suggests dehydration or polycythemia.

Serum transferrin is the most accurate predictor of a patient's protein status. A low serum transferrin level indicates a low protein level.

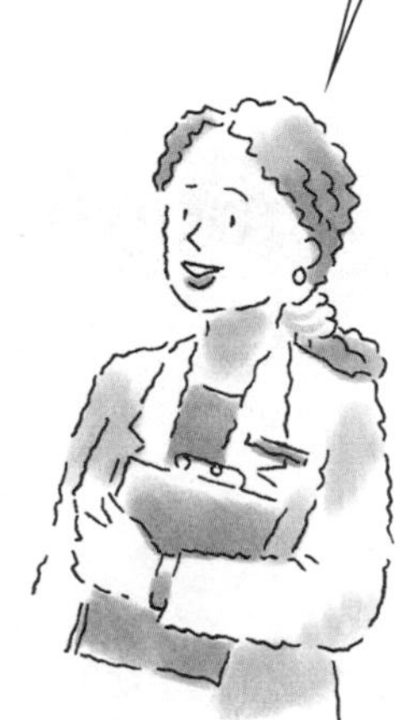

Don't omit hematocrit

Hematocrit reflects the proportion of RBCs in a whole blood sample. This test helps diagnose anemia and dehydration. Decreased values suggest iron deficiency anemia, excessive fluid intake, or excessive blood loss. Increased values suggest severe dehydration or polycythemia.

Carry on with transferrin

Transferrin is a carrier protein that transports iron. The molecule is synthesized mainly in the liver. A serum transferrin level reflects the patient's protein status more accurately than the serum albumin level. The level decreases along with protein levels and indicates depletion of protein stores.

Decreased values may also indicate inadequate protein production resulting from liver damage, protein loss from renal disease, acute or chronic infection, or cancer. Elevated levels may indicate severe iron deficiency.

Next comes nitrogen

A nitrogen balance test involves collecting all urine during a 24-hour period to determine the adequacy of a patient's protein intake. Proteins contain nitrogen. When proteins are broken down into amino acids, nitrogen is excreted in the urine as urea.

Nitrogen intake and excretion should be equal. Nitrogen balance is the difference between nitrogen intake (determined by a calorie count done during the same time frame as the 24-hour urine collection) and excretion. It's calculated using a formula, and the results are interpreted to determine whether the patient is receiving the appropriate amount of protein. Results may vary in patients with such conditions as burns and infection.

Trust in triglycerides

Triglycerides are the main storage form of lipids. Measuring triglyceride levels can help identify hyperlipidemia early. However, increased levels alone aren't diagnostic; further studies such as cholesterol measurements are required.

Patients who consume large amounts of sugar, soda, and refined carbohydrates commonly have elevated triglyceride levels. Decreased triglyceride levels commonly occur in those who are malnourished.

Count the cholesterol

A total cholesterol test measures circulating levels of free cholesterol and cholesterol esters. A diet high in saturated fats raises cholesterol levels by stimulating lipid absorption. Increased levels indicate an increased risk of coronary artery disease. Decreased levels are commonly associated with malnutrition.

Abnormal findings

Patients with nutritional problems may experience such signs and symptoms as excessive weight loss or gain, anorexia, or muscle wasting. Remember that clinical signs of nutritional deficiencies appear late. Also, be aware that patients hospitalized for more than 2 weeks risk developing a nutritional disorder. (See *Nutritional assessment findings*.)

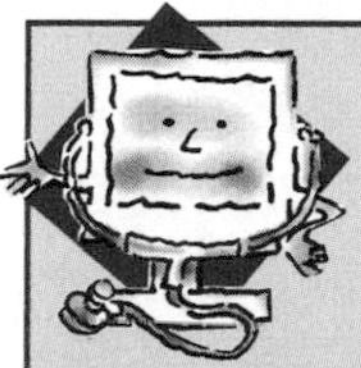

Interpretation station

Nutritional assessment findings

This chart will help you interpret your nutritional assessment findings.

Body system or region	Sign or symptom	Implications
General	• Weakness and fatigue • Weight loss	• Anemia or electrolyte imbalance • Decreased calorie intake, increased calorie use, or inadequate nutrient intake or absorption
Skin, hair, and nails	• Dry, flaky skin • Dry skin with poor turgor • Rough, scaly skin with bumps • Petechiae or ecchymoses • Sore that won't heal • Thinning, dry hair • Spoon-shaped, brittle, or ridged nails	• Vitamin A, vitamin B-complex, or linoleic acid deficiency • Dehydration • Vitamin A or essential fatty acid deficiency • Vitamin C or K deficiency • Protein, vitamin C, or zinc deficiency • Protein or zinc deficiency • Iron deficiency
Eyes	• Night blindness; corneal swelling, softening, or dryness; Bitot's spots (gray triangular patches on the conjunctiva) • Red conjunctiva	• Vitamin A deficiency • Riboflavin deficiency
Throat and mouth	• Cracks at corner of mouth • Magenta tongue • Beefy, red tongue • Soft, spongy, bleeding gums • Swollen neck (goiter)	• Riboflavin or niacin deficiency • Riboflavin deficiency • Vitamin B_{12} deficiency • Vitamin C deficiency • Iodine deficiency
Cardiovascular	• Edema • Tachycardia and hypotension	• Protein deficiency • Fluid volume deficit
GI	• Ascites	• Protein deficiency
Musculoskeletal	• Bone pain and bow leg • Muscle wasting • Pain in calves and thighs	• Vitamin D or calcium deficiency • Protein, carbohydrate, and fat deficiency • Thiamine deficiency
Neurologic	• Altered mental state • Paresthesia	• Dehydration and thiamine or vitamin B_{12} deficiency • Vitamin B_{12}, pyridoxine, or thiamine deficiency

Excessive weight loss

Patients with nutritional deficiencies usually experience weight loss. Weight loss may result from decreased food intake, decreased food absorption, increased metabolic requirements, or a combination of the three. Other possible causes include endocrine, neoplastic, GI, and psychiatric disorders; chronic disease; infection; and neurologic lesions that cause paralysis and dysphagia.

Excessive weight loss may also occur if the patient has a condition that prevents him from consuming a sufficient amount of food, such as painful oral lesions, ill-fitting dentures, or a loss of teeth. In addition, poverty, fad diets, excessive exercise, or certain drugs may contribute to excessive weight loss.

Excessive weight gain

When a person consumes more calories than his body requires for energy, his body stores excess adipose tissue, resulting in weight gain. Emotional factors (such as anxiety, guilt, and depression) as well as social factors can trigger overeating resulting in excessive weight gain. Excessive weight gain is also a primary sign of many endocrine disorders. In addition, patients with conditions that limit activity, such as cardiovascular or respiratory disorders, may also experience excessive weight gain. (See *Overweight children.*)

Anorexia

Defined as a lack of appetite despite a physiologic need for food, anorexia commonly occurs with GI and endocrine disorders. It can also result from anxiety, chronic pain, poor oral hygiene, and changes in taste or smell that normally accompany aging. Short-term anorexia rarely jeopardizes health, but chronic anorexia can lead to life-threatening malnutrition. Anorexia nervosa is a psychological condition in which the patient severely restricts food intake, resulting in excessive weight loss.

Excessive weight gain may be a sign of an endocrine disorder.

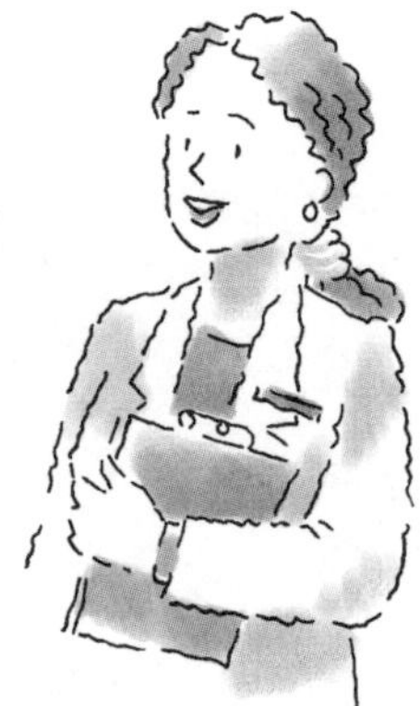

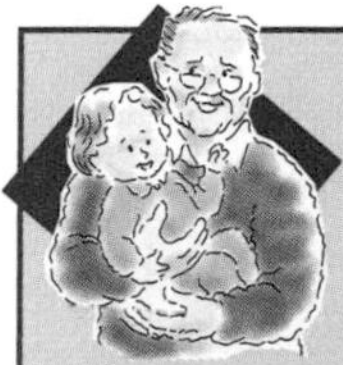

Ages and stages

Overweight children

Like adults, the number of children considered overweight has dramatically increased in recent years. An estimated 15% of children and teens are overweight (as determined by their body mass index); another 15% risk becoming overweight. Most overweight children become overweight or obese adults.

More weight, more risks
Children who are overweight are more likely to have high cholesterol and high blood pressure (risk factors for heart disease) as well as type 2 diabetes. They also tend to suffer from poor self-esteem and depression because of their weight.

Counting causes
During your nutritional assessment, look for these common causes of excessive weight gain in children:
- lack of exercise
- sedentary lifestyle (involving an excessive amount of watching television, using computers, or playing video games)
- unhealthy eating habits.

Healthy habits
Help the child develop an exercise plan and suggest nutritious eating habits to prevent weight gain and promote a healthy lifestyle.

Muscle wasting

Usually a result of chronic protein deficiency, muscle wasting, or *atrophy*, results when muscle fibers lose bulk and length. The muscles involved shrink and lose their normal contour, appearing emaciated or even deformed. Associated symptoms include chronic fatigue, apathy, anorexia, dry skin, peripheral edema, and dull, sparse, dry hair.

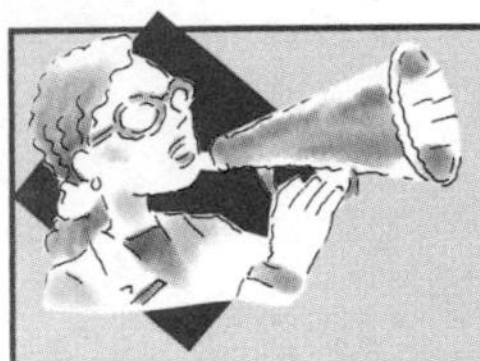

That's a wrap!

Nutritional assessment review

Evaluating nutritional status

- Nutrition is the sum of the processes by which a living organism ingests, digests, absorbs, transports, uses, and excretes nutrients.
- Nutrition includes the adequate intake of proteins, fats, carbohydrates, water, vitamins, and minerals.
- Nutrients can be used for the body's immediate needs, or they may be stored for later use.
- Proteins ensure normal growth and function and maintain body tissues.

Obtaining a nutritional health history

- Determine the patient's chief complaint.
- Obtain the patient's previous medical history, a family history, and a list of his current medications (including vitamins and herbal preparations).
- Ask the patient about his routine activity level and eating habits.
- Ask the patient about what he ate yesterday.

Performing a nutritional physical assessment

- Perform a general inspection.
- Assess key body systems: skin, hair, and nails; eyes, nose, throat, and neck; cardiovascular system; respiratory system; and neuromuscular system.
- Obtain anthropometric measurements: height, weight, and body mass index; when needed, midarm circumference, midarm muscle circumference, and skin-fold thickness.

Evaluating laboratory tests

- Albumin—Decreased levels indicate protein deficiency, liver or renal disease, heart failure, surgery, infection, or cancer.
- Hemoglobin—Decreased levels indicate iron deficiency anemia, overhydration, or excessive blood loss.
- Hematocrit—Decreased values indicate anemia; increased values, dehydration.
- Transferrin—Transferrin levels reflect protein stores.
- Nitrogen—Intake and output should be equal.
- Triglycerides—Triglyceride levels reflect lipid stores.
- Cholesterol—High levels indicate an increased risk of coronary artery disease.

Abnormal nutritional findings

- *Weight loss* reflects decreased food intake, decreased food absorption, increased metabolic requirements, or a combination of the three.
- *Weight gain* occurs when ingested calories exceed body requirements for energy, causing increased adipose tissue storage.
- *Anorexia* refers to a lack of appetite despite the physiologic need for food.
- *Muscle wasting* occurs when muscle fibers lose bulk and length, causing a visible loss of muscle size and contour.

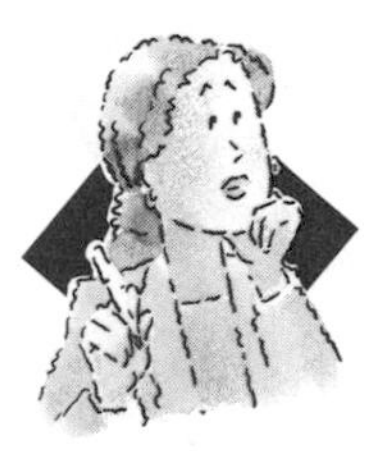

Quick quiz

1. A patient's midarm circumference is measured whenever you:
- A. conduct a basic nutritional assessment.
- B. want to confirm an abnormal protein level.
- C. suspect a serious nutritional problem.
- D. conduct a physical examination.

Answer: C. Midarm circumference isn't measured unless you suspect a serious nutritional problem.

2. A serum albumin test assesses:
- A. protein levels in the body.
- B. the ratio of protein to albumin.
- C. how well the liver metabolizes proteins.
- D. protein anabolism.

Answer: A. A serum albumin test assesses protein levels in the body.

3. The term *nitrogen balance* refers to the difference between:
- A. nitrogen intake and stores.
- B. nitrogen intake and excretion.
- C. nitrogen stores and excretion.
- D. nitrogen stores and metabolism.

Answer: B. The term *nitrogen balance* refers to the difference between nitrogen intake and excretion. It's calculated using a formula and should indicate that nitrogen intake and excretion are equal.

4. During a nutritional assessment, a patient's serum transferrin level helps you assess the patient for:
- A. bleeding disorders.
- B. cardiovascular function.
- C. liver damage.
- D. infection.

Answer: C. Transferrin is a carrier protein that transports iron. It's synthesized mainly in the liver. Decreased values may indicate inadequate protein production resulting from liver damage.

Scoring

☆☆☆ If you answered all four questions correctly, congratulations! Your hunger for nutritional knowledge has been truly satisfied.

☆☆ If you answered three questions correctly, way to go! We're impressed with how you sunk your teeth into this chapter.

☆ If you answered fewer than three questions correctly, don't lose weight over it. Just feast on the facts in this chapter and take the quiz again.

Mental health assessment

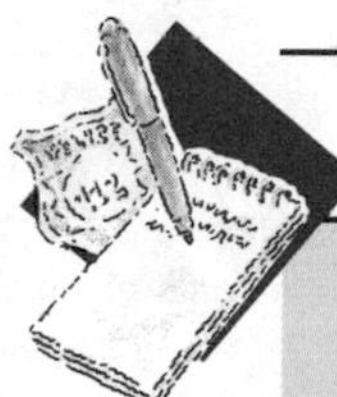

Just the facts

In this chapter, you'll learn:

- methods for establishing a therapeutic relationship with a patient
- ways to obtain important information during the patient interview
- techniques for assessing mental status
- abnormal findings that may be revealed by a mental health assessment
- ways to identify mental health disorders.

A look at mental health assessment

Effective patient care requires consideration of the psychological as well as the physiologic aspects of health. A patient who seeks medical help for chest pain, for example, may also need to be assessed for anxiety and depression. Knowing the brain's basic function and structures will help you perform a comprehensive mental health assessment and recognize abnormalities. (See chapter 15, Neurologic system, for a quick review.)

Any illness can affect a patient's mental outlook. Be sure to include a psychological assessment as part of every patient evaluation.

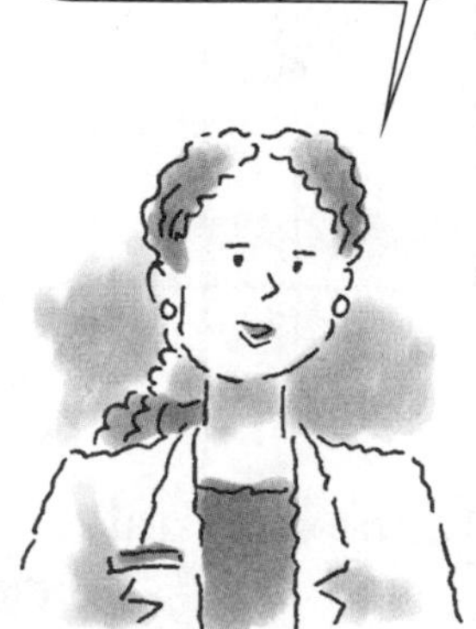

Obtaining a health history

Your assessment begins with a health history. For this assessment to be effective, you need to establish a therapeutic relationship with the patient that's built on trust. You must communicate to him that his thoughts and behaviors are important. Effective communication involves not only speech but also nonverbal communication, such as eye contact, posture, facial expressions, gestures,

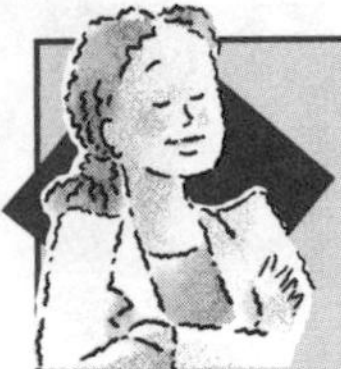

Peak technique

Therapeutic communication techniques

Therapeutic communication is the foundation of any good nurse-patient relationship. Here are some effective techniques for developing that relationship.

Listening

Listening intently to the patient enables the nurse to hear and analyze everything the patient is saying, alerting the nurse to the patient's communication patterns.

Rephrasing

Succinct rephrasing of key patient statements helps ensure that the nurse understands and emphasizes important points in the patient's message. For example, the nurse might say, "You're feeling angry and you say it's because of the way your friend treated you yesterday."

Broad openings and general statements

Using broad openings and general statements to initiate conversation encourages the patient to talk about any subject that comes to mind. These openings allow the patient to focus the conversation and demonstrate the nurse's willingness to interact. An example of this technique is: "Is there something you would like to talk about?"

Clarification

Asking the patient to clarify a confusing or vague message demonstrates the nurse's desire to understand what the patient is saying. It can also elicit precise information crucial to the patient's recovery. An example of clarification is: "I'm not sure I understood what you said."

Focusing

In the technique called *focusing,* the nurse helps the patient redirect attention toward something specific. It fosters the patient's self-control and helps avoid vague generalizations, so the patient can accept responsibility for facing problems. "Let's go back to what we were just talking about," would be one example of this technique.

Silence

Silence has several benefits: It gives the patient time to talk, think, and gain insight into problems. It also allows the nurse to gather more information. The nurse must use this technique judiciously, however, to avoid giving the impression of disinterest or judgment.

Suggesting collaboration

When used correctly, the technique of suggesting collaboration gives the patient the opportunity to explore the pros and cons of a suggested approach. It must be used carefully to avoid directing the patient. An example of this technique is: "Perhaps we can meet with your parents to discuss the matter."

Sharing impressions

In the technique called *sharing impressions,* the nurse attempts to describe the patient's feelings and then seeks corrective feedback from the patient. Doing so allows the patient to clarify any misperceptions and gives the nurse a better understanding of the patient's true feelings. For example, the nurse might say, "Tell me if my perception of what you're telling me agrees with yours."

clothing, affect, and even silence. All convey a powerful message. (See *Therapeutic communication techniques.*)

Peace and quiet

Choose a quiet, private setting for the assessment interview. Interruptions and distractions threaten confidentiality and interfere with effective listening. If you're meeting the patient for the first time, introduce yourself and explain the interview's purpose. Sit a

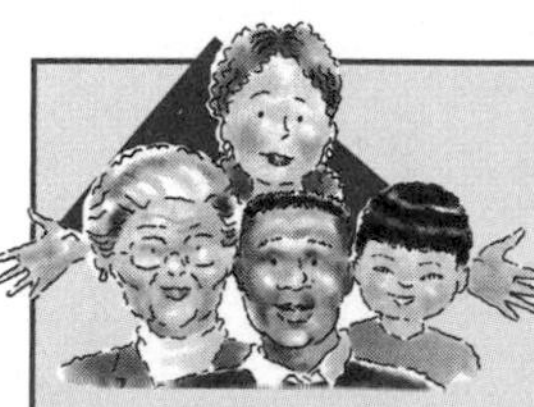

Bridging the gap

Transcultural communication

Communication styles vary among cultures. Qualities viewed as desirable in our culture (such as maintaining eye contact, having a certain degree of openness, offering insight, and portraying emotional expression) may not be considered appropriate in another culture. For example:

- Direct eye contact is considered inappropriate and disrespectful in some in Asian, Black, Native American, and Appalachian cultures.
- Some Middle Eastern cultures focus solely on the present; they usually view the future as something to be accepted as it occurs, rather than planned.
- Some Asians strongly value harmonious interpersonal relationships. As a result, they may nod, smile, and provide answers they feel are expected to maintain harmony rather than expressing their true feelings and concerns.

Avoid making assumptions about a patient's behavior or communication style. An individual's cultural background may explain a communication style you would otherwise deem "inappropriate" or "abnormal."

comfortable distance from the patient and give him your undivided attention. If you're interviewing a patient who has cognitive or memory losses, you may need to reorient him before beginning the interview.

Attitude counts

During the interview, be professional but friendly and maintain eye contact. A calm, nonthreatening tone of voice encourages the patient to talk more openly. Avoid value judgments. Don't rush through the interview; building a trusting therapeutic relationship takes time. (See *Transcultural communication.*)

Patient interview

A patient interview establishes a baseline and provides clues to the underlying or precipitating cause of the patient's current problem. Remember, the patient may not be a reliable source of information, particularly if he has a mental illness or other mental impairment. If possible, verify his responses with family members, friends, or health care personnel. Also, check hospital records for previous admissions, if possible, and compare the patient's past and present behavior, symptoms, and circumstances.

Chief complaint

The patient may not directly voice his chief complaint. Instead, you or others may note that he's having difficulty coping or he's exhibiting unusual behavior. If you note a problem, determine whether the patient is aware of the problem. When documenting the patient's response, write it word for word and enclose it in quotation marks.

Symptom specifics

Find out about the onset of current symptoms. Inquire about the severity and persistence of the symptoms and whether they occurred suddenly or developed over time.

History of psychiatric illnesses

Discuss past psychiatric disturbances — such as episodes of delusions, violence, attempted suicides, drug or alcohol abuse, or depression — and previous psychiatric treatment, if any. Also ask about any family history of psychiatric illness or substance abuse.

Demographic data

Determine the patient's age, ethnic origin, primary language, birthplace, religion, occupation, and marital status. Use this information to establish a baseline and confirm that the patient's record is correct.

Socioeconomic data

Patients suffering hardships are more likely to show symptoms of distress during an illness. Information about your patient's educational level, family, housing conditions, income, and employment status may provide clues to his current problem.

Cultural and religious beliefs

A patient's background and values can affect how he responds to illness and adapts to care. Certain questions and behaviors considered acceptable in one culture may be inappropriate in another.

Always review the patient's medication history, keeping in mind that certain medications can cause symptoms of mental illness.

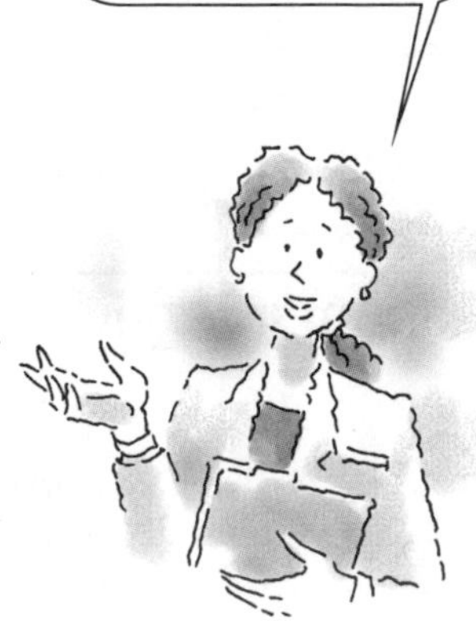

Medication history

Certain drugs can cause symptoms of mental illness. Review any medications the patient is taking, including over-the-counter and herbal preparations, and check for interactions. If he's taking a psychiatric drug, ask if his symptoms have improved, if he's taking the medication as prescribed, and if he has had any adverse reactions.

Physical illnesses

Find out if the patient has a history of medical disorders that may cause distorted thought processes, disorientation, depression, or other symptoms of mental illness. For example, does he have a history of renal or hepatic failure, infection, thyroid disease, increased intracranial pressure, or a metabolic disorder?

Assessing mental status

Most of a mental status assessment can be done during an interview. Assess the patient's appearance, behavior, mood, thought processes and cognitive function, coping mechanisms, and potential for self-destructive behavior. Record your findings.

Initial observations

Much about a patient's mental state can be determined simply by observing his appearance and how he handles himself in your presence.

You seem distracted. Would you like to talk about it?

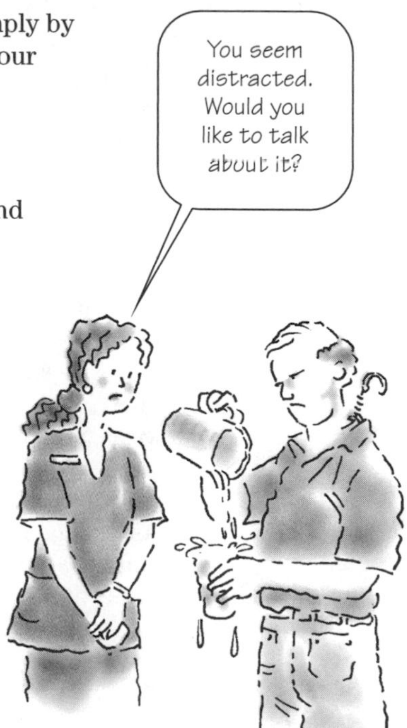

Appearance

The patient's appearance helps to indicate his emotional and mental status. Specifically, note his dress and grooming. Is his appearance clean and appropriate for his age, gender, and situation? Is the patient's posture erect or slouched? Is his head lowered? Observe his gait—is it brisk, slow, shuffling, or unsteady? Does he walk normally? Note his facial expression. Does he look alert, or does he stare blankly? Does he appear sad or angry? Does the patient maintain eye contact? Does he stare at you for long periods?

Behavior

Note the patient's demeanor and overall attitude as well as any extraordinary behavior such as speaking to a person who isn't present. Also, record his mannerisms. Does he bite his nails, fidget, or pace? Does he display any tics or tremors? How does he respond to you? Is he cooperative, friendly, hostile, or indifferent?

Mood

Does the patient appear anxious or depressed? Is he crying, sweating, breathing heavily, or trembling? Ask him to describe his current feelings in concrete terms and to suggest possible reasons for these feelings. Note inconsistencies between body language and mood (such as smiling when discussing an anger-provoking situation).

Thought processes and cognitive function

Evaluate the patient's orientation to time, place, and person, noting any confusion or disorientation. Listen for any indication that the patient might be having delusions, hallucinations, obsessions, compulsions, fantasies, or daydreams.

Attention please

Assess the patient's attention span and ability to recall events in both the distant and recent past. For example, to assess immediate recall, ask him to repeat a series of five or six objects.

Hypothetically speaking

Test his intellectual functioning by asking him to add a series of numbers and test his sensory perception and coordination by having him copy a simple drawing. Inappropriate responses to a hypothetical situation — such as "What would you do if you won the lottery?" — can indicate impaired judgment. Keep in mind that the patient's cultural background will influence his answer.

Spee-eech

Note any speech characteristics that may indicate altered thought processes, including monosyllabic responses, irrelevant or illogical replies to questions, convoluted or excessively detailed speech, slurred speech, repetitious speech patterns, a flight of ideas, and sudden silence without obvious reason.

Insight

Assess the patient's insight by asking if he understands the significance of his illness, the plan of treatment, and the effect the illness will have on his life.

Exploring coping mechanisms

The use of coping, or *defense,* mechanisms helps to relieve anxiety. Common coping strategies include:

- *denial* —the refusal to admit truth or reality
- *displacement*—transferring an emotion from its original object to a substitute
- *fantasy*—the creation of unrealistic or improbable images to escape from daily pressures and responsibilities
- *identification*—the unconscious adoption of another person's personality characteristics, attitudes, values, and behaviors
- *projection*—the displacement of negative feelings onto another person
- *rationalization*—the substitution of acceptable reasons for the real or actual reasons motivating behavior
- *reaction formation*—behaving in a manner opposite from the way the person feels
- *regression*—the return to behavior of an earlier, more comfortable time
- *repression*—the exclusion of unacceptable thoughts and feelings from the conscious mind, leaving them to operate in the subconscious.

Coping mechanisms

The patient who's faced with a stressful situation may adopt coping, or defense, mechanisms—behaviors that operate on an unconscious level to protect the ego. Examples include denial, displacement, fantasy, identification, projection, and repression. Listen for an excessive reliance on these coping mechanisms. (See *Exploring coping mechanisms.*)

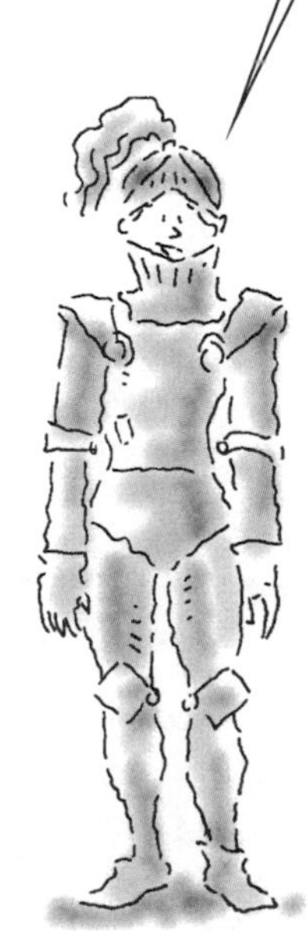

Potential for self-destructive behavior

Mentally healthy people may intentionally take death-defying risks such as participating in dangerous sports. The risks that self-destructive patients take, however, aren't death-defying—they're death-seeking.

Feelin' alive

Not all self-destructive behavior is suicidal in intent. Some patients engage in self-destructive behavior because it makes them feel alive. A patient who has lost touch with reality may cut or mutilate body parts to focus on physical pain, which may be less overwhelming than emotional distress.

Higher risk when they're low

Assess the patient for suicidal tendencies, particularly if he reports symptoms of depression. Not all such patients want to die; however, the incidence of suicide is higher in depressed patients than in patients with other diagnoses. If the patient is actively planning suicide, be prepared to take immediate action to prevent the act from occurring.

Psychological and mental status testing

Although most of a mental status assessment can be done during an interview, you'll also need to evaluate other aspects of your patient's mental status. These aspects can be assessed using psychological and mental status tests. Commonly used tests include:

- *Mini-Mental Status Examination*—measures orientation, registration, recall, calculation, language, and graphomotor function
- *Cognitive Capacity Screening Examination*—measures orientation, memory, calculation, and language
- *Cognitive Assessment Scale*—measures orientation, general knowledge, mental ability, and psychomotor function
- *Beck Depression Inventory*—helps diagnose depression, determine its severity, and monitor the patient's response during treatment
- *Global Deterioration Scale*—assesses and stages primary degenerative dementia based on orientation, memory, and neurologic function
- *Minnesota Multiphasic Personality Inventory*—helps assess personality traits and ego function in adolescents and adults. Test results include information on coping strategies, defenses, strengths, gender identification, and self-esteem; the test pattern may strongly suggest a diagnostic category, point to a suicide risk, or indicate potential violence.

I've never been good at taking tests.

Don't worry. This isn't the type of test on which you'll receive a grade.

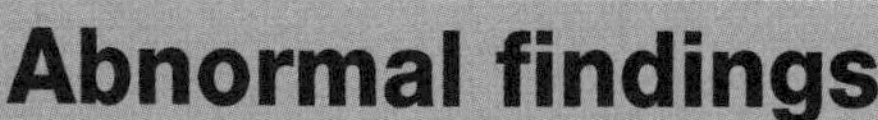

Abnormal findings

During a mental health assessment, you may detect abnormalities in thought processes, thought content, and perception. (See *Mental health assessment findings.*)

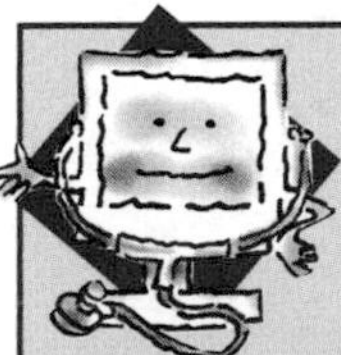

Interpretation station

Mental health assessment findings

Certain findings obtained from your mental health assessment may lead you to suspect a psychiatric disorder. This chart shows assessment findings associated with common psychiatric disorders.

Disorder	Assessment findings
Schizophrenia	• Delusions • Hallucinations • Disorganized speech • Grossly disorganized or catatonic behavior • Flat affect • Inability to speak • Poor eye contact • Distant and unresponsive facial expression • Limited body language
Major depressive disorder	• Severe fatigue • Inability to concentrate or make decisions • Feelings of sadness, worthlessness, or extreme guilt • Appetite changes with either weight loss or gain • Sleep disturbances • Decreased libido
Bipolar I disorder	• Signs and symptoms of major depressive disorder (listed above) • Manic findings, such as euphoria or irritability, delusions of grandeur, flight of ideas, extreme talkativeness, being easily distracted, spending money recklessly

Abnormal thought processes

During the interview, you may identify some of these abnormalities in your patient's thought processes:

- *derailment* — Speech vacillates from one subject to another. (The subjects are unrelated; ideas slip off track between clauses.)
- *flight of ideas* — The patient jumps abruptly from topic to topic in a continuous flow of speech.
- *neologisms* — Words are distorted or invented.

- *confabulation* — The patient fabricates facts or events to fill in the gaps where memory loss has occurred.
- *clanging* — The patient chooses a word based on the sound rather than the meaning.
- *echolalia* — The patient repeats words or phrases that others say.
- *incoherence* — The patient's speech is incomprehensible.

Abnormal thought content

With careful questioning, you may also detect abnormalities in thought content during the interview. Be sure to follow the patient's lead. For example, "You told me a few minutes ago that your mother was responsible for your illness; would you please elaborate?" With this type of questioning, you can find abnormalities in thought content, which may include:

- *obsessions* — recurrent, uncontrollable thoughts, images, or impulses that the patient considers unacceptable
- *compulsions* — repetitive behaviors that result from attempts to alleviate an obsession
- *phobia* — an irrational and disproportionate fear of objects or situations
- *depersonalization* — the feeling that one has become detached from one's mind or body or has lost one's identity
- *delusions* — false, fixed beliefs that aren't shared by others
- *poverty of content* — thoughts that give little information because of vagueness, empty repetition, or obscure phrases.

To detect mental health abnormalities, follow your patient's lead and ask direct questions about his perceptions.

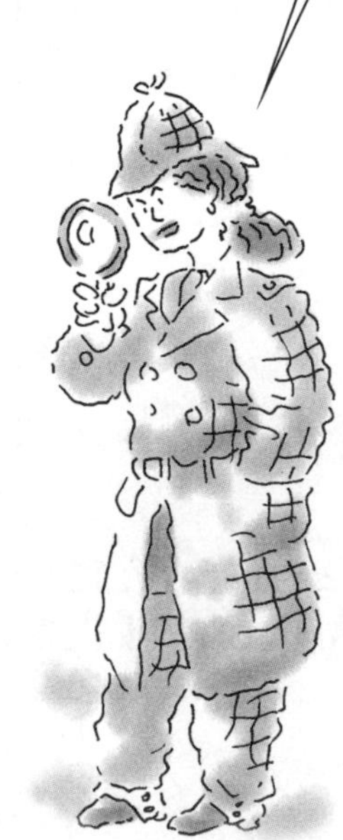

Perception abnormalities

You can assess a patient's perception abnormalities in the same way that you assess his thought content. Ask direct questions about his perceptions, such as "What did the voice say to you when you heard it speaking? How did you feel?" If the patient doesn't speak about abnormal perceptions, you can ask if he ever hears peculiar voices or frightening sounds. Perception abnormalities include:

- *illusions* — misinterpretations of external stimuli
- *hallucinations* — auditory, visual, tactile, somatic, or gustatory sensory perceptions when no external stimuli are present.

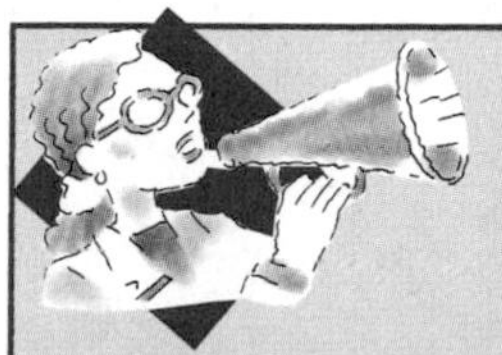

That's a wrap!

Mental health assessment review

Obtaining a mental health history
- Establish a trusting, therapeutic relationship.
- Choose a quiet, private setting.
- Maintain a calm, nonthreatening tone of voice to encourage open communication.
- Determine the patient's chief complaint, using the patient's own words to document it.
- Discuss past psychiatric disturbances and previous psychiatric treatment, if any.
- Obtain the patient's demographic and socioeconomic data.
- Discuss his cultural and religious beliefs.
- Obtain a medication history.
- Ask about a history of medical disorders; some conditions may adversely affect the patient's mental health.

Mental status checklist
- Appearance
- Demeanor and overall attitude
- Extraordinary behavior
- Inconsistencies between body language and mood
- Orientation to time, place, and person
- Confusion or disorientation
- Attention span
- Ability to recall events
- Intellectual function
- Speech characteristics that indicate altered thought processes
- Insight
- Coping or defense mechanisms
- Self-destructive behavior
- Psychological and mental status test results

Abnormal mental health findings
- Abnormal thought processes—derailment, flight of ideas, neologisms, confabulation, clanging, echolalia, incoherence
- Abnormal thought content—obsessions, compulsions, phobia, depersonalization, delusions, poverty of content
- Abnormal perceptions—illusions, hallucinations

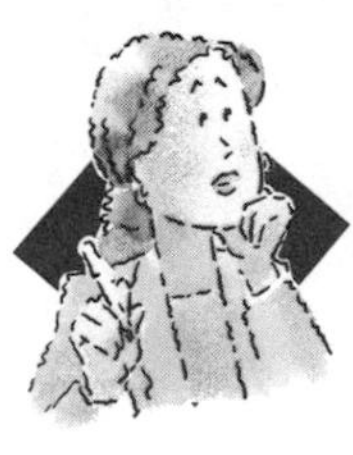

Quick quiz

1. Other sources are needed to validate data from a psychiatric patient's health history because:
   - A. mental status can change abruptly in response to internal or external stimuli.
   - B. personal biases might alter the interpretation of physical findings.
   - C. mental illness may alter the patient's perceptions.
   - D. psychiatric medications impair the patient's memory.

Answer: C. Mental illness can alter the patient's thinking, emotions, and perceptions, making him an unreliable source of information. If possible, verify the patient's responses with family members, friends, or health care personnel.

2. The therapeutic communication technique that involves redirecting the patient's attention toward a specific topic is called:

A. collaboration.
B. clarification
C. rephrasing.
D. focusing.

Answer: D. Focusing redirects the patient to a specific topic to prevent him from making vague generalizations.

3. Which psychological and mental status test helps assess the patient's memory?

A. Cognitive Capacity Screening Examination
B. Minnesota Multiphasic Personality Inventory
C. Beck Depression Inventory
D. Cognitive Assessment Scale

Answer: A. The Cognitive Capacity Screening Examination measures orientation, memory, calculation, and language.

4. You notice that your patient makes up events to fill in memory gaps. You identify this abnormal thought process as:

A. derailment.
B. echolalia.
C. confabulation.
D. clanging.

Answer: C. When a patient makes up events to fill in memory gaps, he's displaying confabulation.

Scoring

☆☆☆ If you answered all four questions correctly, fantastic! We aren't delusional when we say that you're a master of mental health assessments.

☆☆ If you answered three questions correctly, very good! There's nothing abnormal about your thought content when it comes to assessing mental health.

☆ If you answered fewer than three questions correctly, try not to get depressed! After a break to refresh your mental health, try reading the chapter again.

Part II Assessing body systems

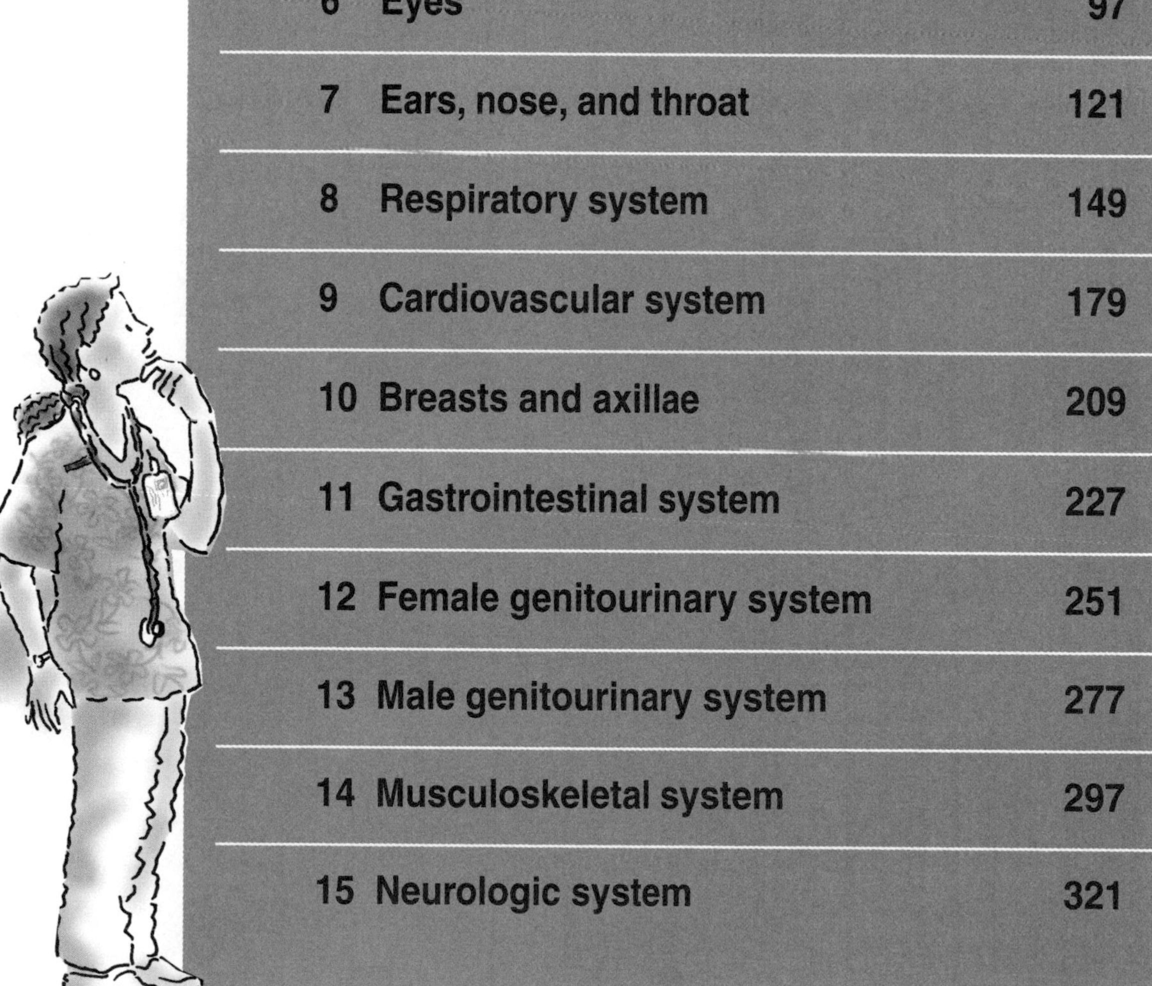

5

Skin, hair, and nails

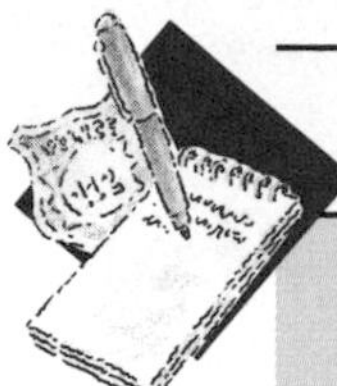

Just the facts

In this chapter, you'll learn:

- components of skin, hair, and nails
- changes in skin, hair, and nails that occur normally with age as well as those that signal a health problem
- questions to ask about skin, hair, and nails during the health history
- techniques for assessing skin, hair, and nails
- abnormalities of skin, hair, and nails and their causes.

A look at skin, hair, and nails

The skin, hair, and nails are like windows into a patient's health.

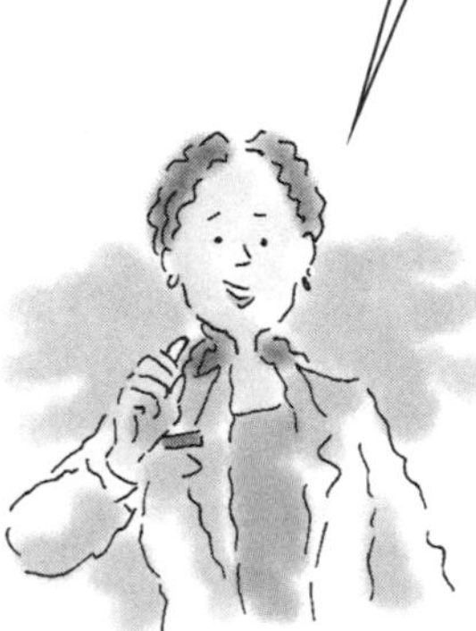

The skin covers the internal structures of the body and protects them from the external world. Along with hair and nails, the skin provides a window for viewing changes taking place inside the body. As a nurse, you observe a patient's skin, hair, and nails regularly, so it's likely that you would be the first to detect abnormalities. Your sharp assessment skills will help supply a reliable picture of the patient's overall health.

Anatomy and physiology of skin, hair, and nails

To perform an accurate physical assessment, you'll need to understand the anatomy and physiology of the skin, hair, and nails. Let's review them one by one.

Skin

Also called the *integumentary system*, the skin is the body's largest organ and has several important functions, including:
- protecting the tissues from trauma and bacteria
- preventing the loss of water and electrolytes from the body
- sensing temperature, pain, touch, and pressure
- regulating body temperature through sweat production and evaporation
- synthesizing vitamin D
- promoting wound repair by allowing cell replacement of surface wounds.

Layers of the skin

The skin consists of two distinct layers: the epidermis and the dermis. Subcutaneous tissue lies beneath these layers. The epidermis—the outer layer—is made of squamous epithelial tissue. It's thin and contains no blood vessels. The two major layers of the epidermis are the stratum corneum—the most superficial layer—and the deeper basal cell layer, or stratum germinativum. (See *What's in your skin.*)

Migrant workers

The stratum corneum is made up of cells that form in the basal cell layer, then migrate to the skin's outer surface, and die as they reach the surface. However, because epidermal regeneration is continuous, new cells are constantly being produced.

The basal cell layer contains melanocytes, which produce melanin and are responsible for skin color. Hormones, the environment, and heredity influence melanocyte production. Because melanocyte production is greater in some people than in others, skin color varies considerably.

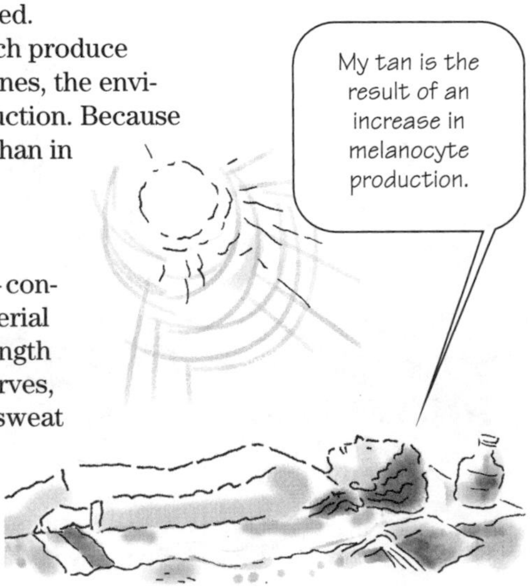

My tan is the result of an increase in melanocyte production.

Laying it on thick

The dermis—the thick, deeper layer of the skin—consists of connective tissue and an extracellular material called *matrix*, which contributes to the skin's strength and pliability. Blood vessels, lymphatic vessels, nerves, and hair follicles are located in the dermis, as are sweat and sebaceous glands. Because it's well supplied with blood, the dermis delivers nutrition to the epidermis. In addition, wound healing and infection control take place in the dermis.

What's in your skin

This cross section of the skin illustrates major skin structures.

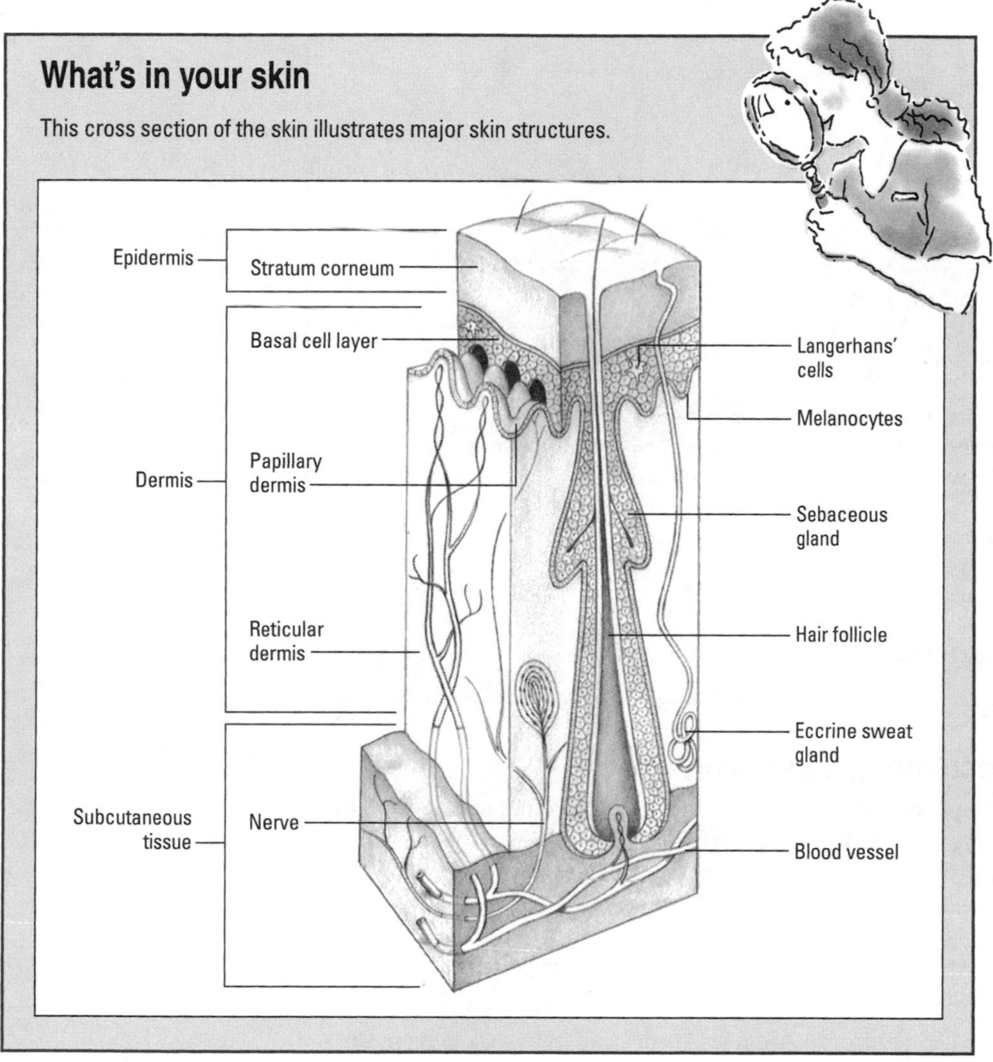

Give the glands a hand!

Sebaceous glands, found primarily in the skin of the scalp, face, upper body, and genital region, are part of the same structure that contains the hair follicles. Their main function is to produce sebum, which is secreted onto the skin or into the hair follicle to make the hair shiny and pliant.

There are two types of sweat glands:

- The eccrine glands, which are located over most of the body, produce a watery fluid that helps regulate body temperature.
- Apocrine glands secrete a milky substance and open into the hair follicle. They're located mainly in the axillae and the genital areas.

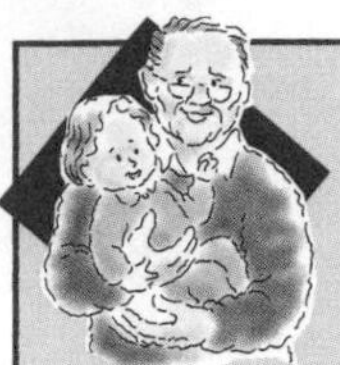

Ages and stages

How skin ages

This table lists skin changes that normally occur with aging.

Change	Findings in elderly people
Pigmentation	• Pale color
Thickness	• Wrinkling, especially on the face, arms, and legs • Parchmentlike appearance, especially over bony prominences and on the dorsal surfaces of the hands, feet, arms, and legs
Moisture	• Dry, flaky, and rough
Turgor	• "Tents" and stands alone, especially if the patient is dehydrated
Texture	• Numerous creases and lines

Affects of aging on skin

As people age, skin functions decline and normal changes occur. As a result, elderly patients are more prone to skin disease, infection, problems with wound healing, and tissue atrophy. (See *How skin ages.*)

Hair

Hair is formed from keratin and produced by matrix cells in the dermal layer. Each hair lies in a hair follicle and receives nourishment from a papilla, a loop of capillaries at the base of the follicle. At the lower end of the hair shaft is the hair bulb. The hair bulb contains melanocytes, which determine hair color. (See *A close look at hair.*)

Each hair is attached at the base to a smooth muscle called the *arrector pili*. This muscle contracts during emotional stress or exposure to cold and elevates the hair, causing goose bumps.

Hair today, gone tomorrow

A neonate's skin is covered with lanugo, a fine, downy growth of hair. Lanugo can be located over the entire body but occurs mostly on the shoulders and back. Most of the lanugo is shed within 2 weeks of birth. The amount of hair on a neonate's head varies, and

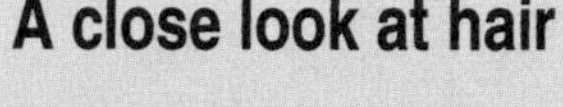

A close look at hair

The illustration below shows a hair shaft and its associated glands.

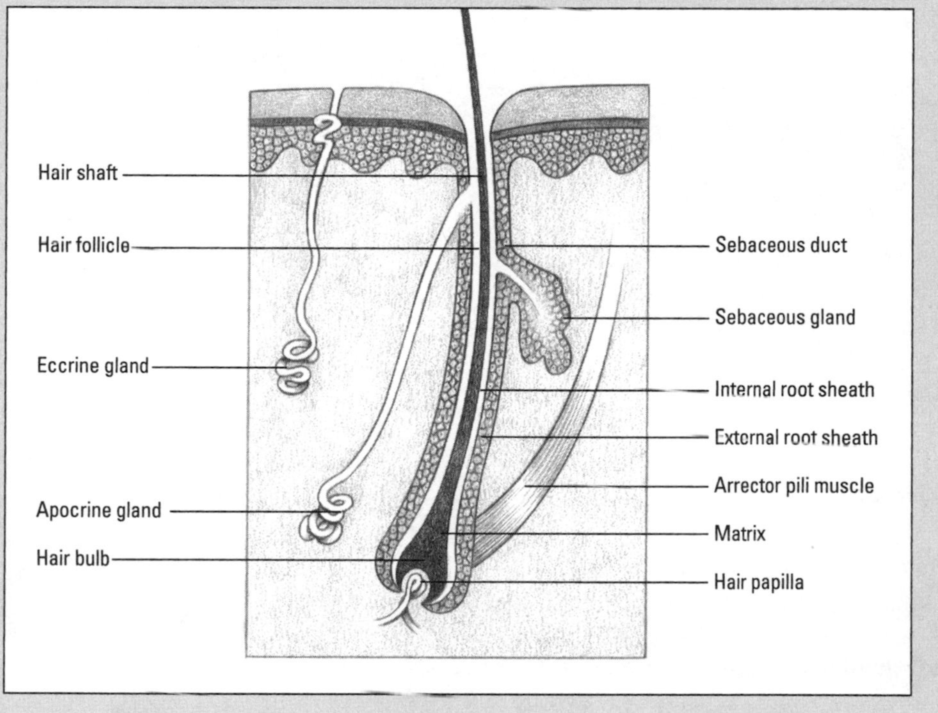

Older adults should anticipate less hair but more gray because hair growth and melanocyte function decline with age.

all of the original hair is lost several weeks after birth. It slowly grows back, sometimes in a different color.

As a person ages, melanocyte function declines, producing light or gray hair, and the hair follicle itself becomes drier as sebaceous gland function decreases. Hair growth declines, so the amount of body hair decreases. Balding, which is genetically determined in younger individuals, occurs in many people as a normal result of aging.

Nails

Nails are formed when epidermal cells are converted into hard plates of keratin. The nails are made up of the nail root (or nail matrix), nail plate, nail bed, lunula, nail folds, and cuticle. (See *Nail anatomy*, page 76.)

Nail anatomy

The illustration below shows the anatomic components of a fingernail.

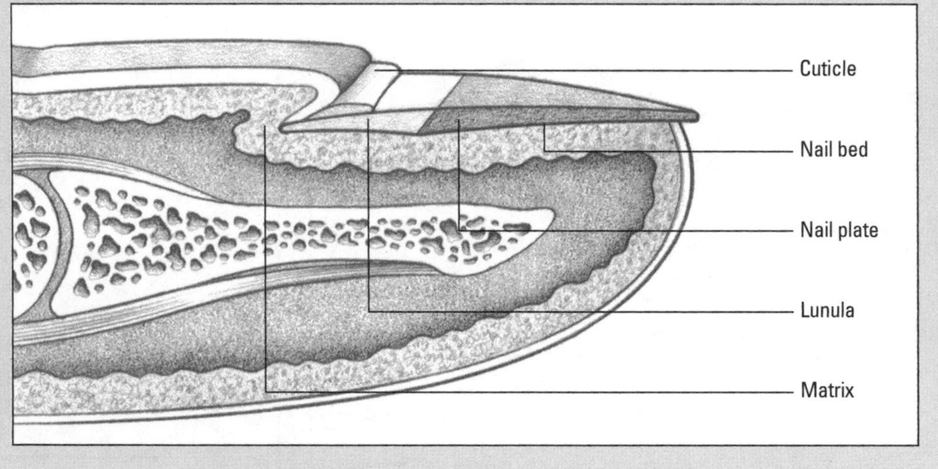

What's on your plate?

The nail plate is the visible, hardened layer that covers the fingertip. The plate is clear with fine longitudinal ridges. The pink color results from blood vessels underlying vascular epithelial cells.

What *is* the matrix?

The nail matrix is the site of nail growth. It's protected by the cuticle. At the end of the matrix is the white, crescent-shaped area, the lunula, which extends beyond the cuticle.

Not hard as nails anymore

With age, nail growth slows and the nails become brittle and thin. Longitudinal ridges in the nail plate become much more pronounced, making the nails prone to splitting. Also, the nails lose their luster and become yellowed.

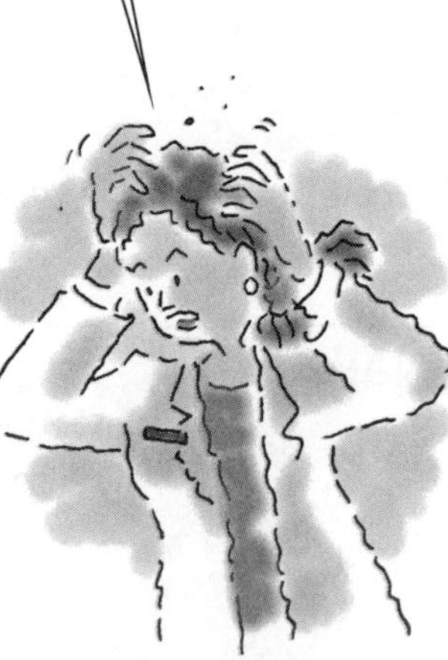

Obtaining a health history

When assessing a problem related to skin, hair, or nails, you need to thoroughly explore the patient's chief complaint, medical history, family history, psychological history, and patterns of daily living. Keep in mind that skin, hair, and nail abnormalities may result from a medical problem related to the patient's chief complaint, but the patient may be overlook or minimize them.

Asking about the skin

Most complaints about the skin involve itching, rashes, lesions, pigmentation abnormalities, or changes in existing lesions.

Skin deep

Typical questions to ask about changes in a patient's skin include:
- How and when did the skin changes occur?
- Are the changes in the form of a skin rash or lesion?
- Is the change confined to one area, or has the condition spread?
- Does the area bleed or have drainage?
- Does the area itch?
- How much time do you spend in the sun, and how do you protect your skin from ultraviolet rays?
- Do you have allergies?
- Do you have a family history of skin cancer or other significant diseases?
- Do you have a fever or joint pain, or have you lost weight?
- Have you had a recent insect bite?
- Do you take any medications or herbal preparations? If so, which ones?
- What changes in your skin have you observed in the past few years?

(See *Additional history questions for infants and children.*)

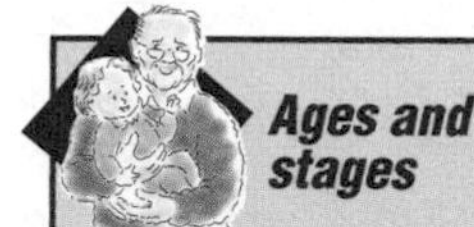

Additional history questions for infants and children

Remember to ask the parents these questions when obtaining a history for infants and children:
- Does the child have any birthmarks?
- When the child was a newborn, did he experience any change in skin color—for example, cyanosis or jaundice?
- Have you noted any rashes, burns, or bruises? If so, where and when, and what was the cause?
- Has the child been exposed to any contagious skin conditions—such as scabies, lice, or impetigo—or communicable diseases?

Asking about the hair

Most concerns about the hair refer either to hair loss or hirsutism, an increased growth and distribution of body hair. Either of these problems can be caused by such factors as skin infections, ovarian or adrenal tumors, increased stress, or systemic diseases, such as hypothyroidism and malignancies.

Getting to the root of the problem

To identify the cause of your patient's hair problem, ask:
- When did you first notice the loss (or gain) of hair? Was it sudden or gradual?
- Did the change occur in just a few spots or all over your body?
- What was happening in your life when the problem started?
- Are you taking any medications or herbal preparations?
- Are you experiencing itching, pain, discharge, fever, or weight loss?
- What serious illnesses, if any, have you had?

Asking about the nails

Most complaints about the nails concern changes in growth or color. Either of these problems may result from infection, nutritional deficiencies, systemic illnesses, or stress.

Nailing down the details

Typical questions to ask about changes in a patient's nails include:

- When did you first notice the changes in your nails?
- What types of changes have you noticed (for example, nail shape, color, or brittleness)?
- Were the changes sudden or gradual?
- Do you have other signs or symptoms, such as bleeding, pain, itching, or discharge?
- What's the normal condition of your nails?
- Do you have a history of serious illness?
- Do you have a history of nail problems?
- Do you bite your nails?
- Have you had nail tips attached?

Assessing skin, hair, and nails

To assess skin, hair, and nails, you'll use the techniques of inspection and palpation. Before beginning the examination, make sure the room is well lit and comfortably warm. Wear gloves during your examination.

Skin

Before you begin your skin assessment, gather these items: a clear ruler with centimeter and millimeter markings, a tongue blade, a penlight or flashlight, a Wood's lamp, and a magnifying glass. This equipment enables you to measure and closely inspect skin lesions and other abnormalities.

The big picture

Start by observing the skin's overall appearance. Such observation can help you identify areas that need further assessment. Inspect and palpate the skin area by area, focusing on color, texture, turgor, moisture, and temperature.

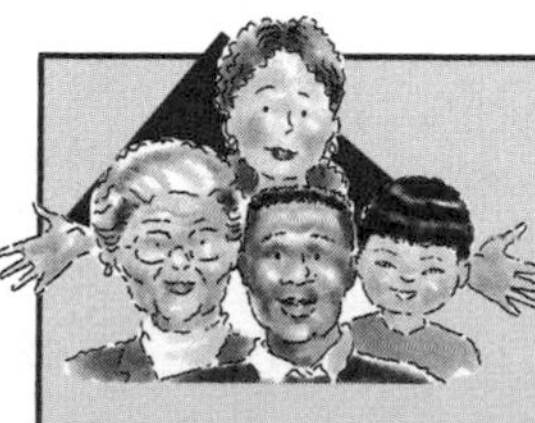

Bridging the gap

Detecting color variations in dark-skinned people

Cyanosis
Examine the conjunctivae, palms, soles, buccal mucosa, and tongue. Look for dull, dark color.

Edema
Examine the area for decreased color and palpate for tightness.

Erythema
Palpate the area for warmth.

Jaundice
Examine the sclerae and hard palate in natural, not fluorescent, light if possible. Look for a yellow color.

Pallor
Examine the sclerae, conjunctivae, buccal mucosa, tongue, lips, nail beds, palms, and soles. Look for an ashen color.

Petechiae
Examine areas of lighter pigmentation such as the abdomen. Look for tiny, purplish red dots.

Rashes
Palpate the area for skin texture changes.

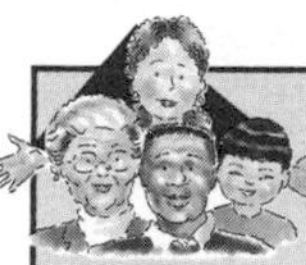

Bridging the gap

Mongolian spots

Mongolian spots are irregularly shaped areas of deep blue pigmentation. They most commonly occur over the sacral and gluteal areas but may also appear on the shoulders, arms, abdomen, or thighs. These bluish discolored areas are normal variations of the skin in children of African, Asian, or Latin descent. In fact, 90% of Black children and 80% of Asian children have Mongolian spots.

Mongolian spots are present at birth and usually remain visible into adulthood, although they may fade over time. They result from deposits of embryonic pigment in the epidermal layer left behind from fetal development.

Mongolian spots are completely benign and require no treatment. When assessing children, be careful not to confuse these spots with bruises, which may cause an erroneous suspicion of child abuse.

Color

Look for localized areas of bruising, cyanosis, pallor, and erythema. Check for uniformity of color and hypopigmented or hyperpigmented areas.

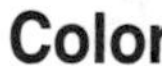

A spotty record

Places exposed to the sun may show a darker pigmentation than other areas. Color changes may vary depending on skin pigmentation. (See *Detecting color variations in dark-skinned people.*) Be aware that some local skin color changes are normal variations that appear in certain cultures. (See *Mongolian spots.*)

Texture and turgor

Inspect and palpate the skin's texture, noting its thickness and mobility. It should look smooth and be intact. Rough, dry skin is common in patients with hypothyroidism, psoriasis, and excessive keratinization. Skin that isn't intact may indicate local irritation or trauma.

Turgor-nomics

Palpation also helps you evaluate the patient's hydration status. Dehydration and edema cause poor skin turgor. Note, however, that because poor skin turgor may also be caused by aging, it may not be a reliable indicator of an elderly patient's hydration status. Overhydration causes skin to appear edematous and spongy. Localized edema also can result from trauma or systemic disease. (See *Evaluating skin turgor*.)

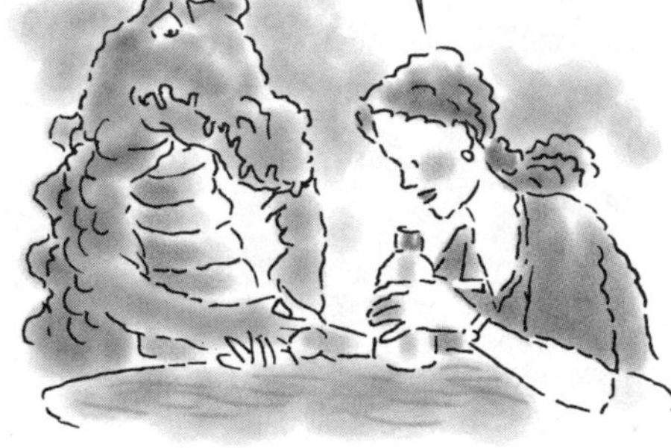

Moisture

Observe the skin's moisture content. The skin should be relatively dry, with a minimal amount of perspiration. Skin-fold areas should also be fairly dry. Overly dry skin appears red and flaky.

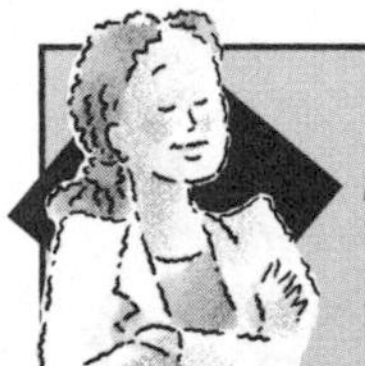

Peak technique

Evaluating skin turgor

To assess skin turgor in an adult, gently squeeze the skin on the forearm or sternal area between your thumb and forefinger, as shown at right. In an infant, roll a fold of loosely adherent abdominal skin between your thumb and forefinger. Then release the skin.

If the skin quickly returns to its original shape, the patient has normal turgor. If it returns to its original shape slowly over 30 seconds or maintains a tented position, as shown at right, the skin has poor turgor.

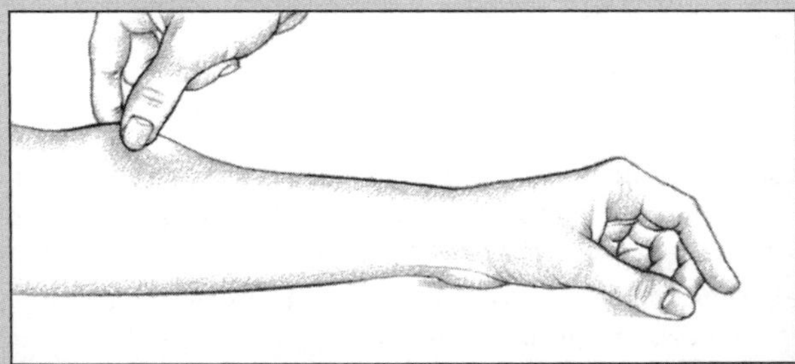

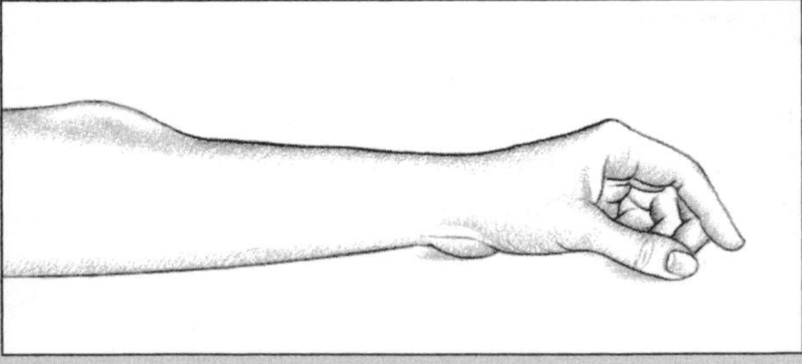

All in a sweat

Overly moist skin can be caused by anxiety, obesity, or an environment that's too warm. Heavy sweating, or diaphoresis, usually accompanies fever; strenuous activity; cardiac, pulmonary, and other diseases; and any activity or illness that elevates metabolic rate.

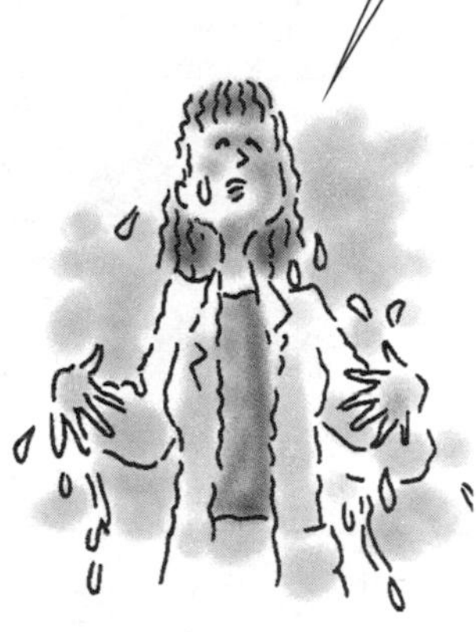

Temperature

Palpate the skin bilaterally for temperature, which can range from cool to warm. Warm skin suggests normal circulation; cool skin, a possible underlying disorder. Distinguish between generalized and localized coolness and warmth. Localized skin coolness can result from vasoconstriction associated with cold environments or impaired arterial circulation to a limb. General coolness can result from such conditions as shock or hypothyroidism. (See *Assessing skin temperature.*)

Hot and bothered

Localized warmth occurs in areas that are infected, inflamed, or burned. Generalized warmth occurs with fever or systemic diseases such as hyperthyroidism. Be sure to check skin temperature bilaterally.

Lesions

During your inspection, you may see normal variations in the skin's texture and pigmentation.

Denoting disease

Red lesions caused by vascular changes include hemangiomas, telangiectases, petechiae, purpura, and ecchymoses and may indicate disease.

Stamp of approval

Normal variations include birthmarks, freckles, and nevi, or moles. Birthmarks are generally flat and range in color from tan to red or brown. They can be found on all areas of the body. Freckles are small, flat macules located primarily on the face, arms, and back. They're usually red brown to brown. Nevi are either flat or raised and may be pink, tan, or dark brown. Like birthmarks, they can be found on all areas of the body.

New or not?

When investigating a lesion, start by classifying it as primary or secondary. A primary lesion is new. Changes in a primary lesion constitute a secondary lesion. Examples of secondary lesions in-

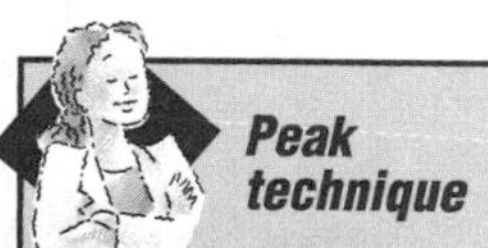

Assessing skin temperature

When you're trying to compare subtle temperature differences in one area of the body to another, use the dorsal surface of your hands and fingers. They're the most sensitive to changes in temperature.

Identifying primary lesions

Are you having trouble identifying your patient's lesion? Here's a quick look at three common lesions. Remember to keep a centimeter ruler handy to accurately measure the size of the lesion.

Macule
Flat, circumscribed area of altered skin color, generally less than ⅜" (1 cm); examples: freckle, flat nevus

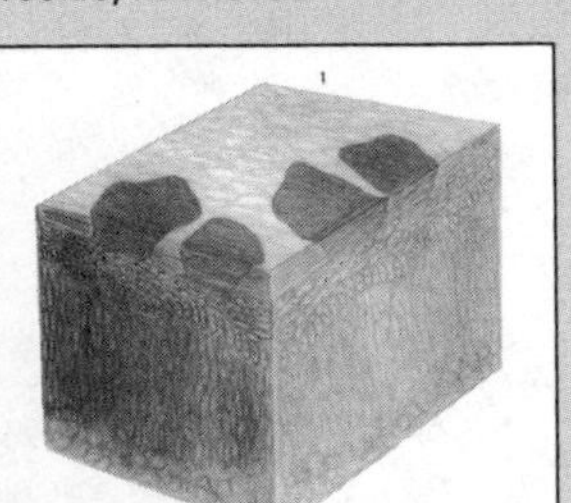

Papule
Raised, circumscribed, solid area; generally less than ⅜"; examples: elevated nevus, wart

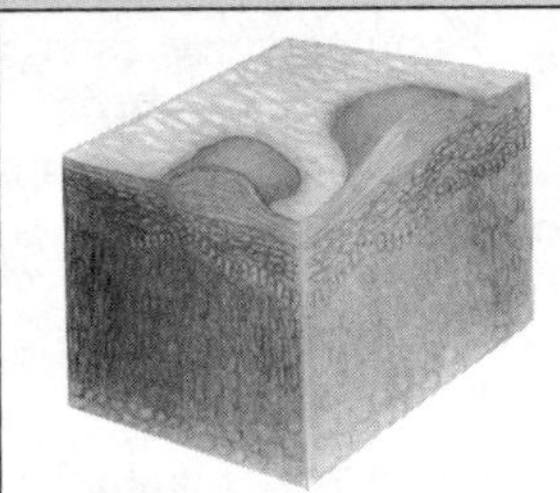

Vesicle
Circumscribed, elevated lesion; contains serous fluid; less than ⅜"; example: early chickenpox

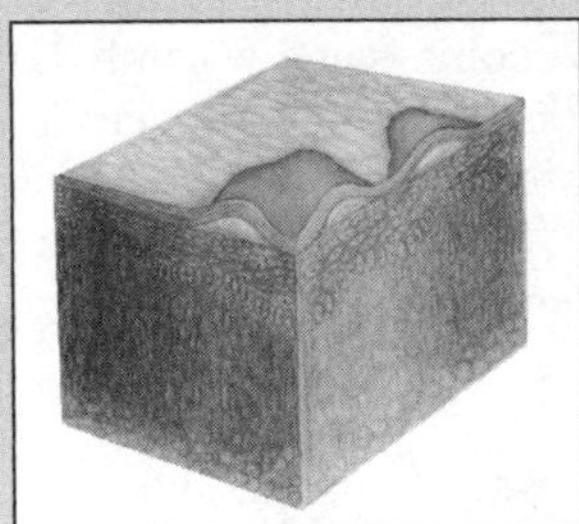

clude fissures, scales, crusts, scars, and excoriations. (See *Identifying primary lesions.*)

It's what's inside that counts

Determine if the lesion is solid or fluid-filled. Macules, papules, nodules, wheals, and hives are solid lesions. Vesicles, bullae, pustules, and cysts are fluid-filled lesions. Use a flashlight or penlight to determine whether a lesion is solid or fluid-filled. (See *Illuminating lesions.*)

Wood you light my lesion?

To identify lesions that fluoresce, use a Wood's lamp, which gives out specially filtered ultraviolet light. Darken the room and shine the light on the lesion. If the lesion looks bluish green, the patient has a fungal infection.

Lesion lowdown

After you've identified the type of lesion, you'll need to describe its characteristics, pattern, location, and distribution. A detailed description can help you determine whether the lesion is a normal or pathologic skin change.

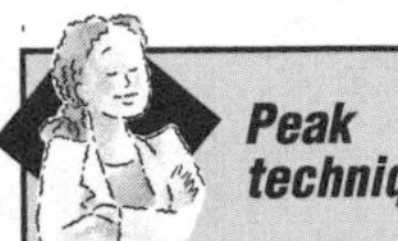

Peak technique

Illuminating lesions

Illuminating a lesion can help you see it better and learn more about its characteristics. Here are two techniques worth perfecting.

Macule or papule?
To determine whether a lesion is a macule or a papule, use this technique: Reduce the direct lighting and shine a penlight or flashlight at a right angle to the lesion. If the light casts a shadow, the lesion is a papule. Macules are flat and don't produce shadows.

Solid or fluid-filled?
To determine whether a lesion is solid or fluid-filled, use this technique: Place the tip of a flashlight or penlight against the side of the lesion. Solid lesions don't transmit light. Fluid-filled lesions transilluminate with a red glow.

Border patrol

Examine the lesion to see if it looks the same on both sides. Also, check the borders to see if they're regular or irregular. An asymmetrical lesion with an irregular border may indicate malignancy.

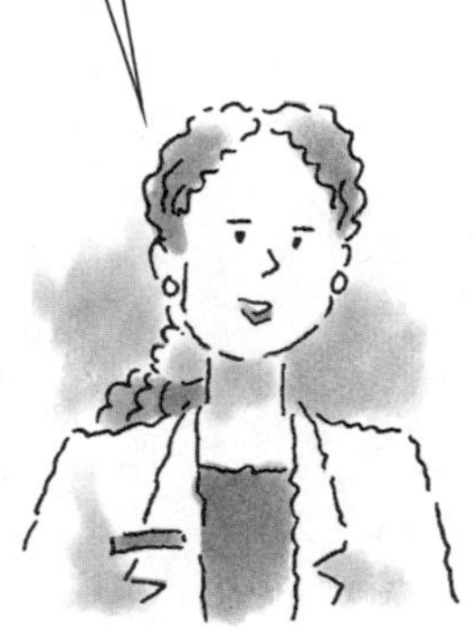

A horse of a different color

Lesions occur in various colors and can change color over time. Therefore, watch for such changes in your patient. For example, if a lesion such as a mole (nevus) has changed from tan or brown to multiple shades of tan, dark brown, black, or a mixture of red, white, and blue, the lesion might be malignant.

Follow the pattern

Pay close attention as well to the configuration and distribution of the lesions. Many skin diseases have typical configuration patterns. Identifying those patterns can help you determine the cause of the problem. (See *Recognizing common lesion configurations*, page 84.)

Sizing up the situation

Measure the diameter of the lesion using a millimeter-centimeter ruler. If you estimate the diameter, you may not be able to determine subtle changes in size. An increase in the size or elevation of a mole over many years is common and probably normal. Still, be sure to take note of moles that rapidly change size, especially moles that are 6 mm or larger.

If you note drainage, document the type, color, and amount. Also note if the lesion has a foul odor, which can indicate a superimposed infection.

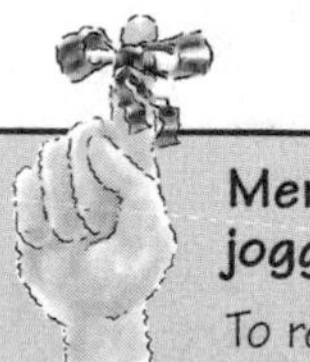

Memory jogger

To remember what to assess when evaluating a lesion, think of the letters **ABCDE.**

Asymmetry

Border

Color and **C**onfiguration

Diameter and **D**rainage

Evolution or progression of the lesion

Hair

Start by inspecting and palpating the hair over the patient's entire body, not just on his head. Note the distribution, quantity, texture, and color. The quantity and distribution of head and body hair vary between patients. However, hair should be evenly distributed over the entire body.

Too much or too little?

Check for patterns of hair loss and growth. If you notice patchy hair loss, look for regrowth. Also, examine the scalp for erythema, scaling, and encrustation. Excessive hair loss with scalp crusting may indicate ringworm infestation. The only way to detect scalp crusting is by using a Wood's lamp. Also, note areas of excessive hair growth, which may indicate a hormone imbalance or be a sign of a systemic disorder such as Cushing's syndrome.

Recognizing common lesion configurations

Identify the configuration of your patient's skin lesion by matching it to one of these diagrams.

Discrete
Individual lesions are separate and distinct.

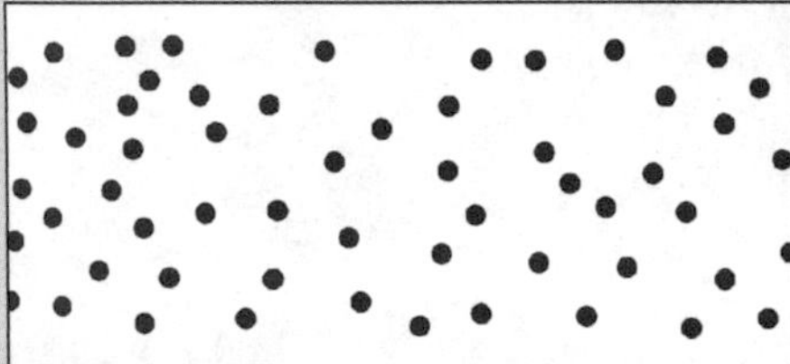

Annular
Lesions are arranged in a single ring or circle.

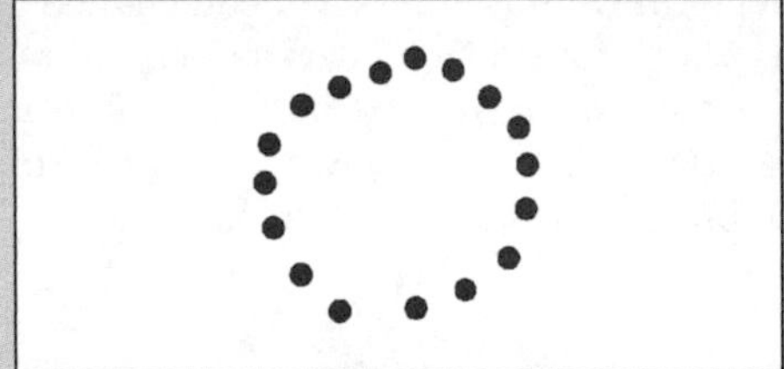

Grouped
Lesions are clustered together.

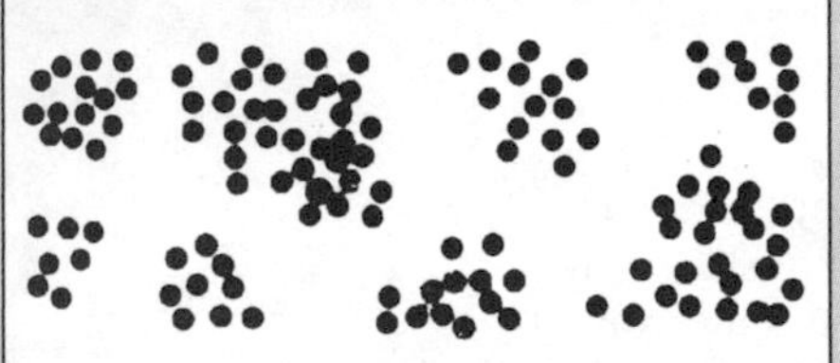

Polycyclic
Lesions are arranged in multiple circles.

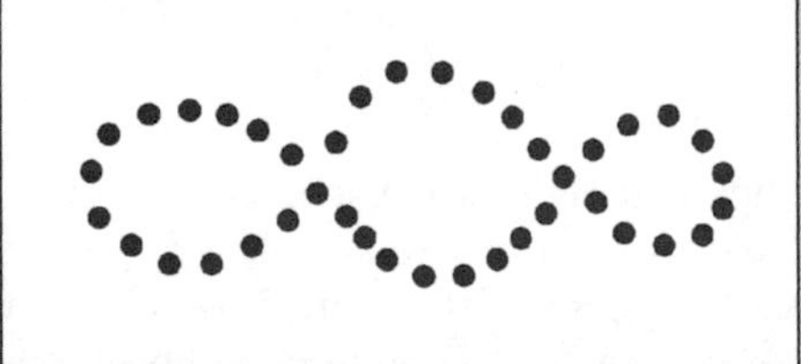

Confluent
Lesions merge so that individual lesions aren't visible or palpable.

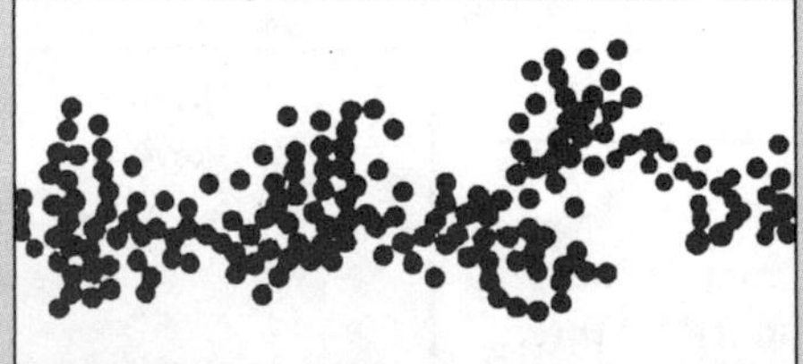

Arciform
Lesions form arcs or curves.

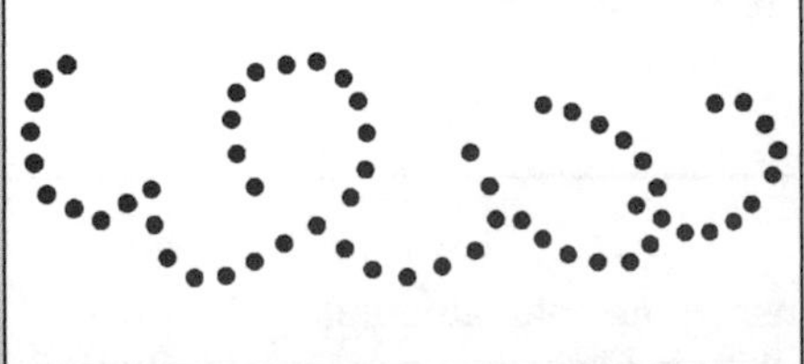

Linear
Lesions form a line.

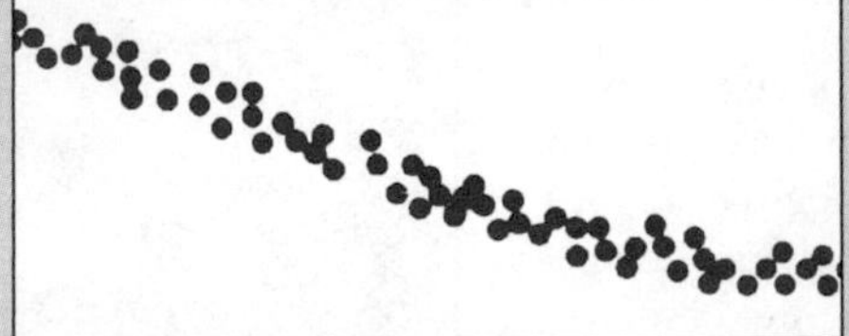

Reticular
Lesions form a meshlike network.

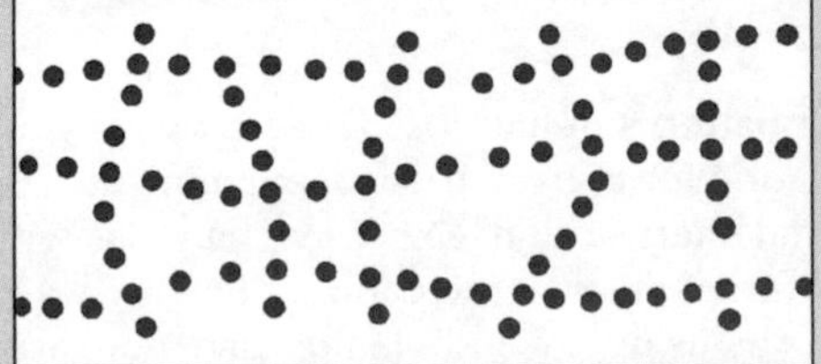

Having a bad hair day?

The texture of scalp hair also varies between patients. As a rule, hair should be shiny and smooth, not dry or brittle. Differences in grooming and hairstyling may affect the hair's texture and quality. Dryness or brittleness can result from the use of harsh hair treatments or hair care products or can be caused by a systemic illness. Extreme oiliness is usually related to excessive sebum production or poor grooming habits.

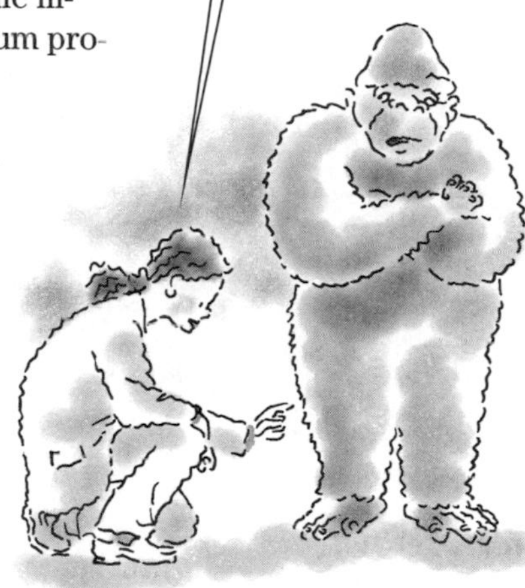

Nails

Assessing the nails is vital for two reasons: The appearance of the nails can be a critical indicator of systemic illness, and their overall condition tells you a lot about the patient's grooming habits and ability to care for himself. Examine the nails for color, shape, thickness, consistency, and contour.

Nail that color

First, look at the color of the nails. Light-skinned people generally have pinkish nails. Dark-skinned people generally have brown nails. Brown-pigmented bands in the nail beds are normal in dark-skinned people and abnormal in light-skinned people. Yellow nails may occur in smokers as a result of nicotine stains.

Circulation check

Nail beds can be used to assess a patient's peripheral circulation. Press on the nail bed and then release, noting how long the color takes to return. It should return immediately, or at least within 3 seconds.

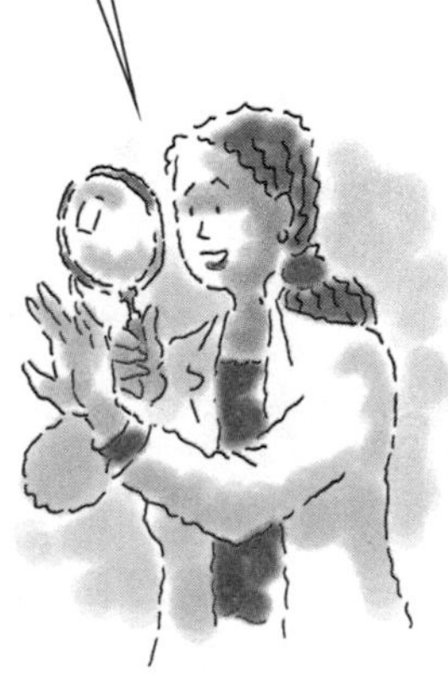

What shapely nails!

Next, inspect the shape and contour of the nails. The surface of the nail bed should be either slightly curved or flat. The edges of the nail should be smooth, rounded, and clean.

What's the angle?

The angle of the nail base is normally less than 180 degrees. An increase in the nail angle suggests clubbing. Curved nails are a normal variation. They may appear to be clubbed until you notice that the nail angle is still less than 180 degrees.

Thick and strong?

Finally, palpate the nail bed to check the thickness of the nail and the strength of its attachment to the bed.

Abnormal findings

Are you feeling self-conscious about your nails?

Various abnormalities may be found when assessing the skin, hair, and nails. Because these abnormalities may be visible to others, the patient may experience some degree of emotional stress. Carefully document all abnormal findings, pertinent health history, and as much information as possible from the physical examination. (See *Skin, hair, and nail abnormalities.*)

Skin abnormalities

The signs and symptoms you detect during your assessment may be caused by a wide variety of disorders. This section describes the most common skin abnormalities. You can also refer to the chart *Skin color variations*, page 89, and the color photographs on pages C1 to C4 for more on skin abnormalities.

Café-au-lait spots

Café-au-lait spots appear as flat, light brown, uniformly hyperpigmented macules or patches on the skin surface. They usually appear during the first 3 years of life but may develop at any age.

Coffee, anyone?

Café-au-lait spots can be differentiated from freckles and other benign birthmarks by their larger size and irregular shape. They usually have no significance; however, six or more café-au-lait spots may be associated with an underlying neurologic disorder such as neurofibromatosis.

Cherry angiomas

Cherry angiomas are tiny, bright red, round papules that may become brown over time. These clinically insignificant lesions occur in virtually everyone older than age 30 and increase in number with age.

Papular rash

A papular rash consists of small, raised, circumscribed — and perhaps discolored (red to purple) — lesions known as *papules.* It may erupt anywhere on the body in various configurations and may be acute or chronic. Papular rashes characterize skin disorders; they may also result from allergies and from infectious, neoplastic, and systemic disorders.

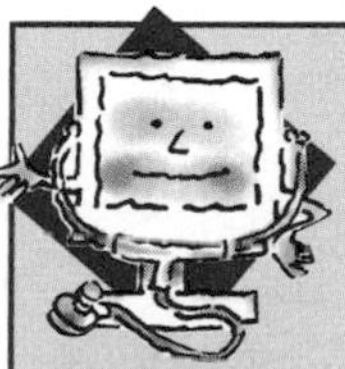

Interpretation station

Skin, hair, and nail abnormalities

After you assess the patient, a group of findings may lead you to suspect a particular disorder. The chart below shows common groups of findings for the signs and symptoms of the integumentary system, along with their probable causes.

Sign or symptom and findings	Probable cause
Alopecia	
• Patchy alopecia, typically on the lower extremities • Thin, shiny, atrophic skin • Thickened nails • Weak or absent peripheral pulses • Cool extremities • Paresthesia	Arterial insufficiency
• Translucent, charred or ulcerated skin • Pain	Burns
• Loss of the outer third of the eyebrows • Thin, dull, coarse, brittle hair on the face • Fatigue • Constipation • Cold intolerance • Weight gain • Puffy face, hands, and feet	Hypothyroidism
Clubbing	
• Anorexia • Malaise • Dyspnea • Tachypnea • Diminished breath sounds • Pursed-lip breathing • Barrel chest • Peripheral cyanosis	Emphysema
Clubbing *(continued)*	
• Wheezing • Dyspnea • Fatigue • Neck vein distention • Palpitations • Unexplained weight gain • Dependent edema • Crackles on auscultation	Heart failure
• Hemoptysis • Dyspnea • Wheezing • Chest pain • Fatigue • Weight loss • Fever	Lung and pleural cancer
Pruritus	
• Intense, severe pruritus • Erythematous rash on dry skin at flexion points • Possible edema, scaling, and pustules	Atopic dermatitis
• Scalp excoriation from scratching • Matted, foul-smelling, lusterless hair • Occipital and cervical lymphadenopathy • Oval, gray-white nits on hair shafts	Pediculosis capitis (head lice)

(continued)

Skin, hair, and nail abnormalities *(continued)*

Sign or symptom and findings	Probable cause
***Pruritus** (continued)*	
• Gradual or sudden pruritus • Ammonia breath odor • Oliguria or anuria • Fatigue • Irritability • Muscle cramps	Chronic renal failure
Urticaria	
• Rapid eruption of diffuse urticaria and angioedema, with wheals ranging from pinpoint to palm-size or larger • Pruritic, stinging lesions • Profound anxiety • Weakness • Shortness of breath • Nasal congestion • Dysphagia • Warm, moist skin	Anaphylaxis
***Urticaria** (continued)*	
• Nonpitting, nonpruritic edema of an extremity of the face • Possibly acute laryngeal edema	Hereditary angioedema
• Erythema chronicum migrans that results in urticaria • Constant malaise and fatigue • Fever • Chills • Lymphadenopathy • Neurologic and cardiac abnormalities • Arthritis	Lyme disease

Port-wine hemangiomas

Port-wine hemangiomas, commonly called *port-wine stains*, are usually present at birth and commonly appear on the face and upper body as flat purple marks.

Pruritus

Commonly provoking scratching to obtain relief, this unpleasant itching sensation is the most common symptom of skin disorders.

I've got you under my skin

Pruritus may also result from a local or systemic disorder, drug use, emotional upset, or contact with skin irritants. Pruritus may be exacerbated by increased skin temperature, poor skin turgor, local vasodilation, dermatoses, and stress.

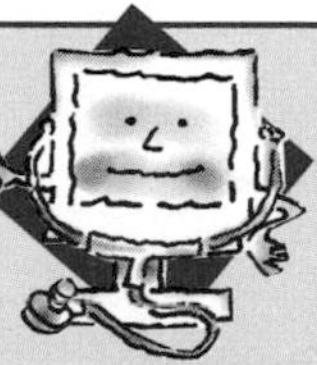

Interpretation station

Skin color variations

To interpret skin color variation findings faster, refer to this chart.

Color	Distribution	Possible cause
Absent	• Small, circumscribed areas • Generalized	• Vitiligo • Albinism
Blue	• Around lips, buccal mucosa, or generalized	• Cyanosis (*Note:* In blacks, blue gingivae are normal.)
Deep red	• Generalized	• Polycythemia vera (increased red blood cell count)
Pink	• Local or generalized	• Erythema (superficial capillary dilation and congestion)
Tan to brown	• Facial patches	• Chloasma of pregnancy; butterfly rash of lupus erythematosus
Tan to brown-bronze	• Generalized (not related to sun exposure)	• Addison's disease
Yellow to yellowish brown	• Sclera or generalized	• Jaundice from liver dysfunction (*Note:* In blacks, yellowish brown pigmentation of sclera is normal.)
Yellowish orange	• Palms, soles, and face; not sclera	• Carotenemia (carotene in the blood)

Purpuric lesions

Purpuric lesions are caused by red blood cells and blood pigments in the skin, so they don't blanch under pressure.

On the spot

The three types of purpuric lesions are:
- petechiae — red or brown pinpoint lesions generally caused by capillary fragility; diseases associated with the formation of microemboli or bleeding, such as subacute bacterial endocarditis and thrombocytopenia, can cause petechiae
- ecchymoses — bluish or purplish discolorations resulting from blood accumulation in the skin after injury to the vessel walls
- hematomas — masses of blood that accumulate in a tissue, organ, or body space after a break in a blood vessel.

Cruisin' for a bruisin'

Purpuric lesions also produce deep red or reddish purple bruising that may be caused by bleeding disorders such as disseminated intravascular coagulation.

Telangiectases

Telangiectases are permanently dilated, small blood vessels that typically form a weblike pattern. For example, spider hemangiomas, a type of telangiectasis, are small, red lesions arranged in a weblike configuration. They usually appear on the face, neck, and chest and may be normal or associated with pregnancy or cirrhosis.

Urticaria

Urticaria is a vascular skin reaction characterized by the eruption of transient pruritic wheals — smooth, slightly elevated patches with well-defined erythematous margins and pale centers of various shapes and sizes.

Remember: In addition to allergies, stress and environmental factors can cause urticaria.

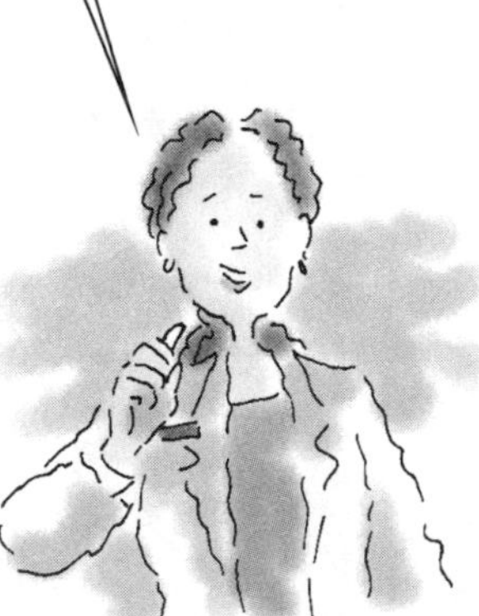

Allergy alert

Urticaria lesions, also called *hives*, are produced by the local release of histamine or other vasoactive substances as part of a hypersensitivity reaction, commonly to certain drugs, foods, insect bites, inhalants, or contact with certain substances. Urticaria may also result from emotional stress or environmental factors.

Vesicular rash

A vesicular rash is a scattered or linear distribution of blisterlike lesions — sharply circumscribed and filled with clear, cloudy, or bloody fluid. The lesions, which are usually less than 0.5 cm in diameter, may occur singly or in groups. They sometimes occur with bullae — fluid-filled lesions larger than 0.5 cm in diameter.

A vesicular rash may be mild or severe and temporary or permanent. It can result from infection, inflammation, or allergic reactions.

Hair abnormalities

Typically stemming from other problems, hair abnormalities can cause patients emotional distress. Among the most common hair abnormalities are alopecia and hirsutism.

(Text continues on page 91.)

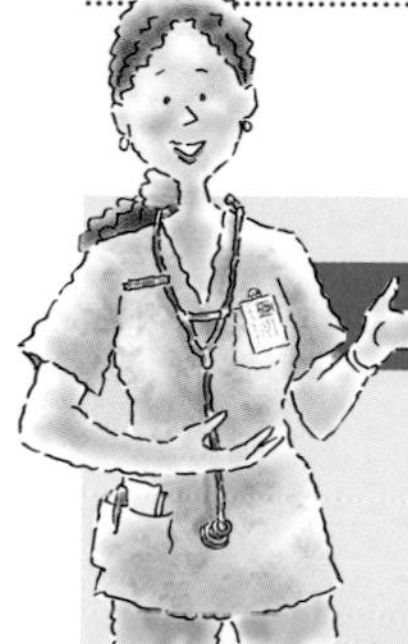

Recognizing common skin disorders

On this page and the pages that follow, you'll find photos of common skin disorders along with brief descriptions of each. Use the photos to guide your assessment of abnormal skin findings.

Basal cell carcinoma

The most common type of skin cancer, basal cell carcinoma results from sun exposure. It usually appears as a small waxy-looking nodule that ulcerates and forms a central depression. Basal cell carcinoma usually starts as a skin-colored papule (may be deeply pigmented) with a translucent top and overlying telangiectases. It rarely metastasizes and commonly appears on the head and neck.

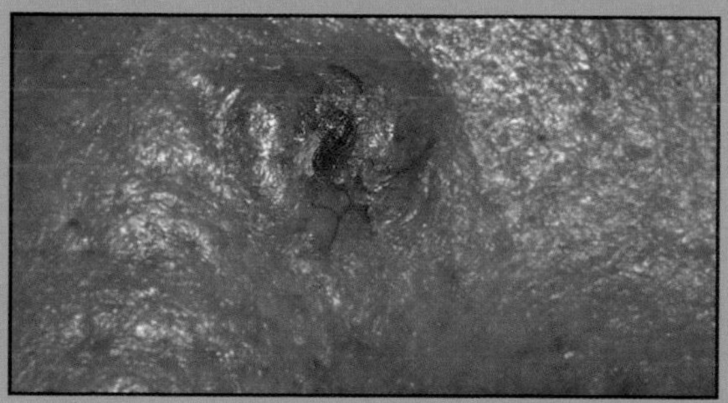

Malignant melanoma

Malignant melanoma can occur anywhere on the body and can arise from a preexisting mole. Its border, color, and surface are usually irregular. The lesion is usually black or purple, although some may be pink, red, or whitish blue. The lesion may be accompanied by scaling, flaking, or oozing.

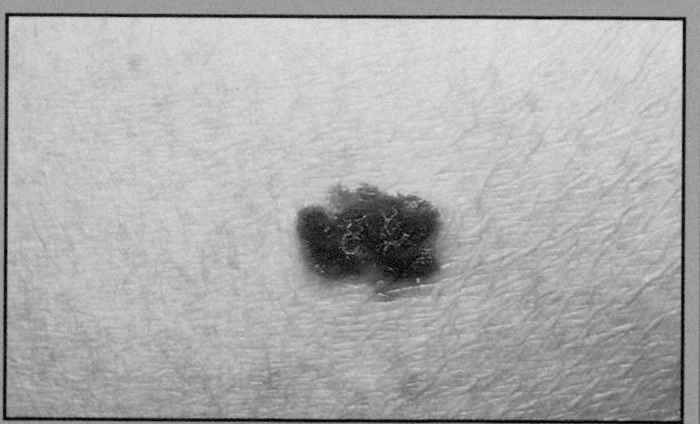

Squamous cell carcinoma

Squamous cell carcinoma results from sun exposure and can metastasize. It appears as a raised border with a central ulcer and may be rough, thickened, or scaly. It most commonly appears on the face and neck as an erythematous scaly patch with sharp edges.

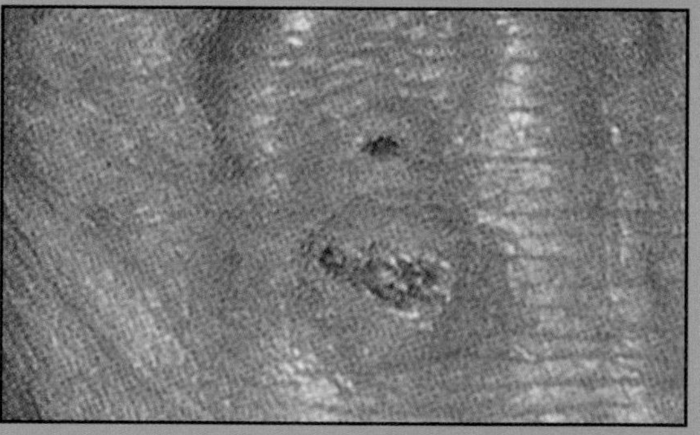

Kaposi's sarcoma

Kaposi's sarcoma tends to appear first on the lower legs, but lesions may develop anywhere. Initially, you'll note multiple brown or bluish red nodules of varying shapes and sizes. These nodules develop into larger plaques. The lesions may open and drain or cause edema of the legs.

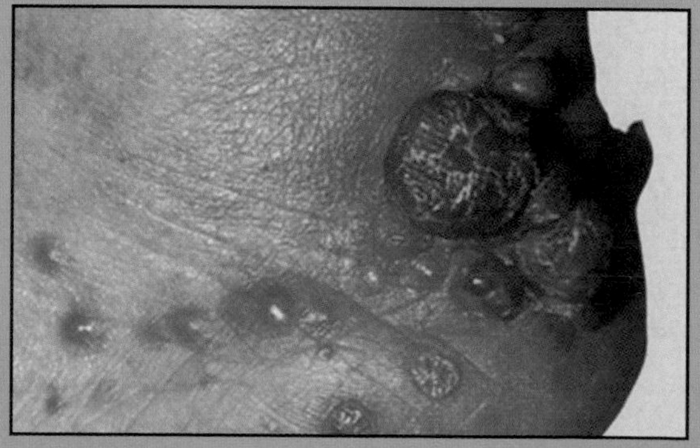

(continued)

Recognizing common skin disorders *(continued)*

Lupus erythematosus (discoid or systemic)

The typical sign of lupus erythematosus appears as a red, scaly, sharply demarcated, butterfly-shaped rash over the cheeks and nose. The rash may extend to other areas of the face or to other exposed areas, such as the ears and neck.

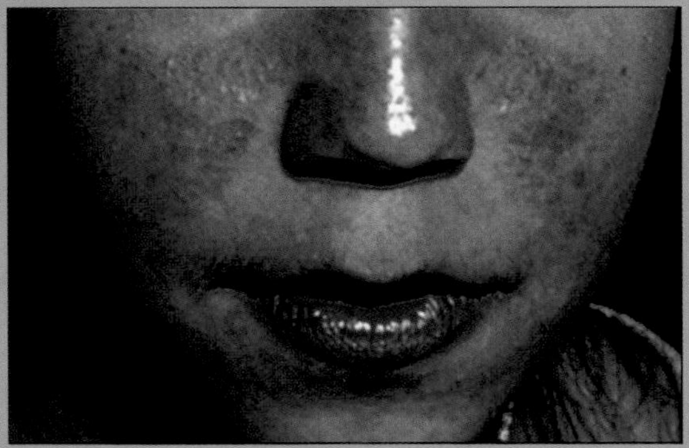

Scabies

Mites, which can be picked up from an infested person, burrow under the skin and cause scabies lesions. The lesions appear in a straight or zigzagging line about ⅜″ (1 cm) long with a black dot at the end. Commonly seen between the fingers, at the bend of the elbow and knee, and around the groin, abdomen, or perineal area, scabies lesions itch and may cause a rash.

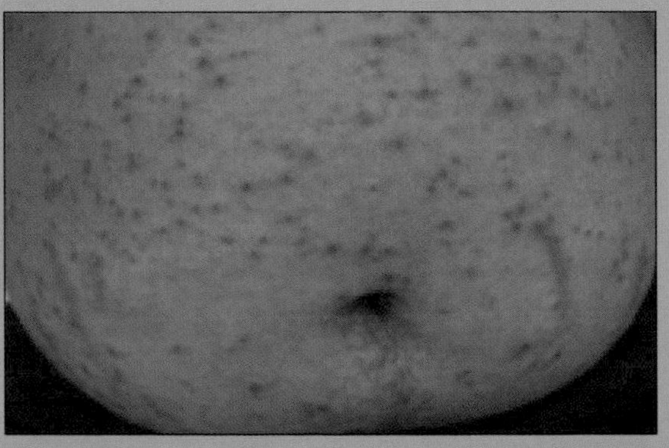

Telangiectasia

Formed by dilation of small blood vessels, telangiectasia blanches when pressure is applied. This type of lesion may be a normal finding in an elderly person or may be associated with cirrhosis or lupus erythematosus.

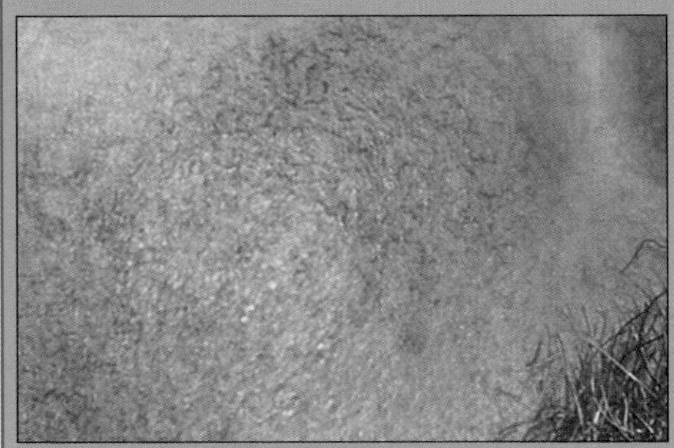

Vitiligo

Vitiligo is a slowly progressive disease of hypopigmentation that causes irregular areas of pigmented skin around milk-colored patches. These areas commonly appear on the face, hands, and feet.

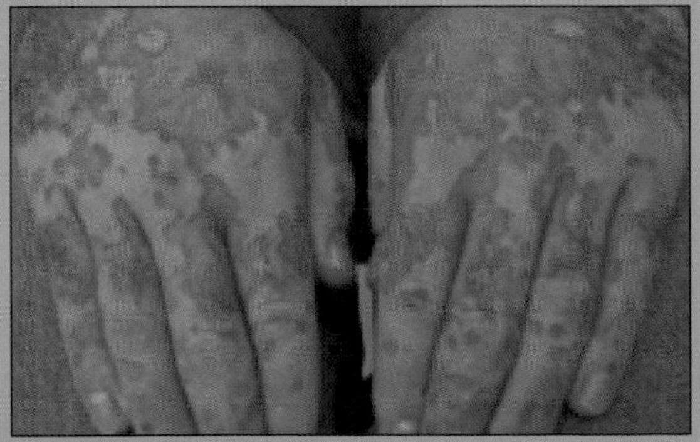

Psoriasis

Psoriasis is a chronic disease of marked epidermal thickening. Plaques are symmetrical and generally appear as red bases topped with silvery scales. The lesions, which may connect with one another, occur most commonly on the scalp, elbows, and knees.

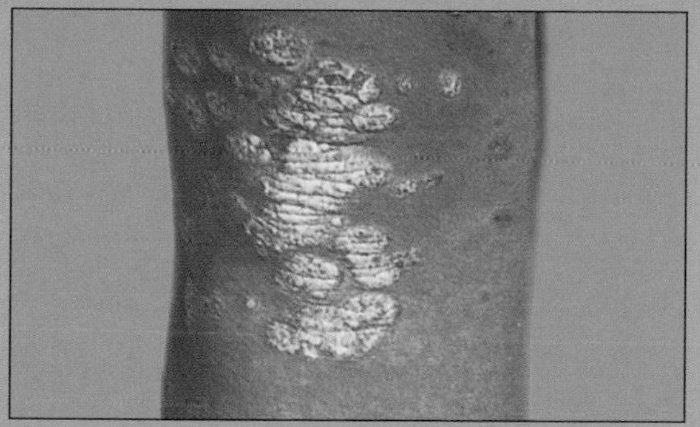

Urticaria (hives)

Occurring as an allergic reaction, urticaria appears suddenly as pink, edematous papules or wheals (round elevations of the skin). Itching is intense. The lesions may become large and contain vesicles.

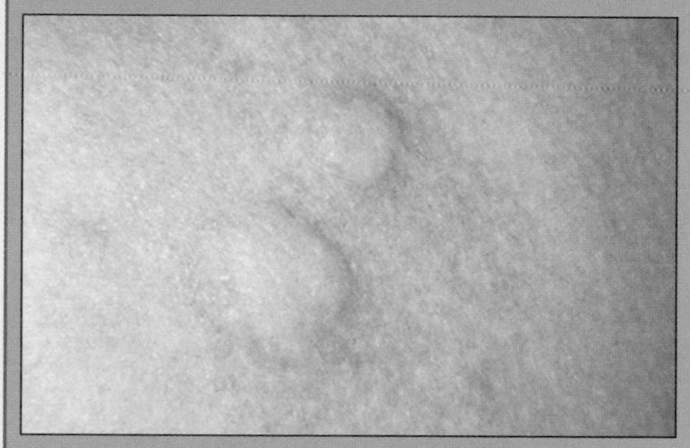

Contact dermatitis

Contact dermatitis is an inflammatory disorder that results from contact with an irritant. Primary lesions include vesicles, large oozing bullae, and red macules that appear at localized areas of redness. These lesions may itch and burn.

Eczema

Eczema may be acute or chronic and may be accompanied by severe itching. Mostly affecting the antecubital and popliteal areas, these lesions may be red and papular, vesicular, or pustular. Lesions cause blisters, oozing, and crusting. Thickening, excoriation, and extreme dryness of the skin can also occur.

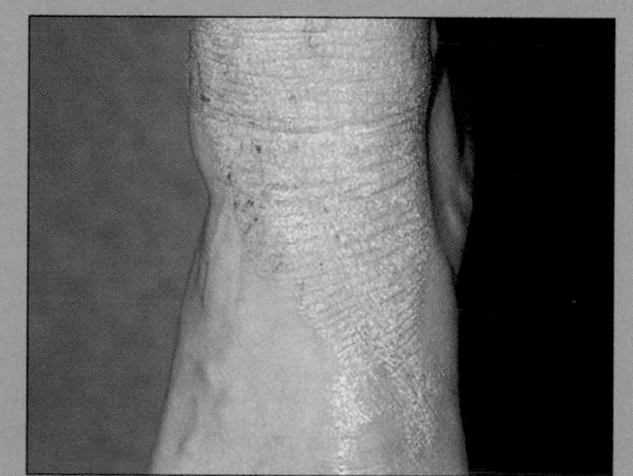

(continued)

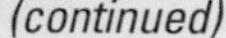

Recognizing common skin disorders *(continued)*

Herpes zoster

Herpes zoster appears as a group of vesicles or crusted lesions along a nerve root. The vesicles are usually unilateral and appear mostly on the face, hands, and neck. These lesions cause pain but not itching or rash.

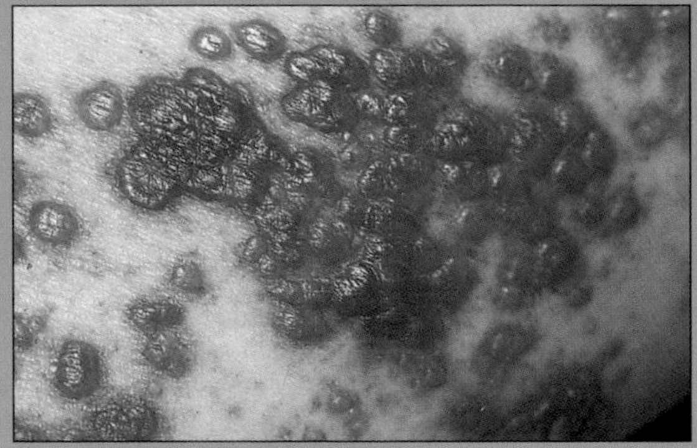

Tinea corporis (ringworm)

Tinea corporis is characterized by round, red, scaly lesions that are accompanied by intense itching. These lesions have slightly raised, red borders consisting of tiny vesicles. Individual rings may connect to form patches with scalloped edges. They usually appear on exposed areas of the body.

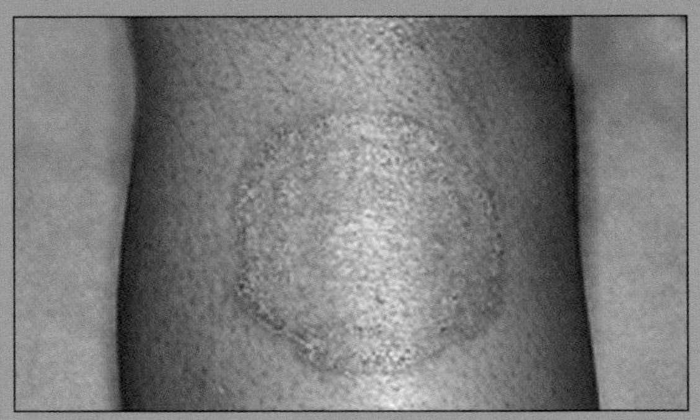

Candidiasis

Candidiasis is a fungal infection that produces erythema and a scaly, papular rash. Because the fungus thrives in moist environments, it most commonly occurs under the breasts and in the axillae.

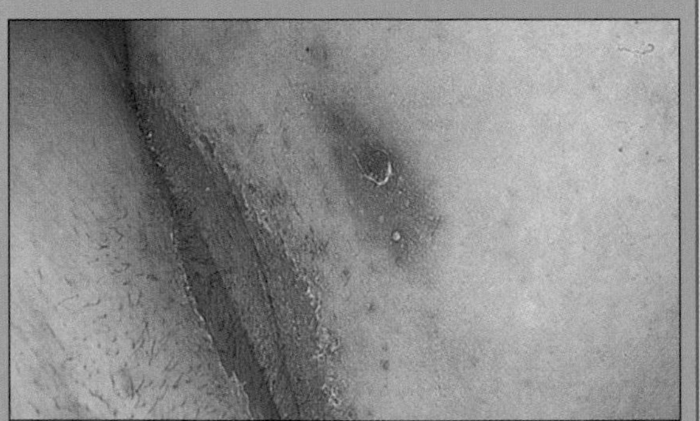

Impetigo

Impetigo is a rash that usually appears on the face. It's caused by a bacterial infection. When ruptured, fragile vesicles in the rash ooze a honey-colored fluid and crusts may form.

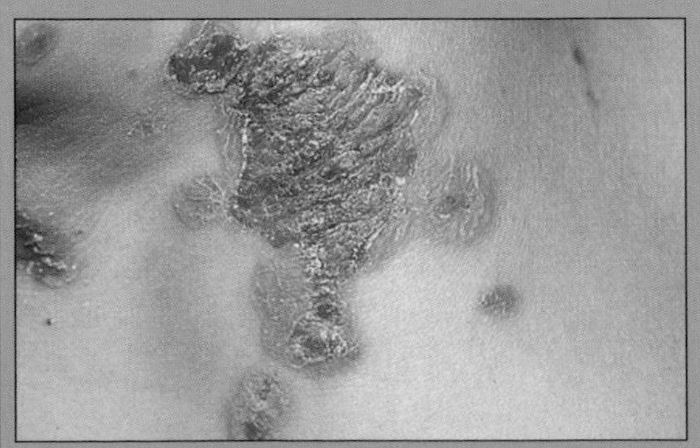

Alopecia

Alopecia occurs more commonly and extensively in men than in women. Diffuse hair loss, although commonly a normal part of aging, may occur as a result of pyrogenic infections, chemical trauma, ingestion of certain drugs, and endocrinopathy and other disorders. Tinea capitis, trauma, and third-degree burns can cause patchy hair loss.

Hirsutism

Excessive hairiness in women, or hirsutism, can develop on the body and face, affecting the patient's self-image. Localized hirsutism may occur on pigmented nevi. Generalized hirsutism can result from certain drug therapy or from such endocrine problems as Cushing's syndrome and acromegaly.

Nail abnormalities

Although many nail abnormalities are harmless, some point to serious underlying problems. Common nail problems include Beau's lines, clubbing, koilonychia, onycholysis, paronychia, and Terry's nails.

Beau's lines

Beau's lines are transverse depressions in the nail that extend to the nail bed. They occur with acute illness, malnutrition, anemia, and trauma that temporarily impairs nail function. A dent appears first at the cuticle and then moves forward as the nail grows.

This isn't the type of clubbing I was looking for!

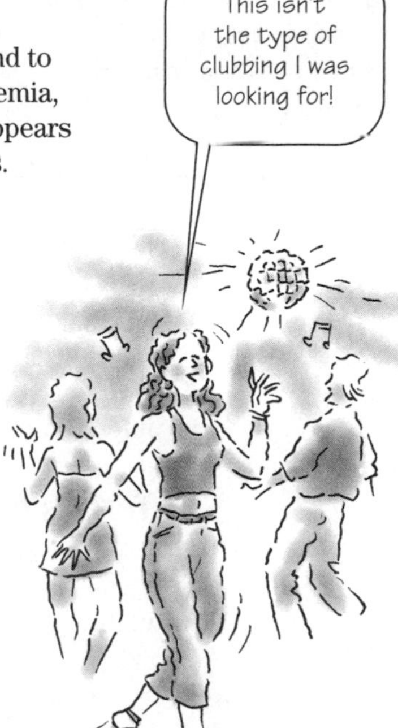

Clubbing

With clubbed fingers, the proximal edge of the nail elevates so the angle is greater than 180 degrees. The nail is also thickened and curved at the end, and the distal phalanx looks rounder and wider than normal. To check for clubbing, view the index finger in profile and note the angle of the nail base. (See *Evaluating clubbed fingers*, page 92.)

Koilonychia

Koilonychia refers to thin, spoon-shaped nails with lateral edges that tilt upward, forming a concave profile. The nails are white and opaque. This condition is associated with hypochromic anemia, chronic infections, Raynaud's disease, and malnutrition.

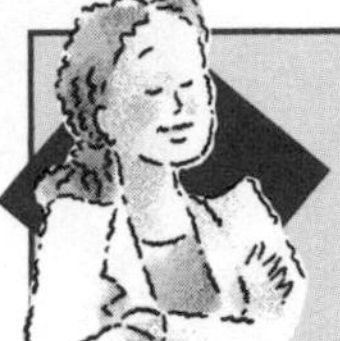

Peak technique

Evaluating clubbed fingers

Think hypoxia when you see a patient whose fingers are clubbed. To quickly examine a patient's fingers for early clubbing, gently palpate the bases of his nails. Normally, they'll feel firm, but in early clubbing, they'll feel springy.

To evaluate late clubbing, have the patient place the first phalanges of the forefingers together. Normal nail bases are concave and create a small, diamond-shaped space when the first phalanges are opposed, as shown at top right.

In late clubbing, the now convex nail bases can touch without leaving a space, as shown at bottom right. This condition is associated with pulmonary and cardiovascular disease. When you spot clubbed fingers, think about the possible causes, such as emphysema, chronic bronchitis, lung cancer, and heart failure.

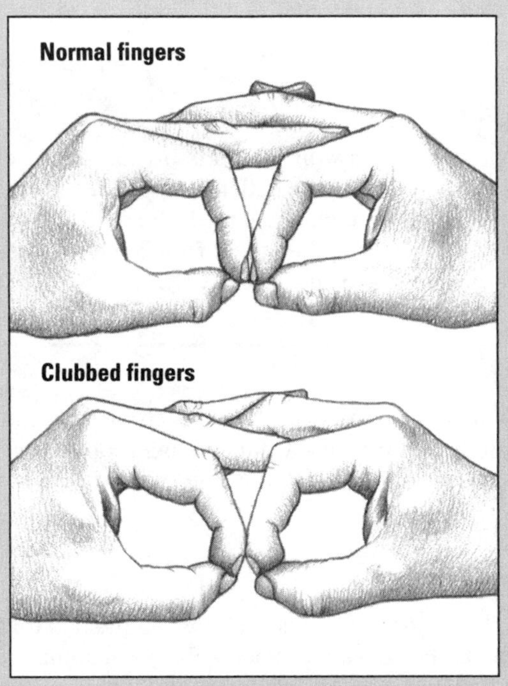

Onycholysis

Onycholysis is the loosening of the nail plate with separation from the nail bed, which begins at the distal groove. It's associated with minor trauma to long fingernails and such disease processes as psoriasis, contact dermatitis, hyperthyroidism, and *Pseudomonas* infections.

Terry's nails

Terry's nails are characterized by transverse bands of white that cover the nail, except for a narrow zone at the distal end. Terry's nails are associated with hypoalbuminemia.

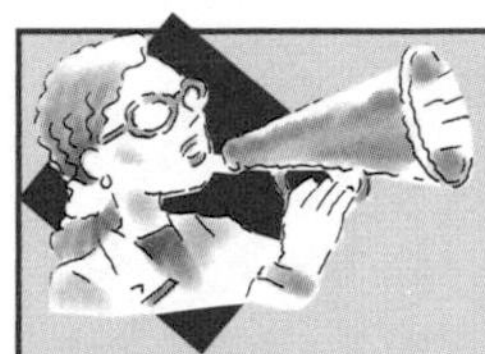

That's a wrap!

Skin, hair, and nails review

Health history
- Determine the patient's chief complaint.
- Ask him about skin changes, the presence of lesions, and exposure to sun.
- Ask about a family history of allergies or skin cancer.
- Ask about hair loss or gain, and about sudden or gradual nail changes.
- Ask about associated signs and symptoms, such as discharge, fever, weight loss, and joint pain.
- Determine which medications the patient takes, including herbal preparations.

Skin

Structures
- Epidermis—thin outer layer composed of epithelial tissue
- Dermis—thick, deeper layer that contains blood vessels, lymphatic vessels, nerves, hair follicles, and sweat and sebaceous glands
- Subcutaneous tissue—innermost layer

Functions
- Protects tissues
- Prevents water and electrolyte losses
- Senses temperature, pain, touch, and pressure
- Regulates body temperature
- Synthesizes vitamin D
- Promotes wound repair

Assessment
- Inspect and palpate the texture—it should be smooth and intact.
- Observe for moisture content—it should be dry with a minimal amount of perspiration.
- Palpate the skin for temperature, checking each side for localized temperature changes.
- Observe for skin lesions.

Lesion assessment
- Classify the lesion as primary or secondary.
- Determine if it's solid or fluid-filled.
- Check the borders to see if they're regular or irregular.
- Note the lesion's color as well as its pattern, location, and distribution.
- Measure the lesion's diameter using a millimeter-centimeter ruler.
- Describe any drainage, noting the type, color, amount, and odor.

Abnormal findings
- Café-au-lait spots—flat, light brown, uniformly hyperpigmented macules or patches on the skin surface
- Cherry angiomas—tiny, bright red, round papules that may become brown over time
- Papular rash—small, raised, circumscribed, and perhaps discolored (red to purple) lesions appearing in various configurations
- Port-wine hemangiomas—flat, purple marks usually present at birth that may appear on the face and upper body
- Pruritus—unpleasant itching sensation
- Purpuric lesions—petechiae (brown, pinpoint lesions); ecchymoses (bluish or purplish discolorations); hematomas (masses of accumulated blood)
- Telangiectases—permanently dilated, small blood vessels typically in a weblike pattern
- Urticaria—vascular skin reaction of transient pruritic wheals
- Vesicular rash—scattered or linear distribution of blisterlike lesions filled with clear, cloudy, or bloody fluid

(continued)

Skin, hair, and nails review *(continued)*

Hair
- Formed from keratin
- Lies in a hair follicle, receiving nourishment from the papilla, and is attached at the base by the arrector pili

Assessment
- Inspect and palpate the hair over the patient's entire body, noting distribution, quantity, texture, and color.
- Check for patterns of hair loss and growth.
- Inspect the scalp for erythema, scaling, and encrustations.

Abnormal findings
- Alopecia—hair loss
- Hirsutism—excessive hairiness in women

Nails
Structures
- Nail root (or nail matrix)—site of nail growth
- Nail plate—visible, hardened layer that covers the fingertip
- Lunula—white, crescent-shaped area that extends beyond the cuticle

Assessment
- Examine the nails for color, shape, thickness, and consistency.

Abnormal findings
- Beau's lines—transverse depressions in the nail extending to the bed
- Clubbing—proximal end of the nail elevates so the angle is greater than 180 degrees
- Koilonychia—thin, spoon-shaped nails with lateral edges that tilt upward
- Onycholysis—nail plate loosening with separation from the nail bed
- Terry's nails—transverse bands of white that cover the nail

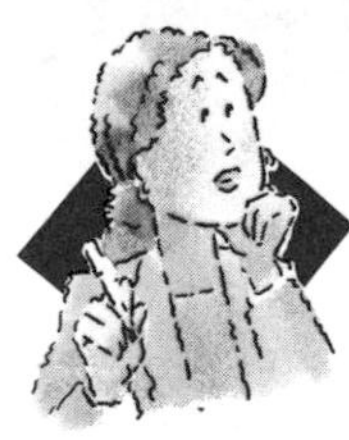

Quick quiz

1. If your patient has a skin rash, you should ask specific questions to determine whether either of the patient's parents has a history of:

A. allergies.
B. emphysema.
C. Kaposi's sarcoma.
D. impetigo.

Answer: A. A family history of allergic disorders might predispose the patient to allergies, including skin rashes.

2. A Wood's lamp is used to identify:
   A. folliculitis.
   B. skin exudates.
   C. ringworm infestation.
   D. acne.

Answer: C. A Wood's lamp is used to identify lesions that fluoresce and is the only way to identify ringworm infestation.

3. Asymmetric borders on a lesion suggest a:
   A. benign lesion.
   B. malignant lesion.
   C. normal variation.
   D. purpuric lesion.

Answer: B. Asymmetric borders are significant and typically signal malignancy.

4. Skin temperature is best assessed with the:
   A. fingertips.
   B. wrist.
   C. palm of the hand.
   D. back of the hand.

Answer: D. The dorsal surface of the hand is the most sensitive to temperature changes.

5. A dark band is a normal finding on the nails of:
   A. elderly people.
   B. pregnant women.
   C. dark-skinned people.
   D. children.

Answer: C. Dark bands are normal in dark-skinned people and abnormal in light-skinned people.

6. As you assess your patient, you note clubbed fingers. This is a sign of:
   A. malnutrition.
   B. hypoxia.
   C. bacterial infection.
   D. allergic reaction.

Answer: B. Clubbed fingers are typically a sign of hypoxia. Clubbing may also be found in patients with thyroid dysfunction, colitis, or cirrhosis.

Scoring

☆☆☆ If you answered all six questions correctly, fabulous! You really nailed this chapter.

☆☆ If you answered four or five questions correctly, good work! We aren't splitting hairs when we say your assessment skills are growing.

☆ If you answered fewer than four questions correctly, don't despair. Take a little more time to get the skinny on this topic.

6 Eyes

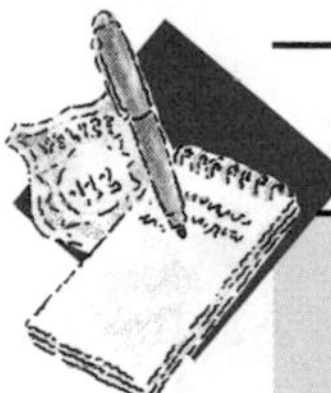

Just the facts

In this chapter, you'll learn:

- the importance of eye assessments
- eye structures and their functions
- questions to ask about the eyes during the health history
- techniques for assessing the eyes
- ways to recognize normal and abnormal variations in the eyes.

A look at the eyes

About 70% of all sensory information reaches the brain through the eyes. Disorders in vision can interfere with a patient's ability to function independently, perceive the world, and enjoy beauty.

A thorough assessment of your patient's eyes and vision can help you identify problems that can affect the patient's health and quality of life. In many cases, early detection can lead to successful, sight-saving treatment.

The eyes transmit 70% of all sensory information reaching the brain. Now, that's an eyeful!

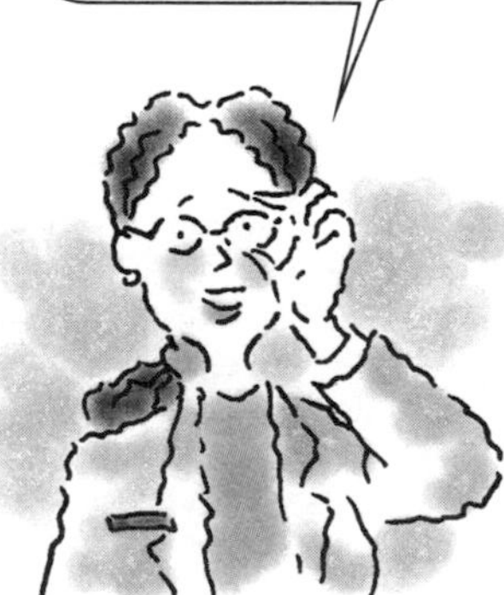

The eyes have it!

Fewer people lose their sight from infections or injuries today than they did in the past. Still, the overall incidence of blindness is rising as the population ages. Primary causes of vision loss include diabetic retinopathy, glaucoma, cataracts, and macular degeneration — conditions more common in elderly patients than in younger ones.

Young people can lose their sight because of opportunistic infections associated with human immunodeficiency virus (HIV) and acquired immunodeficiency syndrome. The opportunistic infections toxoplasmosis and cytomegalovirus retinitis commonly cause blindness as well. Other vision disorders that may limit a person's ability to function include strabismus, amblyopia, and refractory errors.

Structures of the eye

In this section, we'll look at the external (extraocular) structures as well as the internal (intraocular) structures of the eye. (See *A close look at the eye.*)

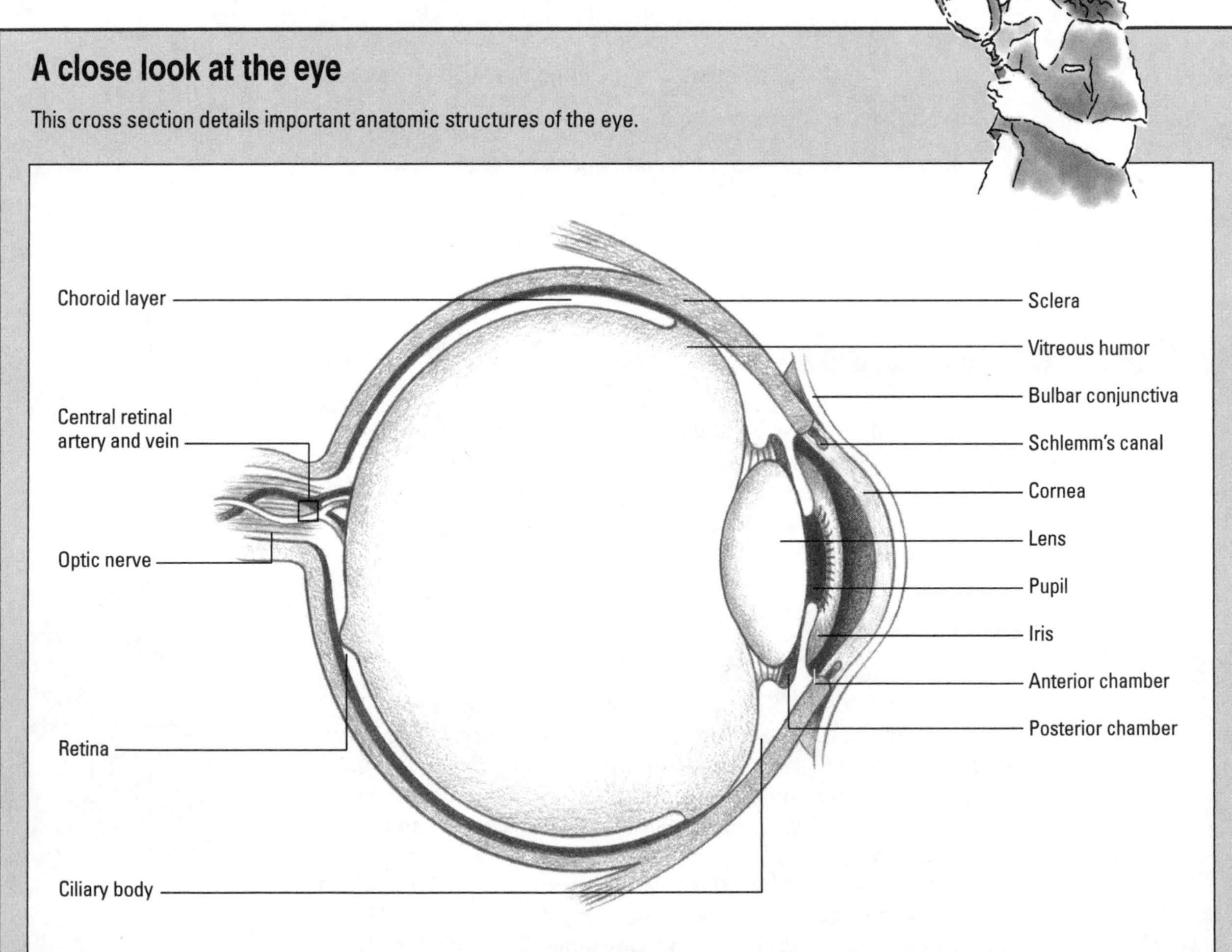

A close look at the eye

This cross section details important anatomic structures of the eye.

Extraocular structures

The eyes are delicate sensory organs equipped with many protective structures. On the outside, the bony orbits protect the eyes from trauma. Eyelids (or *palpebrae*), lashes, and the lacrimal apparatus protect the eyes from injury, dust, and foreign bodies.

Muscling in

Also included in extraocular structures are six extraocular muscles. Innervated (stimulated) by the cranial nerves, these muscles control the movement of the eyes. The coordinated actions of those muscles allow the eyes to move in tandem, ensuring clear vision.

Intraocular structures

The eye contains multiple structures that function together to provide vision. Some structures are easily visible, whereas others can only be viewed with special instruments. Here's a brief review of these structures.

Sclera and choroid

The white coating on the outside of the eyeball, the sclera, maintains the eye's size and shape. The choroid, which lines the recessed portion of the eyeball and lies between the sclera and the retina, contains a network of arteries and veins that maintain blood supply to the back of the eye.

Bulbar conjunctiva

A thin, transparent membrane, the bulbar conjunctiva lines the eyelid. It also covers and protects the anterior portion of the white sclera.

Cornea

The cornea is a smooth, avascular, transparent tissue that merges with the sclera at the limbus. It refracts, or bends, light rays entering the eye. Located in front of the pupil and iris, the cornea is fed by the ophthalmic branch of cranial nerve V (the trigeminal nerve). Stimulation of this nerve initiates a protective blink, the corneal reflex.

Iris

The iris is a circular, contractile diaphragm that contains smooth and radial muscles and is perforated in the center by the pupil. Varying amounts of pigment granules within the smooth-muscle fibers give it color. Its posterior portion contains involuntary muscles that control pupil size and regulate the amount of light entering the eye.

Ciliary body

The ciliary body lies just beneath the iris. The suspensory ligaments of the ciliary body attach to the lens, controlling its shape for close and distant vision. The ciliary body also continuously produces aqueous humor. Aqueous humor is a clear, watery fluid in the front of the eye that fills the anterior and posterior chambers. It gives the front of the eye its shape and provides nourishment to the cornea and lens.

Pupil

The iris's central opening, the pupil is normally round and equal in size to the opposite pupil. The pupil permits light to enter the eyes. Depending on the patient's age, pupil diameter can range from 3 to 5 mm. Small and unresponsive to light at birth, the pupil enlarges during childhood and then progressively decreases in size throughout adulthood.

Anterior and posterior chambers

The anterior chamber is filled with clear aqueous humor. The amount of fluid in the chamber varies to maintain pressure in the eye. Fluid drains from the anterior chamber through collecting channels into Schlemm's canal.

The posterior chamber, located between the iris and the lens, is filled with aqueous humor. This fluid bathes the lens capsule as it flows through the pupil into the anterior chamber.

I can tell by the shape of your eyeball that you clearly have a great sense of aqueous humor.

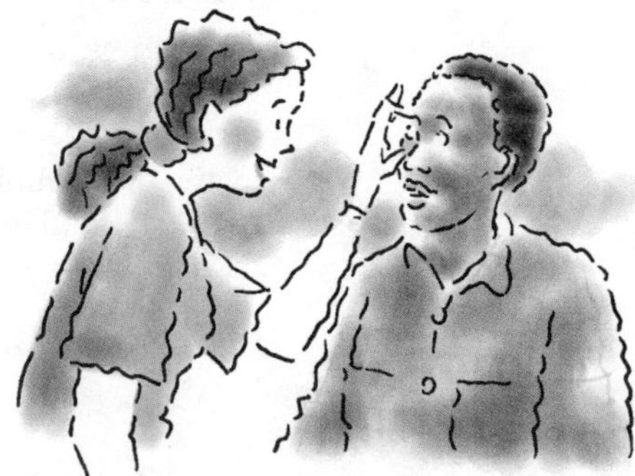

Lens

Located directly behind the iris at the pupillary opening, the lens consists of avascular, transparent fibrils in an elastic membrane called the *lens capsule.* The lens refracts and focuses light onto the retina.

Vitreous chamber

The vitreous chamber, located behind the lens, occupies four-fifths of the eyeball. This chamber is filled

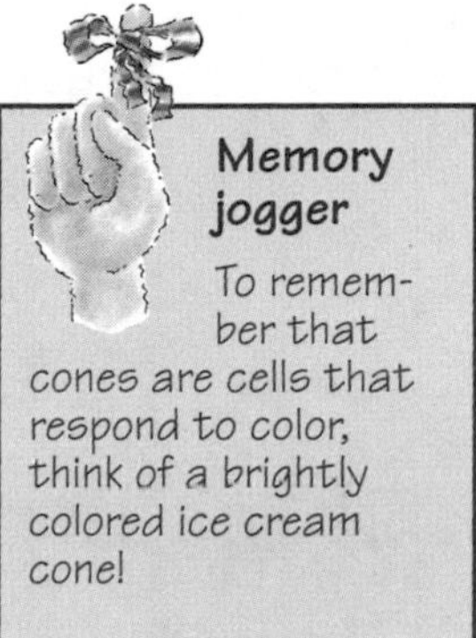

with vitreous humor, a thick, gelatinous substance that fills the center of the eye and maintains the placement of the retina and the shape of the eyeball.

Retina

The innermost region of eyeball, the retina receives visual stimuli and transmits images to the brain for processing.

Various vessels

There are four sets of retinal blood vessels — the superonasal, inferonasal, superotemporal, and inferotemporal. These vessels are visible through an ophthalmoscope. Each set of vessels contains a transparent arteriole and vein. As the vessels leave the optic disk, they become progressively thinner, intertwining as they extend to the periphery of the retina.

Optic disk and physiologic cup

A well-defined, round or oval area measuring less than ⅛″ (0.3 cm) within the retina's nasal portion, the optic disk is the opening through which the ganglion nerve axons (fibers) exit the retina to form the optic nerve. This area is called the *blind spot* because no light-sensitive cells (photoreceptors) are located there.

Cup and cover

The physiologic cup is a light-colored depression within the temporal side of the optic disk where blood vessels enter the retina. It covers one-fourth to one-third of the disk but doesn't extend completely to the margin.

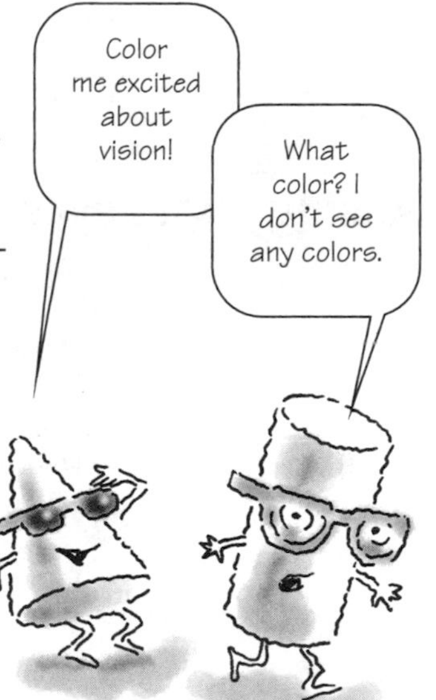

Color me excited about vision!
What color? I don't see any colors.

Photoreceptor neurons

Photoreceptor neurons make up the retina's visual receptors. Not visible through the ophthalmoscope, these receptors — some shaped like rods and some like cones — are responsible for vision. Rods respond to low-intensity light, but they don't provide sharp images or color vision. Cones respond to bright light and provide high-acuity color vision.

Macula and fovea centralis

Located laterally from the optic disk, the macula is slightly darker than the rest of the retina and contains no visible retinal vessels. Because its borders are poorly defined, the macula is difficult to see on an ophthalmologic examination. It's best identified by having the patient look straight at the ophthalmoscope's light.

Cone container

The fovea centralis, a slight depression in the macula, appears as a bright reflection when examined with an ophthalmoscope. Because the fovea contains the heaviest concentration of cones, it acts as the eye's clearest vision and color receptor.

Obtaining a health history

Now that you're familiar with the normal anatomy and physiology of the eyes, you're ready to obtain a health history of them. The most common eye-related complaints are double vision (diplopia), visual floaters, photophobia (light sensitivity), vision loss, and eye pain. Other complaints include decreased visual acuity or clarity, defects in color vision, and difficulty seeing at night.

Even if the patient's chief complaint isn't eye-related, you still need to question him about his eyes and vision.

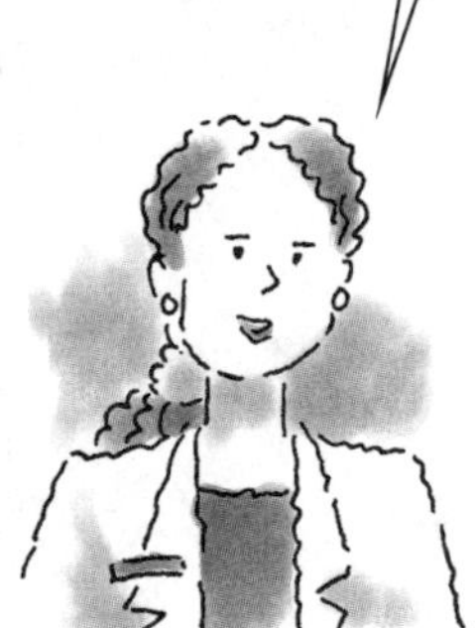

Ask anyway

Even if a patient's reason for seeking care or previous diagnosis isn't eye-related, you'll need to question him about his eyes and vision. Keep in mind that poor vision can affect the patient's ability to comply with treatment.

Asking about eyes

To obtain an accurate history, first ask the patient questions specific to his eyes:

- Does he wear corrective lenses for distance or for reading?
- Has he experienced blurred vision, blind spots, floaters, double vision, discharge, or unusual sensitivity to light?
- Does he having trouble seeing at night?
- Has he ever had an eye injury or eye surgery?
- Did he ever have a lazy eye?
- Does he have allergies?
- When was his last eye examination?
- Does he complain of eye pain or headaches?
- Does he squint to see objects at a distance?
- Does he hold objects close to his eyes to see them?

Asking about general health

Now that you've asked the patient questions about his eyes, broaden your assessment to include questions about other diseases, medications, work issues, and smoking habits.

Family matters

Ask the patient if he has a history of hypertension, diabetes, stroke, multiple sclerosis, syphilis, or HIV. Find out if anyone in his family has glaucoma, cataracts, vision loss, or retinitis. Because a family history may predispose the patient to these conditions, he'll need frequent testing.

Drug connection

Ask the patient which medications he takes. Some drugs can affect vision. For example, digoxin (Lanoxin) overdose can cause a patient to see yellow halos around bright lights. Remember to ask about over-the-counter drugs, herbal preparations, eyedrops, and eyewashes, too.

All in a day's work

Ask the patient what kind of work he does and what he does for recreation. Is he exposed to chemicals, fumes, flying debris, or infectious agents? If so, does he wear eye protection? Caution all patients to wear protective eyewear when working with substances that may injure the eye.

Igniting a problem

If your patient smokes, warn him that smoking increases the risk of vascular disease, which can lead to blindness and can damage vision.

A view of the situation

If your patient is elderly or has impaired vision, ask him how well he can manage activities of daily living. Assess whether he and his family need assistance in learning to use adaptive devices or a referral to an agency that helps people with impaired vision.

Kiddin' around

If your patient is a young child, the interview will vary slightly because you'll be asking the parents the questions. As a result, you may receive only objective answers, not subjective responses. (See *Seeing things differently*, page 104.)

Assessing the eyes

A complete eye assessment involves inspecting the external eye and lids, testing visual acuity, assessing eye muscle function, palpating the nasolacrimal sac, and examining intraocular structures with an ophthalmoscope.

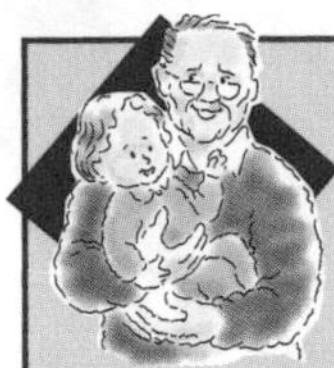

Ages and stages

Seeing things differently

You'll need to modify your health history for a child or an aging adult.

Young ones
If your patient is a child, ask the parents these questions:
- Was the child delivered vaginally or by cesarean birth? If he was delivered vaginally, did his mother have a vaginal infection at the time? (Inform the parents that infections such as chlamydia, gonorrhea, genital herpes, or candidiasis can cause eye problems in infants.)
- Did he have erythromycin ointment instilled in his eyes at birth?
- Has he passed the normal developmental milestones?
- Does he know how to hold and care for sharp objects such as scissors?

The oldies
If your patient is an aging adult, ask him these questions:
- Have you had any difficulty climbing stairs or driving?
- Have you ever been tested for glaucoma? If so, when and what was the result?
- If you have glaucoma, has your doctor prescribed eyedrops for you? If so, what kind?
- How well can you instill your eyedrops?
- Do your eyes ever feel dry? Do they burn? If so, how do you treat the problem?

Gather your gear

Before starting your examination, gather the necessary equipment, including a good light source, a penlight, one or two opaque cards, an ophthalmoscope, vision-test cards, gloves, tissues, and cotton-tipped applicators. Make sure that the patient is seated comfortably and that you're seated at eye level with him.

Inspecting the eyes

Start your assessment by observing the patient's face. With the scalp line as the starting point, check that his eyes are in a normal position. They should be about one-third of the way down the face and about one eye's width apart from each other. Then assess the eyelid, conjunctiva, cornea, anterior chamber, iris, and pupil.

Eyelid

Each upper eyelid should cover the top quarter of the iris so the eyes look alike. Check for an excessive amount of visible sclera above the limbus (corneo-scleral junction). Ask the patient to open and close his eyes to see if they close completely. If the downward movement of the upper eyelid in down gaze is delayed, the patient has a condition known as *lid lag,* which is a common sign of hyperthyroidism.

Assess the lids for redness, edema, inflammation, or lesions. Check for a stye, or hordeolum, a common eyelid lesion.

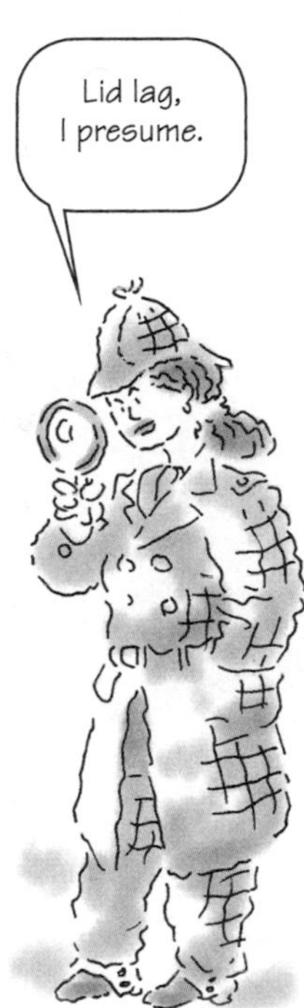

Eye opener

Protrusion of the eyeball, called *exophthalmos* or *proptosis,* commonly occurs in patients who have hyperthyroidism.

Crying or drying?

Inspect the eyes for excessive tearing or dryness. The eyelid margins should be pink, and the eyelashes should turn outward. Observe whether the lower eyelids turn inward toward the eyeball, called *entropion*, or outward, called *ectropion.* Examine the eyelids for lumps.

Pressing the point

Before palpating the nasolacrimal sac, explain the procedure to the patient. Then put on examination gloves. With the patient's eyes closed, gently palpate the area below the inner canthus, noting tenderness, swelling, or discharge through the lacrimal point, which could indicate blockage of the nasolacrimal duct.

Conjunctiva

To inspect the bulbar conjunctiva (the delicate mucous membrane that covers the exposed surface of the sclera) have your patient look up. Gently pull the lower eyelid down. The bulbar conjunctiva should be clear and shiny. Note excessive redness or exudate.

True colors

With the lid still secured, inspect the bulbar conjunctiva for color changes, foreign bodies, and edema. Also, observe the sclera's color, which should be white to buff. In black patients, you may see flecks of tan. A bluish discoloration may indicate scleral thinning.

Getting an eye lift

To examine the palpebral conjunctiva (the membrane that lines the eyelids), have the patient look down. Then lift the upper lid, holding the upper lashes against the eyebrow with your finger. The palpebral conjunctiva should be uniformly pink. In patients with a history of allergies, the palpebral conjunctiva may have a cobblestone appearance.

Cornea

Examine the cornea by shining a penlight first from both sides and then from straight ahead. The cornea should be clear and without lesions. Test corneal sensitivity by lightly touching the cornea with a wisp of cotton. (See *Tips for assessing corneal sensitivity.*)

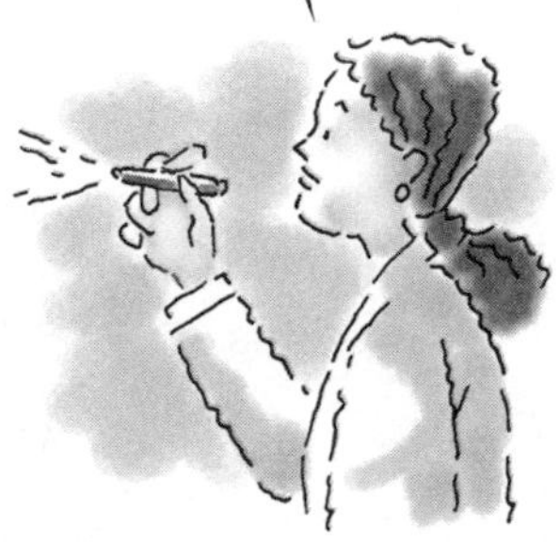

Anterior chamber and iris

The anterior chamber of the eye is bordered anteriorly by the cornea and posteriorly by the iris. The iris should appear flat, and the cornea should appear convex. Excess pressure in the eye—such as that caused by acute angle-closure glaucoma—may push the iris forward, making the anterior chamber appear very small. The irises should be the same size, color, and shape.

Pupil

Each pupil should be equal in size, round, and about one-fourth the size of the iris in normal room light. About one person in four has asymmetrical pupils without disease. Unequal pupils generally indicate neurologic damage, iritis, glaucoma, or therapy with certain drugs. A fixed pupil that doesn't react to light can be an ominous neurologic sign.

In perfect agreement

Test the pupils for direct and consensual response. In a slightly darkened room, hold a penlight about 20″ (50.8 cm) from the patient's eyes, and direct the light at the eye from the side. Note the reaction of the pupil you're testing (direct response) and the opposite pupil (consensual response). They should both react the same way. Also, note sluggishness or inequality in the response. Repeat the test with the other pupil. *Note:* If you shine the light in a blind eye, neither pupil will respond. If you shine the light in a seeing eye, the pupils will respond consensually.

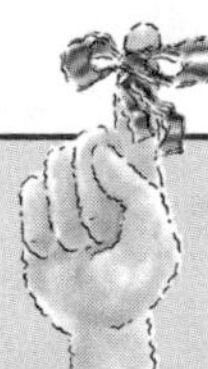

Memory jogger

To make sure that your pupil assessment is complete, think of the acronym PERRLA.

Pupils
Equal
Round
Reactive
Light-reacting
Accommodation

Willing to accommodate

To test the pupils for accommodation, place your finger approximately 4″ (10.2 cm) from the bridge of the patient's nose. Ask the patient to look at a fixed object in the distance and then to look at your finger. His pupils should constrict and his eyes converge as he focuses on your finger.

Testing visual acuity

To test your patient's far and near vision, use a Snellen chart and a near-vision chart. To test his peripheral vision, use confrontation.

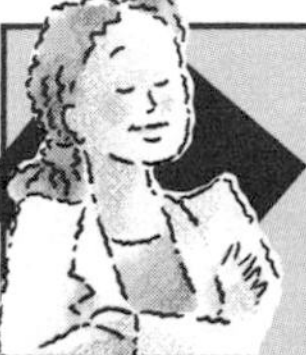

Peak technique

Tips for assessing corneal sensitivity

To test corneal sensitivity, touch a wisp of cotton from a cotton ball to the cornea, as shown below.

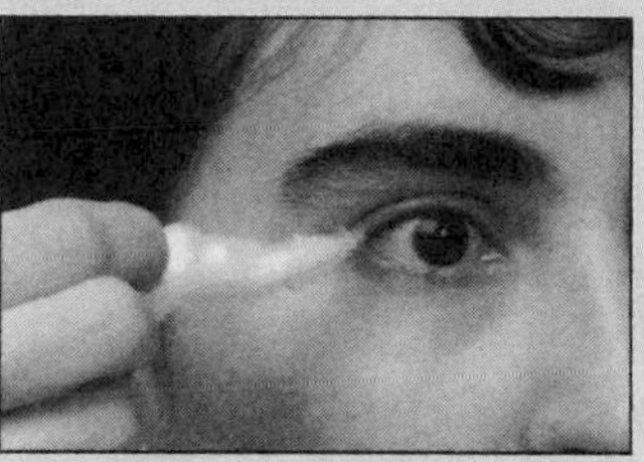

The patient should blink. If he doesn't, he may have suffered damage to the sensory fibers of cranial nerve V or to the motor fibers controlled by cranial nerve VI.

Keep in mind that people who wear contact lenses may have reduced sensitivity because they're accustomed to having foreign objects in their eyes.

Just a wisp

Remember that a wisp of cotton is the only safe object to use for this test. Even though a 4″ × 4″ gauze pad or tissue is soft, it can cause corneal abrasions and irritation.

Before each test, ask the patient to remove corrective lenses, if he wears them.

Snellen chart

Have the patient sit or stand 20′ (6.1 m) from the chart, and then cover his left eye with an opaque object. Ask him to read the letters on one line of the chart and then to move downward to increasingly smaller lines until he can no longer discern all of the letters. Have him repeat the test covering his right eye. Finally, have him read the smallest line he can read with both eyes uncovered to test his binocular vision.

One more time

If the patient wears corrective lenses, have him repeat the test wearing them. Record the vision with and without correction.

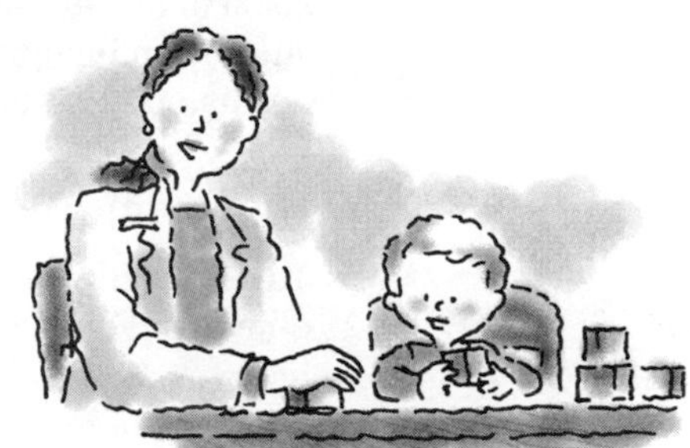

The Big E

Use the Snellen E chart to test visual acuity in young children and other patients who can't read. Cover the patient's left eye to check the right eye, point to an E on the chart, and ask the patient to indicate which

Visual acuity charts

The most commonly used charts for testing vision are the Snellen alphabet chart (left) and the Snellen E chart (right), which is used for young children and adults who can't read. Both charts are used to test distance vision and measure visual acuity. The patient reads each chart at a distance of 20′ (6.1 m).

Recording results

Visual acuity is recorded as a fraction. The top number (20) is the distance between the patient and the chart. The bottom number is the distance from which a person with normal vision could read the line. The larger the bottom number, the poorer the patient's vision.

Age differences

In adults and children age 6 and older, normal vision is measured as 20/20. For children age 3 and younger, normal vision is 20/50; for children age 4, 20/40; and for children age 5, 20/30.

Snellen alphabet chart

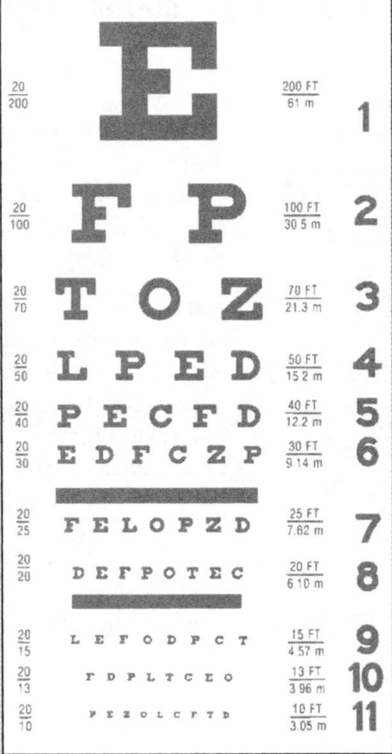

Snellen E chart

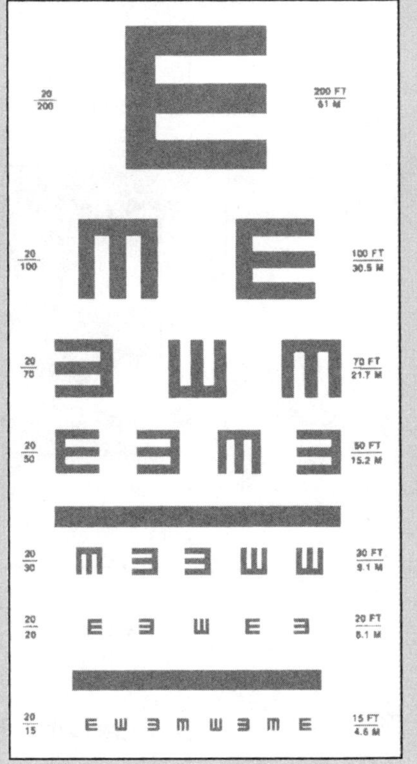

way the letter faces. Repeat the test with the left eye. (See *Visual acuity charts.*)

Eye-catching values

If the test values between the two eyes differ by two lines, such as 20/30 in one eye and 20/50 in the other, suspect an abnormality such as amblyopia (reduced vision in an eye that appears normal during ophthalmoscopic examination)—especially in children.

Near-vision chart

To test near vision, cover one of the patient's eyes with an opaque object and hold a Rosenbaum near-vision card 14″ (35.6 cm) from his eyes. Have him read the line with the smallest letters he can distinguish. Repeat the test with the other eye. If the patient wears

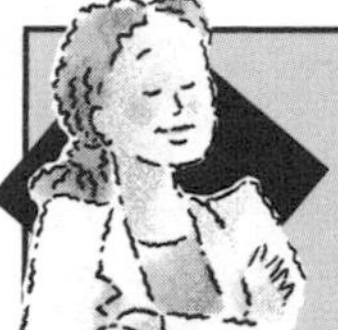

Peak technique

Using confrontation

Follow these steps to assess peripheral vision with confrontation:

- Sit directly across from the patient and have her focus her gaze on your eyes.
- Place your hands on either side of the patient's head at the level of her ears so that they're about 2′ apart (as shown).
- Tell the patient to focus her gaze on you as you gradually bring your wiggling fingers into her visual field.
- Instruct the patient to tell you as soon as she can see your wiggling fingers; she should see them at the same time you do.
- Repeat the procedure while holding your hands at the superior and inferior positions.

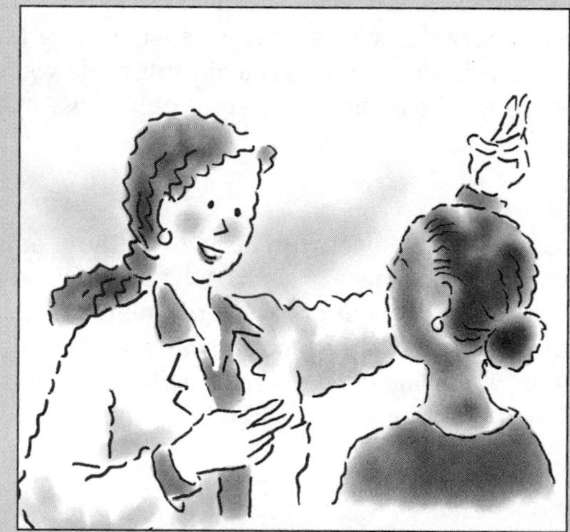

corrective lenses, have him repeat the test while wearing them. Record the visual accommodation with and without lenses.

Confrontation

To assess peripheral vision, use a method known as *confrontation.* This test can help identify abnormalities such as homonymous hemianopsia and bitemporal hemianopsia. (See *Using confrontation.*)

Assessing eye muscle function

A thorough assessment of the eyes includes an evaluation of the extraocular muscles. To evaluate these muscles, you'll need to assess the corneal light reflex and the cardinal positions of gaze, and then perform the cover-uncover test.

Corneal light reflex

To assess the corneal light reflex, ask the patient to look straight ahead; then shine a penlight on the bridge of his nose from about 12″ to 15″ (30.5 cm to 38 cm) away. The light should fall at the same spot on each cornea. If it doesn't, the eyes aren't being held in the same plane by the extraocular muscles. This commonly occurs in a patient who lacks muscle coordination, a condition called *strabismus.*

Cardinal positions of gaze

Cardinal positions of gaze evaluate the oculomotor, trigeminal, and abducent nerves as well as the extraocular muscles. To perform this test, ask the patient to remain still while you hold a pencil or other small object directly in front of his nose at a distance of about 18″ (45 cm).

Eyeballs on the move

Ask him to follow the object with his eyes, without moving his head. Then move the object to each of the six cardinal positions, returning to the midpoint after each movement. The patient's eyes should remain parallel as they move. Note abnormal findings such as nystagmus and amblyopia, the failure of one eye to follow an object. (See *Cardinal positions of gaze.*)

Cardinal positions of gaze

The illustration below identifies the six cardinal positions of gaze.

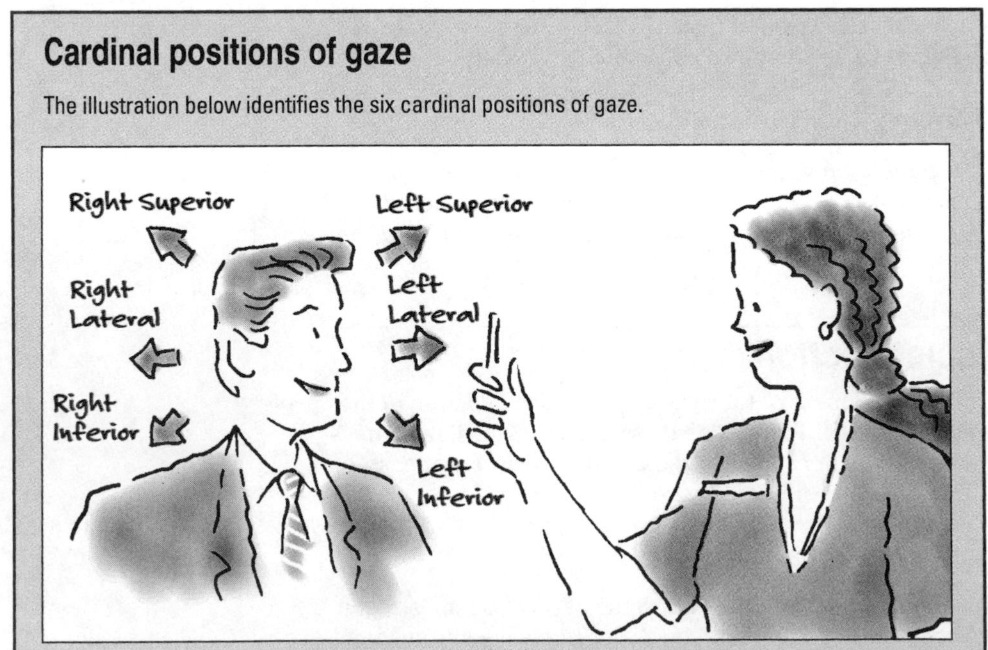

Cover-uncover test

The cover-uncover test usually isn't done unless you detect an abnormality when assessing the corneal light reflex and cardinal positions of gaze. To perform a cover-uncover test, have the patient stare at a wall on the other side of the room. Cover one eye and watch for movement in the uncovered eye. Remove the eye cover and watch for movement again. Repeat the test with the other eye.

When you cover and then uncover the patient's eye, his eye should remain still. Any movement is considered abnormal.

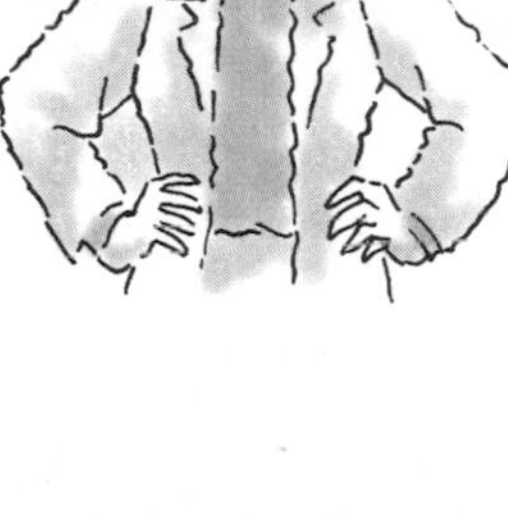

On the move

Eye movement while covering or uncovering the eye is considered abnormal. It may result from weak or paralyzed extraocular muscles, which may be caused by cranial nerve impairment.

Examining intraocular structures

The ophthalmoscope allows you to directly observe the eye's internal structures. To see those structures properly, you'll need to adjust the lens dial. Use the green, positive numbers on the dial to focus on near objects such as the patient's cornea and lens. Use the red, minus numbers to focus on distant objects such as the retina.

Before the examination, have the patient remove his contact lenses (if they're tinted) or eyeglasses, and darken the room to dilate his pupils and make your examination easier. Ask the patient to focus on a point behind you. Tell him that you'll be moving into his visual field and blocking his view. Also, explain that you'll be shining a bright light into his eye, which may be uncomfortable but not harmful. (See *Seeing eye to eye.*)

Seeing eye to eye

This illustration shows the correct position for the examiner and the patient when an ophthalmoscope is used to examine the eye's internal structures.

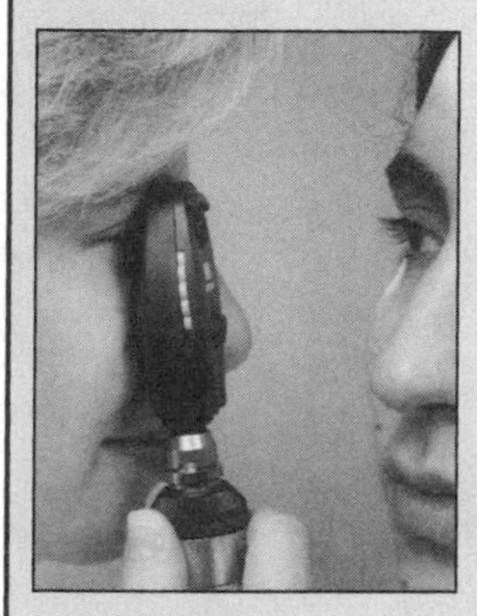

Closing in on the cornea

Set the lens dial at zero, hold the ophthalmoscope about 4″ (10 cm) from the patient's eye, and direct the light through the pupil to elicit the red reflex, a reflection of light off the choroid. Check the red reflex for depth of color.

Now, move the ophthalmoscope closer to the eye. Adjust the lens dial so you can focus on the anterior chamber and lens. Look for clouding, foreign matter, or opacities. If the lens is opaque, indicating cataracts, you may not be able to complete the examination.

Rotating to the retinal structures

To examine the retina, start with the dial turned to zero. Rotate the lens-power dial to adjust for your refractive correction and the patient's refractive error. Now, observe the vitreous body for clarity. The first retinal structures you'll see are the blood vessels. Rotating the dial into the negative numbers will bring the blood vessels into focus. The arteries will look thinner and brighter than the veins.

Pick a vessel and follow it

Follow one of the vessels along its path toward the nose until you reach the optic disk, where all vessels in the eye originate. Examine arteriovenous crossings for arteriovenous nicking (localized constrictions in the retinal vessels), which might be a sign of hypertension.

Diggin' the disk and depression

The optic disk is a creamy pink to yellow-orange structure with clear borders and a round-to-oval shape. With practice, you'll be able to identify the physiologic cup, a small depression that occupies about one-third of the disk's diameter. The disk may fill or exceed your field of vision. If you don't see it, follow a blood vessel toward the center until you do. The nasal border of the disk may be somewhat blurred.

Riveting on the retina

Completely scan the retina by following four blood vessels from the optic disk to different peripheral areas. The retina should have a uniform color and be free from scars and pigmentation. As you scan, note any lesions or hemorrhages. (See *A close look at the retina.*)

Movin' in on the macula

Finally, move the light laterally from the optic disk to locate the macula, the part of the eye most sensitive to light. It appears as a darker structure, free from blood vessels. Your view may be fleeting because most patients can't tolerate having a beam of light fall on the macula. If you locate it, ask the patient to shift his gaze into the light.

The macula is the part of the eye that's most sensitive to light.

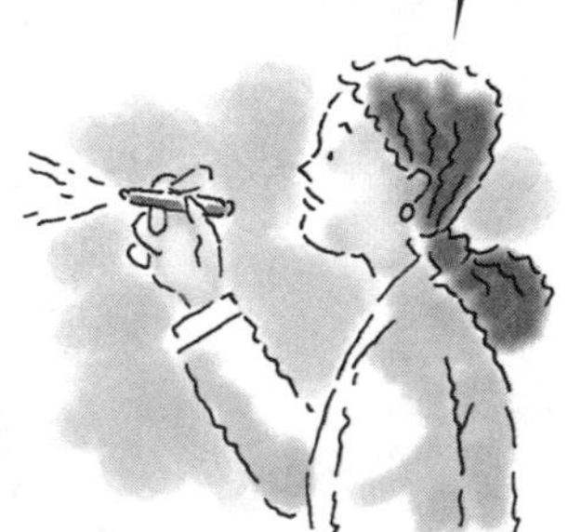

Abnormal findings

Common abnormalities you may detect during an eye assessment include arteriolar narrowing, decreased visual acuity, diplopia, eye discharge, eye pain, periorbital edema, ptosis, strabismus, vision loss, visual floaters, and visual halos. (See *Eye abnormalities*, page 114.)

A close look at the retina

This illustration shows the complex anatomy of the retina and its structures.

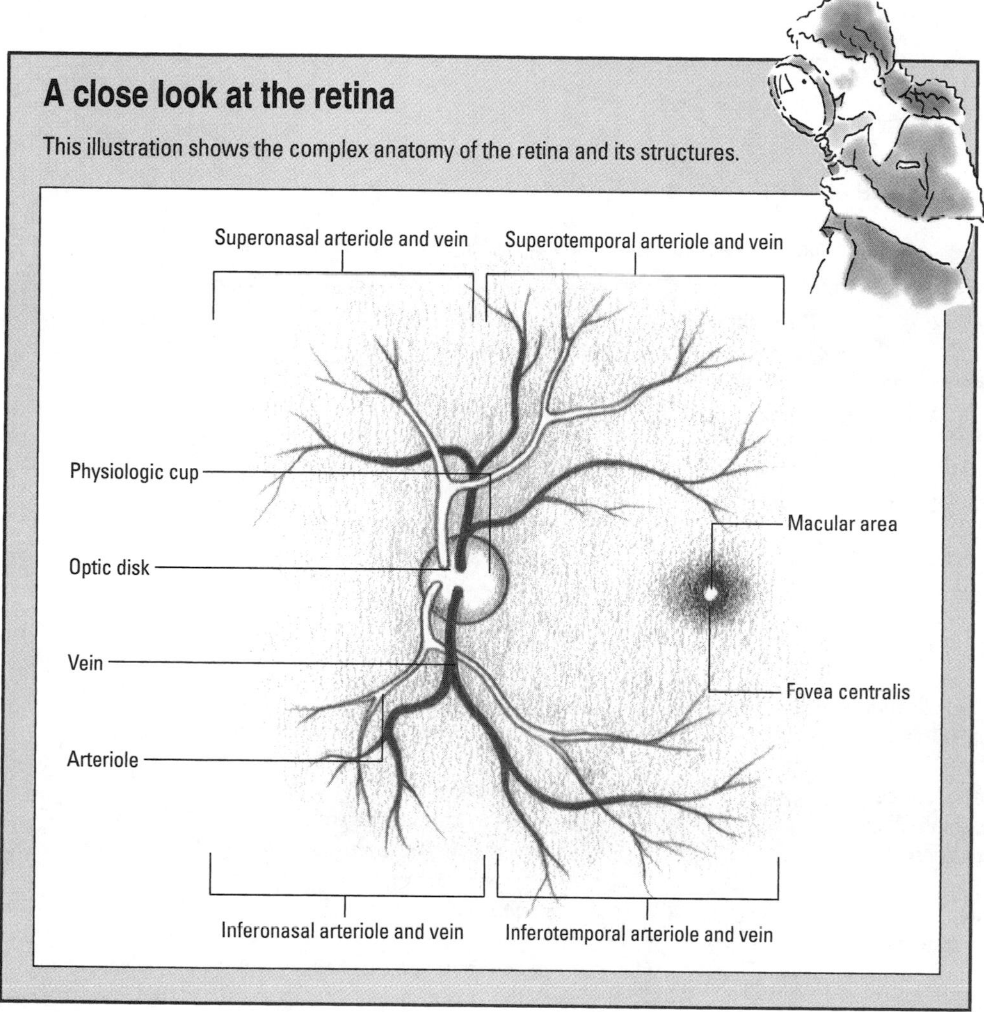

Arteriolar narrowing

Typically, arterioles of the inner eye are between two-thirds and three-fourths the width of veins and have a brighter appearance. When these minute arteries narrow, they appear to be about one-half as wide as veins. Arteriolar narrowing commonly occurs in patients who have hypertension.

Decreased visual acuity

Decreased visual acuity — the ability to see clearly — commonly occurs with refractive errors. In nearsightedness, or myopia, the eye focuses the visual image in front of the retina, causing objects in close view to be seen clearly while those at a distance appear

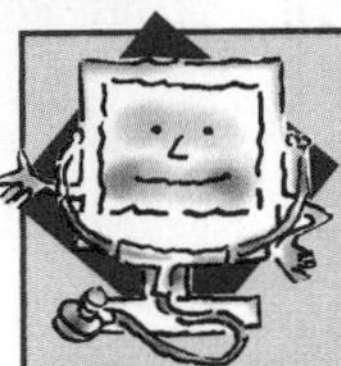

Interpretation station

Eye abnormalities

This chart shows common groups of findings for signs and symptoms of the eyes along with their probable causes.

Sign or symptom and findings	Probable cause
Eye discharge	
• Purulent or mucopurulent, greenish white discharge that occurs unilaterally • Sticky crusts that form on the eyelids during sleep • Itching and burning • Excessive tearing • Sensation of a foreign body in the eye	Bacterial conjunctivitis
• Scant but continuous purulent discharge that's easily expressed from the tear sac • Excessive tearing • Pain and tenderness near the tear sac • Eyelid inflammation and edema noticeable around the lacrimal punctum	Dacryocystitis
• Continuous frothy discharge • Chronically red eyes with inflamed lid margins • Soft, foul-smelling, cheesy yellow discharge elicited by pressure on the meibomian glands	Meibomianitis
Decreased visual acuity	
• Gradual visual blurring • Halo vision • Visual glare in bright light • Progressive vision loss • Gray pupil that later turns milky white	Cataract
Decreased visual acuity *(continued)*	
• Constant morning headache that decreases in severity during the day • Possible severe, throbbing headache • Restlessness • Confusion • Nausea and vomiting • Seizures • Decreased level of consciousness	Hypertension
• Paroxysmal attacks of severe, throbbing unilateral or bilateral headache • Nausea and vomiting • Sensitivity to light and noise • Sensory or visual auras	Migraine headache
Visual floaters	
• Sudden onset of spots or flashing lights • Curtainlike loss of vision • Black retinal vessels	Retinal detachment
• Onset of spots or flashing lights • Gradual development of eye pain • Photophobia • Blurred vision • Conjunctival injection	Posterior uveitis

blurry. In farsightedness, or hyperopia, the eye focuses the visual image behind the retina, causing objects in close view to appear blurry while those at a distance seem clear. Both problems result from an abnormal shape of the eyeball.

Diplopia

When the extraocular muscles are misaligned, the visual axes aren't directed at the object of sight at the same time. This results in double vision, or diplopia.

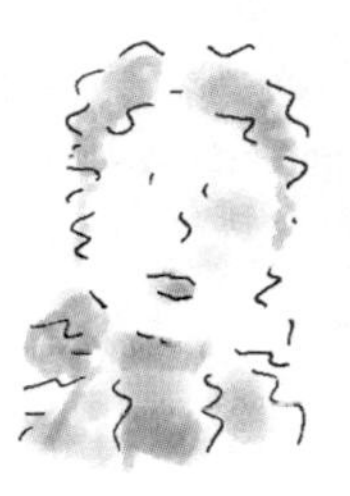

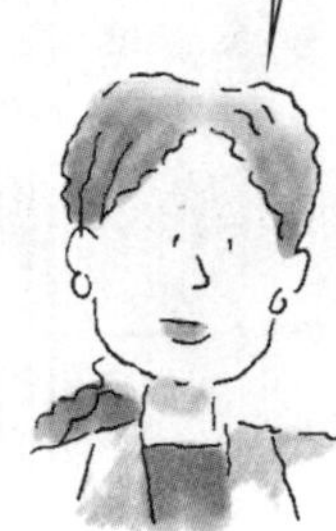

Discharge

The excretion of any substance from the eyes other than tears is known as a *discharge.* A common finding, discharge may occur in one or both eyes and may be scant or copious. The discharge may be purulent, frothy, mucoid, cheesy, serous, clear, or have a stringy, white appearance. Eye discharge commonly results from inflammatory and infectious eye disorders, such as conjunctivitis, but it may also occur in certain systemic disorders.

Pain

Eye pain may signal an emergency and requires immediate attention. Diseases causing eye pain include acute angle-closure glaucoma and conjunctivitis. Corneal damage caused by a foreign body or abrasions as well as trauma to the eye can also cause eye pain.

Periorbital edema

Swelling around the eyes, or periorbital edema, may result from allergies, local inflammation, fluid-retaining disorders, or crying.

Ptosis

Ptosis, or a drooping upper eyelid, may be caused by an interruption in sympathetic innervation to the eyelid, muscle weakness, or damage to the oculomotor nerve. (See *Recognizing periorbital edema and ptosis.*)

Strabismus

In strabismus, the eyes deviate from their normal gazing position. This condition may result from extraocular weakness or paralysis as a result of poor vision in one eye. It may also result from thyroid ophthalmopathy. Although adults may develop strabismus, it

Recognizing periorbital edema and ptosis

During an eye examination, you may observe any of a number of abnormalities. These illustrations show periorbital edema and ptosis.

Periorbital edema

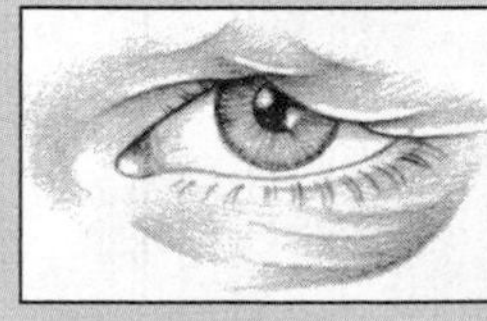

Ptosis

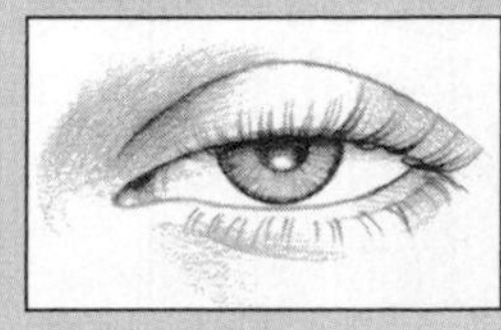

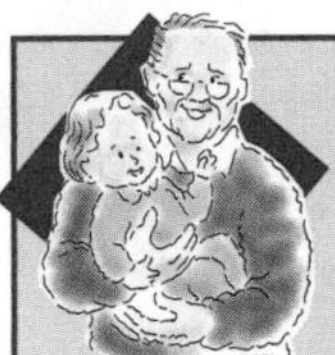

Ages and stages

Strabismus in children

Strabismus is the most common abnormal eye movement in children. Although severe strabismus is readily apparent, mild strabismus must be confirmed by tests for misalignment, such as the corneal light reflex test and the cover-uncover test. Such testing is crucial because early corrective measures help preserve binocular vision—which is normally achieved by age 3 to 4 months—and cosmetic appearance. Also, mild strabismus may indicate retinoblastoma, a tumor that may produce no symptoms before age 2 except for a characteristic whitish reflex in the pupil.

most commonly occurs in children. Detected early, it can be corrected without surgery. (See *Strabismus in children.*)

Vision loss

Disorders of any structure of the eye can result in vision loss. Types of vision loss include central vision loss, peripheral vision loss, or a blind spot in the middle of an area of normal vision (scotoma).

The degree and location of blindness depends on the disease causing the problem as well as the location of the lesion. The major causes of blindness in the United States include glaucoma, untreated cataracts, retinal disease, and macular degeneration.

Visual halos may indicate glaucoma, corneal edema, or a fluctuation in blood glucose levels.

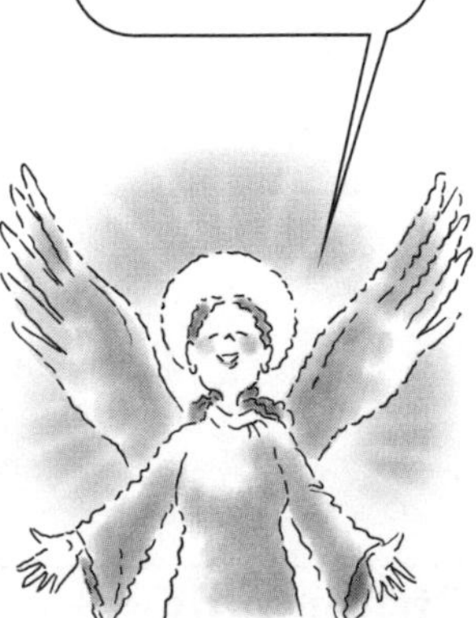

Visual floaters

Visual floaters are specks of varying shape and size that float through the visual field and disappear when the patient tries to look at them. Caused by small cells floating in the vitreous humor, visual floaters may signal vitreous hemorrhage or retinal separation and therefore require further investigation. A large, black floater that appears suddenly may indicate retinal detachment.

Visual halos

Increased intraocular pressure, which occurs in glaucoma, causes the patient to see halos and rainbows around bright lights. Other possible causes include corneal edema as a result of prolonged contact lens wear or a fluctuation in blood glucose levels.

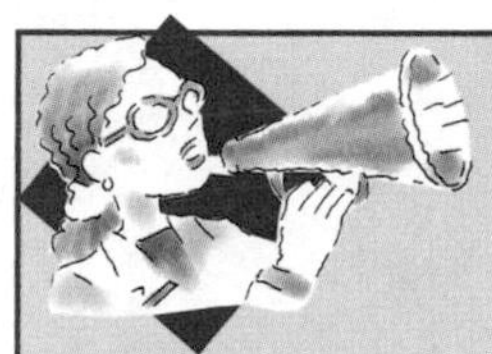

That's a wrap!

Eye review

Eye structures and functions
- Sclera—maintains the eye's size and shape
- Choroid—maintains blood supply to the eye
- Vitreous humor—maintains the placement of the retina and the eyeball's spherical shape
- Cornea—refracts, or bends, light rays entering the eye
- Iris—contains pigment granules that give the eye its color; contains involuntary muscles that control pupil size
- Pupil—permits light to enter the eye
- Lens—refracts and focuses light onto the retina
- Retina—receives visual stimuli and transmits images to the brain for processing

Health history
- Determine the patient's chief complaint.
- Ask if the patient wears corrective lenses.
- Obtain his past medical history. Be sure to ask about disorders that may affect vision, such as hypertension, diabetes, or stroke.
- Ask about a family history of glaucoma, cataracts, or vision loss.
- Obtain a medication history. Some medications, such as digoxin (Lanoxin), can affect vision.
- Ask a patient with vision impairment how he manages activities of daily living and assess his support system.

Assessment
- Note the position of the eyes.
- Check eyelids for closure and for redness, edema, inflammation, or lesions.
- Inspect for excessive tearing or dryness.
- Palpate the nasolacrimal sac.
- Examine the bulbar and palpebral conjunctiva.
- Inspect the cornea and assess corneal sensitivity using a wisp of cotton.
- Evaluate each iris for size, color, and shape.
- Examine the pupils for equal size, shape, and reactivity.

Tests for visual acuity
- Snellen chart, Snellen E chart, and near-vision chart—test near and distance vision and measure visual acuity
- Confrontation—tests peripheral vision and assesses visual fields

Tests for extraocular muscle function
- Corneal light reflex—light should fall at the same spot on each cornea
- Cardinal positions of gaze—eyes should remain parallel and move smoothly through the six cardinal positions
- Cover-uncover test—eye shouldn't move while covering or uncovering it

Ophthalmoscopic examination
- Have patient remove his corrective lenses; darken the room.
- Check for the presence and depth of the red reflex.
- Examine the lens for clouding, foreign matter, or opacities.
- Examine the retina: Observe the vitreous body for clarity; note the characteristics of the blood vessels; identify the optic disk, noting color, shape, and borders; and locate the light-sensitive macula.

(continued)

Eye review *(continued)*

Abnormal findings

- Arteriolar narrowing — arterioles of the inner eye narrow to a width of about one-half that of vein width
- Decreased visual acuity — the inability to see clearly
- Diplopia — double vision
- Discharge — excretion of any substance other than tears
- Pain — may demand immediate attention
- Periorbital edema — swelling around the eyes
- Ptosis — a drooping upper eyelid
- Strabismus — eyes deviate from their normal gazing position
- Vision loss — may be central or peripheral
- Visual floaters — specks of varying shape and size that float through the visual field but disappear when the patient tries to look at them
- Visual halos — rings or halos seen when looking at bright lights

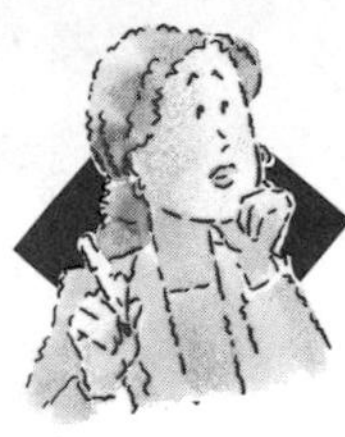

Quick quiz

1. The normal reaction to a corneal sensitivity test is:

A. blinking.
B. coughing.
C. pupil dilation.
D. pupil contraction.

Answer: A. The normal response to a corneal sensitivity test is blinking.

2. In addition to trauma, unequal pupils can result from:

A. a cataract.
B. an iridectomy.
C. severe conjunctivitis.
D. strabismus.

Answer: B. During an iridectomy, part of the iris is excised, resulting in an irregular pupil.

3. Cone receptors are mainly responsible for sensing:

A. light.
B. color.
C. shapes.
D. black and white.

Answer: B. Cones, which are located in the fovea centralis, aid in color recognition.

4. To determine a patient's visual acuity, you would use the:

A. Snellen chart.
B. cover-uncover test.
C. corneal light reflex test.
D. cardinal positions of gaze.

Answer: A. The Snellen chart tests visual acuity by having the patient read a series of letters. The Snellen E chart contains only the letter *E* and can be used for children and patients who can't read.

5. The red reflex seen during an ophthalmoscope examination is the result of:

A. an increase in intraocular pressure.
B. incorrect adjustment of the diopter.
C. light from the scope reflecting back from the choroid.
D. arteriolar narrowing.

Answer: C. The red reflex results from light reflecting off the choroid. To test for the reflex, shine the ophthalmoscope light at the patient's pupil from a distance of about 4″ (10 cm) and at a slight angle.

6. Compared with the size of a child's pupils, the size of an adult's pupils is:

A. smaller.
B. larger.
C. the same throughout life.
D. wider.

Answer: A. Pupils are small and unresponsive to light at birth. They enlarge during childhood and progressively decrease in size throughout adulthood and into old age.

7. Which item is used to test corneal sensitivity?

A. Wisp of cotton
B. Tissue
C. Gauze pad
D. Ophthalmoscope

Answer: A. A wisp of cotton is the only safe object to use for assessing corneal sensitivity. Even though a gauze pad or tissue is soft, it can cause corneal abrasions and irritation.

Scoring

☆☆☆ If you answered all seven questions correctly, terrific! You're a star pupil.

☆☆ If you answered five or six questions correctly, good job! You really have vision.

☆ If you answered fewer than five questions correctly, don't lose focus. Becoming an assessment whiz requires lots of practice.

Ears, nose, and throat

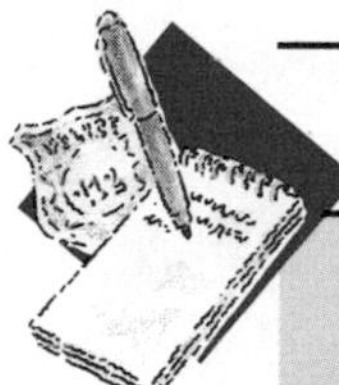

Just the facts

In this chapter, you'll learn:

- structures of the ears, nose, and throat and their functions
- questions to ask about the ears, nose, and throat during the health history
- techniques for assessing the ears, nose, and throat
- ear, nose, and throat abnormalities and their causes.

A look at the ears, nose, and throat

The ability to hear, smell, and taste allows us to communicate with others, connect with the world around us, and take pleasure in life. Because these senses play such vital roles in daily life, you'll need to thoroughly assess a patient's ears, nose, and throat.

Clues for you

Besides revealing impairments in hearing, smell, and taste, your assessment also can uncover important clues to physical problems in the patient's integumentary, musculoskeletal, cardiovascular, respiratory, immune, and neurologic systems.

Anatomy and physiology of the ears, nose, and throat

To perform an accurate physical assessment, you'll need to understand the anatomy and physiology of the ears, nose, and throat.

Ears

The ear is divided into three parts: external, middle, and inner. The anatomy and physiology of each part play separate but equally important roles in hearing. (See *A close look at the ear.*)

External ear

The flexible external ear consists mainly of elastic cartilage. This part of the ear contains the ear flap, also known as the *auricle* or

A close look at the ear

Use this illustration to review the structures of the ear.

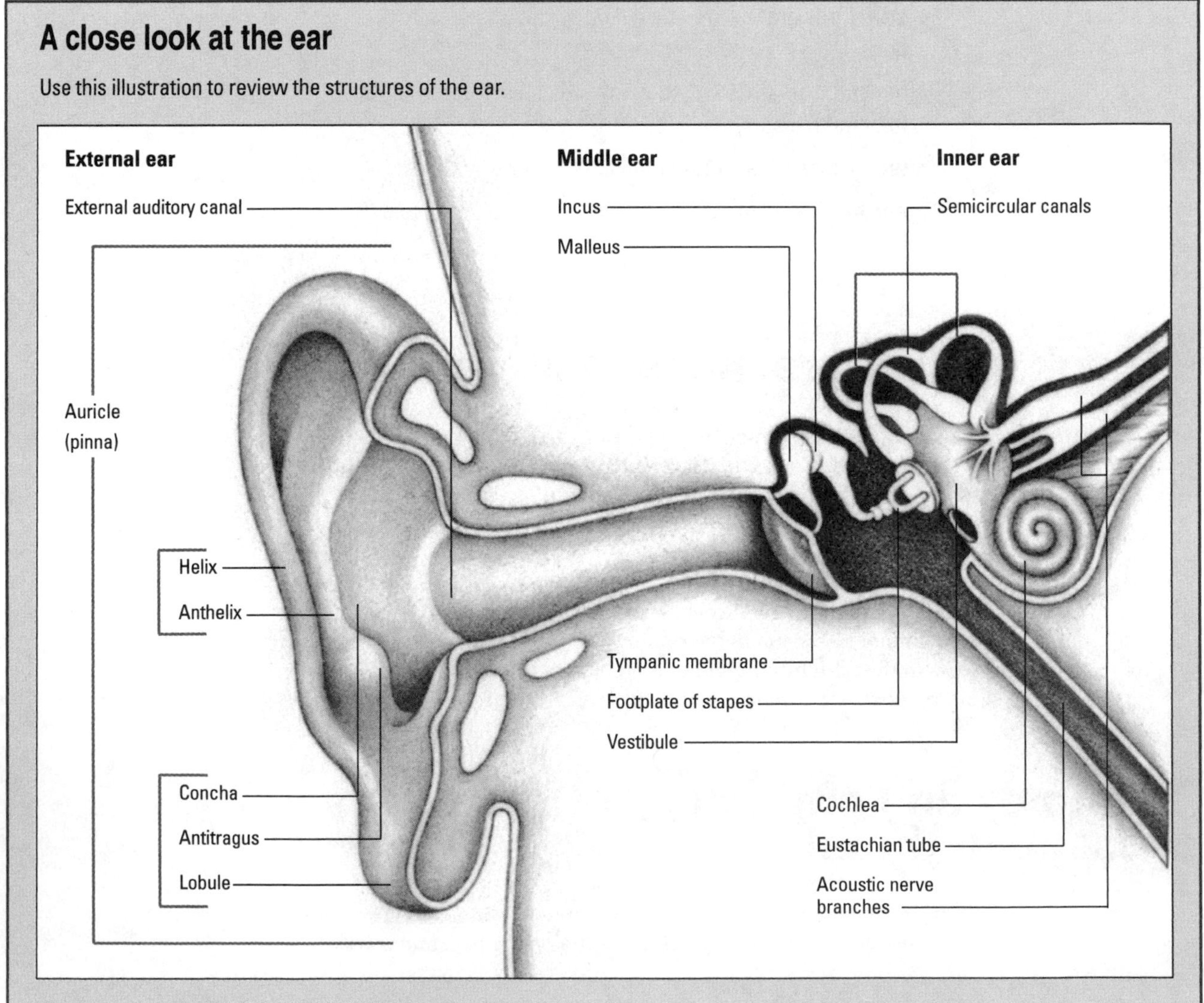

pinna, and the auditory canal. The outer third of this canal has a bony framework. Coarse hair may be visible in the canal in elderly men. The external ear and ear canal collect sounds and transmit them to the middle ear.

Middle ear

The tympanic membrane separates the external and middle ear. This pearl gray structure consists of three layers: skin, fibrous tissue, and a mucous membrane. Its upper portion, the pars flaccida, has little support; its lower portion, the pars tensa, is held taut. The center, or umbo, is attached to the tip of the long process of the malleus on the other side of the tympanic membrane.

A small, air-filled structure, the middle ear performs three vital functions:

- It transmits sound vibrations across the bony ossicle chain to the inner ear.
- It protects the auditory apparatus from intense vibrations.
- It equalizes the air pressure on both sides of the tympanic membrane to prevent it from rupturing.

Those bones, those bones, those wee small bones

The middle ear contains three small bones of the auditory ossicles: the malleus, or hammer; the incus, or anvil; and the stapes, or stirrup. These bones are linked like a chain and vibrate in place. The long process of the malleus fits into the incus, forming a true joint, and allows the two structures to move as a single unit. The proximal end of the stapes fits into the oval window, an opening that joins the middle and inner ear.

A tube with connections

The eustachian tube connects the middle ear with the nasopharynx, equalizing air pressure on either side of the tympanic membrane. This tube also connects the ear's sterile area to the nasopharynx.

A normally functioning eustachian tube keeps the middle ear free from contaminants from the nasopharynx. It opens during yawning or swallowing. Upper respiratory tract infections and allergies can block the tube, obstructing middle ear drainage and possibly causing otitis media or effusion.

Did you hear me? The eustachian tube keeps contaminants away from the middle ear!

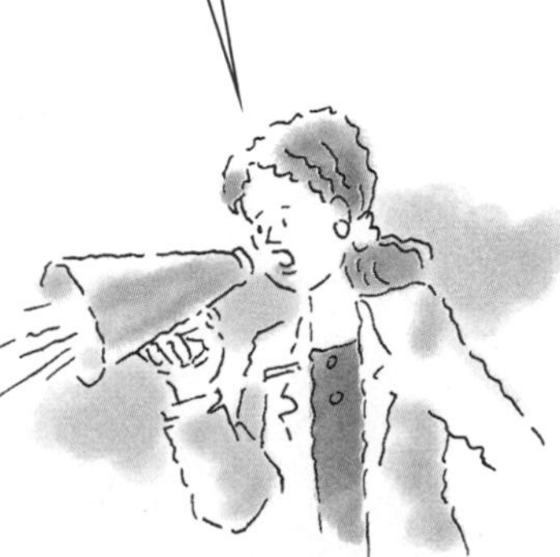

Inner ear

The inner ear consists of closed, fluid-filled spaces within the temporal bone. It contains the bony labyrinth, which includes three connected structures: the vestibule, the semicircular canals, and the cochlea. These structures are lined with the membranous labyrinth. A fluid called *perilymph* fills the space between the bony labyrinth and the membranous labyrinth, cushioning these sensitive organs.

The vestibule and semicircular canals help maintain equilibrium. The cochlea, a spiral chamber that resembles a snail shell, is the organ of hearing. The organ of Corti, part of the membranous labyrinth, contains hair cells that receive auditory sensations.

I heard it through the...sound waves

When sound waves reach the external ear, structures there transmit the waves through the auditory canal to the tympanic membrane, where they cause a chain reaction of vibrations along the structures of the middle and inner ear. Finally, the cochlear branch of the acoustic nerve (cranial nerve VIII) transmits the vibrations to the temporal lobe of the cerebral cortex, where the brain interprets the sound.

Double duty

In addition to controlling hearing, structures in the middle and inner ear control balance. The semicircular canals of the inner ear contain cristae—hairlike structures that respond to body movements. Endolymph fluid bathes the cristae.

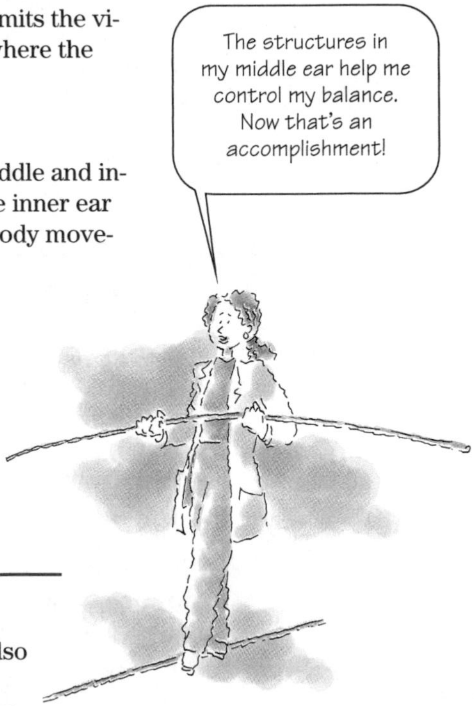

Balancing act

When a person moves, the cristae bend, releasing impulses through the vestibular portion of the acoustic nerve to the brain, which controls balance. When a person is stationary, nerve impulses to the brain orient him to this position, and the pressure of gravity on the inner ear helps him maintain balance.

Nose

The nose is more than the sensory organ of smell. It also plays a key role in the respiratory system by filtering, warming, and humidifying inhaled air. When you assess the nose, you'll commonly assess the paranasal sinuses, too.

Inside and out

The lower two-thirds of the external nose consist of flexible cartilage, and the upper one-third is rigid bone. Posteriorly, the internal nose merges with the pharynx. Anteriorly, it merges with the external nose.

Dividing line

The internal and external nose are divided vertically by the nasal septum, which is straight at birth and in early life but becomes slightly deviated or deformed in almost every adult. Only the posterior end, which separates the posterior nares, remains constantly in the midline.

Nosebleed central

Kiesselbach's area, the most common site of nosebleeds, is located in the anterior portion of the septum.

Just nosing around

Air entering the nose passes through the vestibule, which is lined with coarse hair that helps filter dust. Olfactory receptors lie above the vestibule in the roof of the nasal cavity and the upper one-third of the septum. Known as the *olfactory region*, this area is rich in capillaries and mucus-producing goblet cells that help warm, moisten, and clean inhaled air.

Breathe easy

Farther along the nasal passage are the superior, middle, and inferior turbinates. Separated by grooves called *meatus*, the curved bony turbinates and their mucosal covering ease breathing by further warming, filtering, and humidifying inhaled air.

Singling out the sinuses

Four pairs of paranasal sinuses open into the internal nose, including the:

- maxillary sinuses, located on the cheeks below the eyes
- frontal sinuses, located above the eyebrows
- ethmoidal and sphenoidal sinuses, located behind the eyes and nose in the head.

The sinuses serve as resonators for sound production and provide mucus. You'll be able to assess the maxillary and frontal sinuses, but the ethmoidal and sphenoidal sinuses aren't readily accessible. (See *A close look at the nose and mouth*, page 126.)

The small openings between the sinuses and the nasal cavity can easily become obstructed because they're lined with mucous membranes that can become inflamed and swollen.

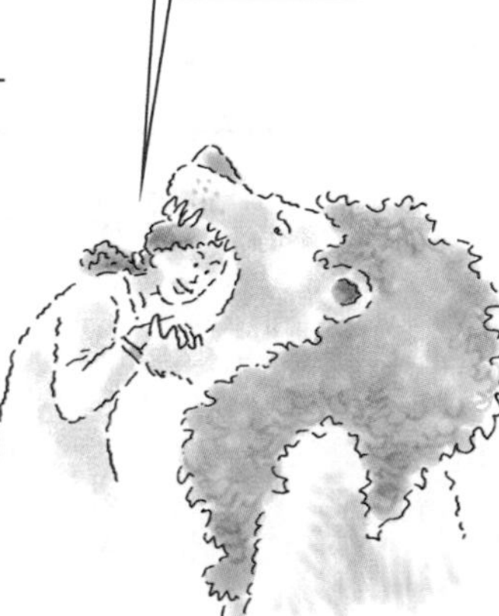

Throat

The throat, or pharynx, is divided into the nasopharynx, oropharynx, and laryngopharynx. Located within the throat are the hard and soft palates, the uvula, and the tonsils. The mucous

A close look at the nose and mouth

These illustrations show the anatomic structures of the nose and mouth.

Nose and mouth

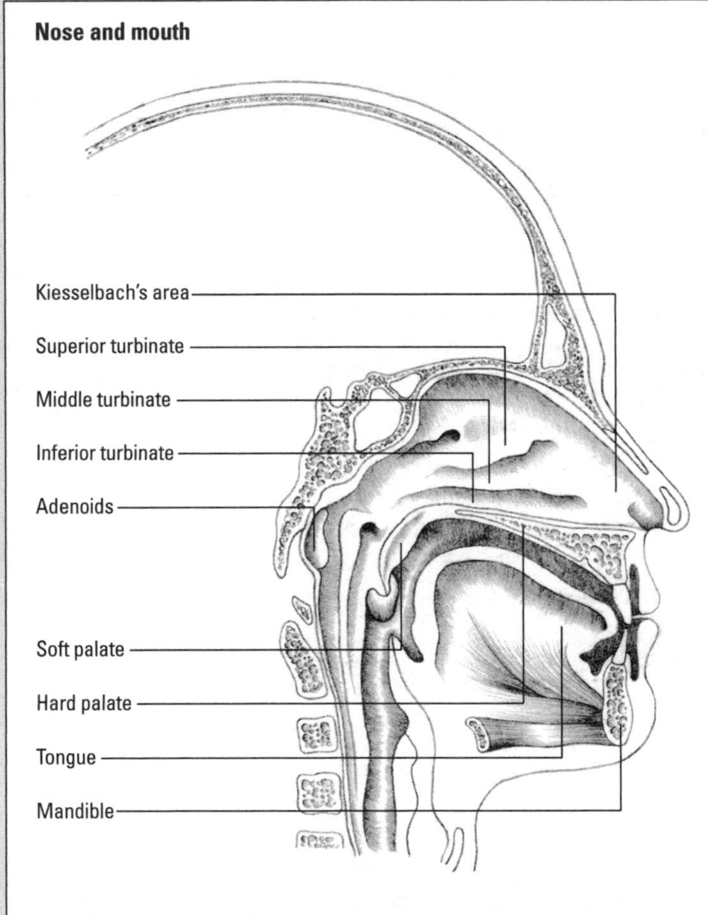

Mouth and oropharynx

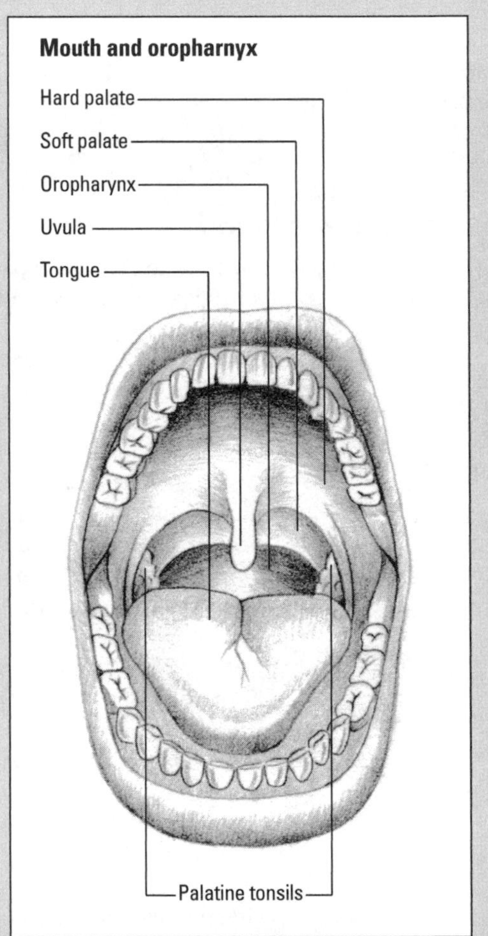

membrane lining the throat is usually smooth and bright pink to light red.

Running neck and neck

The neck is formed by the cervical vertebrae, the major neck and shoulder muscles, and their ligaments. Other important structures of the neck include the trachea, thyroid gland, and chains of lymph nodes.

Grand gland

The thyroid gland lies in the anterior neck, just below the larynx. Its two cone-shaped lobes are located on either side of the trachea and are connected by an isthmus below the cricoid cartilage, which gives the gland its butterfly shape. The largest endocrine gland, the thyroid produces the hormones triiodothyronine and thyroxine, which affect the metabolic reactions of every cell in the body.

Obtaining a health history

To investigate a complaint about the ears, nose, or throat, ask about the onset, location, duration, and characteristics of the symptom as well as what aggravates and relieves it.

Asking about the ears

The most common ear complaints are hearing loss, tinnitus, pain, discharge, and dizziness. Ask the patient if he has any associated symptoms. Have him describe the color and consistency of any ear discharge, and ask about a history of head injury. Ask the patient if he has had feelings of abnormal movement or vertigo (spinning). Determine when the episodes occur, how frequently they occur, and whether they're associated with nausea, vomiting, or tinnitus.

Ask the patient if he has previously had an ear problem or injury, or if anyone in his family has ear or hearing problems. Also, ask if he has been ill recently or if he has a chronic disorder. For example, diabetes can cause hearing loss, and hypertension can cause high-pitched tinnitus.

Ask about current treatments and medications. Certain antibiotics and other medications can cause hearing loss and tinnitus.

Nothing to sneeze at

Ask the patient if he has allergies. Serous otitis media, or inflammation of the middle ear, is common in people with environmental or seasonal allergies. Otitis externa, or inflammation of the external ear, can be caused by allergic reactions to hair dyes, cosmetics, perfumes, and other personal care products.

My seasonal allergies always seem to trigger an ear infection. Ah-choo!

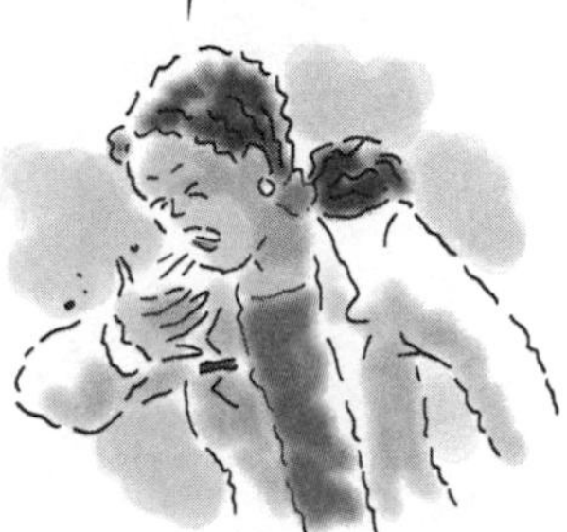

Asking about the nose

The most common complaints about the nose include nasal stuffiness, nasal discharge, and epistaxis, or nosebleed. Ask if the patient has had any of these problems. Also ask about frequent colds, hay fever, headaches, and sinus trouble. Determine whether certain conditions or places seem to cause or aggravate the patient's problem. Ask if he has ever had nose or head trauma.

Allergens all around

Environmental allergies can cause nasal stuffiness and discharge, and stagnant nasal discharge can act as a culture medium and lead to sinusitis and other infections. Also, inquire about the color and consistency of the discharge.

Asking about the mouth, throat, and neck

Ask the patient if he has bleeding or sore gums, mouth or tongue ulcers, a bad taste in his mouth, bad breath, toothaches, loose teeth, frequent sore throats, hoarseness, or facial swelling. Also ask whether he smokes or uses other types of tobacco. If the patient is having neck problems, ask if he has neck pain or tenderness, neck swelling, or trouble moving his neck.

Asking about general health

After asking specific questions about the ears, nose, mouth, throat, and neck, ask about the patient's general health. Be alert for responses that might indicate a thyroid disorder. Hyperthyroidism can cause heat intolerance, weight loss, and a short menstrual pattern with scant flow. Hypothyroidism can cause cold intolerance, weight gain, an increase in menstrual pattern and flow and, in extreme cases, bradycardia and dyspnea from low cardiac output.

Get specific

Ask the patient these questions pertaining to signs and symptoms:
- Have you noticed changes in the way you tolerate hot and cold weather?
- Has your weight changed recently?
- Do you have breathing problems or feel as if your heart is skipping beats?
- Have you noticed a change in your menstrual pattern?
- Have you noticed any tremors, agitation, or difficulty concentrating or sleeping?

Assessing the ears, nose, and throat

Examining the ears, nose, and throat mainly involves using the techniques of inspection, palpation, and auscultation. An ear assessment also requires the use of an otoscope and the administration of hearing acuity tests.

Examining the ears

To assess your patient's ears, you'll need to inspect and palpate the external structures, perform an otoscopic examination of the ear canal, and test his hearing acuity.

External observations

Begin by observing the ears for position and symmetry. The top of the ear should line up with the outer corner of the eye, and the ears should look symmetrical, with an angle of attachment of no more than 10 degrees. The face and ears should be the same shade and color.

Ear-y situation

Auricles that protrude from the head, or "lop" ears, are fairly common and don't affect hearing ability. However, low-set ears commonly accompany congenital disorders, including kidney problems.

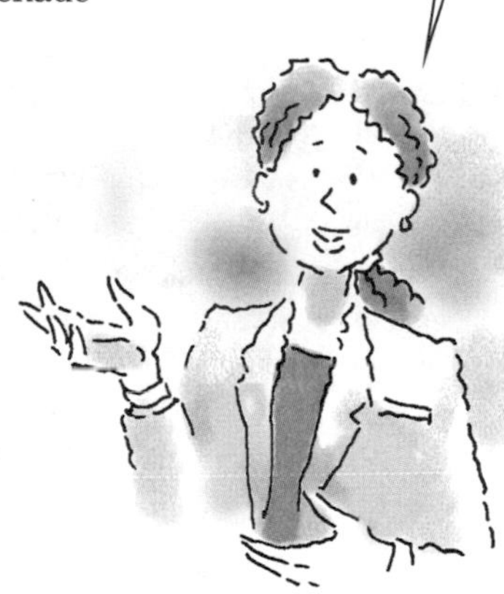

An auricle oracle

Inspect the auricle for lesions, drainage, nodules, or redness. Pull the helix back and note if it's tender. If pulling the ear back hurts the patient, he may have otitis externa. Then inspect and palpate the mastoid area behind each auricle, noting tenderness, redness, or warmth.

Conclude with the canal

Finally, inspect the opening of the ear canal, noting discharge, redness, odor, or the presence of nodules or cysts. Patients normally have varying amounts of hair and cerumen (earwax) in the ear canal.

Otoscopic examination

The next part of your ear assessment involves examining the patient's auditory canal, tympanic membrane, and malleus with the otoscope. Before inserting the speculum into the patient's ear

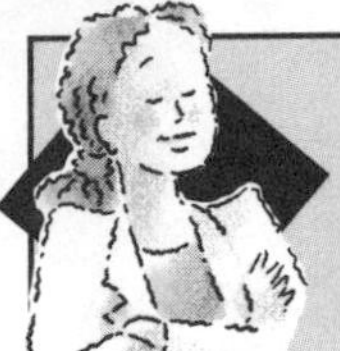

Peak technique

Using an otoscope

Here's how to use an otoscope to examine the ears.

Inserting the speculum

Before inserting the speculum into the patient's ear, straighten the ear canal by grasping the auricle and pulling it up and back, as shown below.

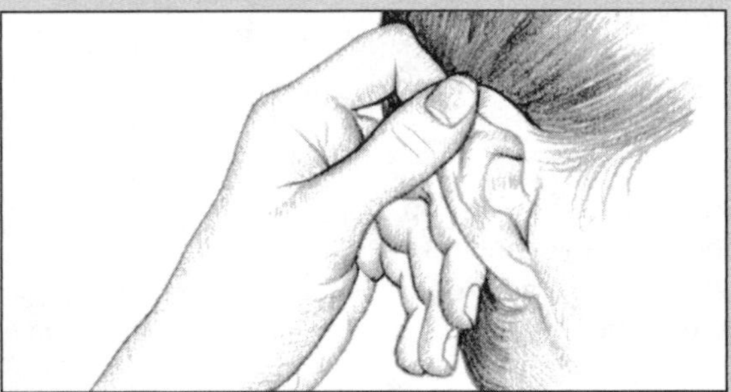

Positioning the scope

To examine the ear's external canal, hold the otoscope with the handle parallel to the patient's head, as shown below. Bracing your hand firmly against his head keeps you from hitting the canal with the speculum.

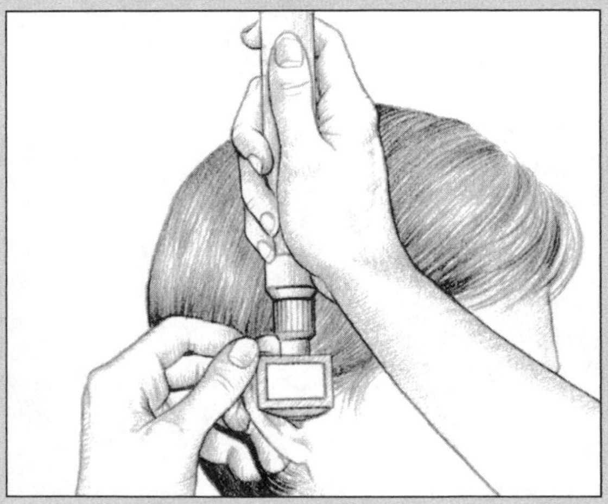

Viewing the structures

When the otoscope is positioned properly, you should see the tympanic membrane structures shown here.

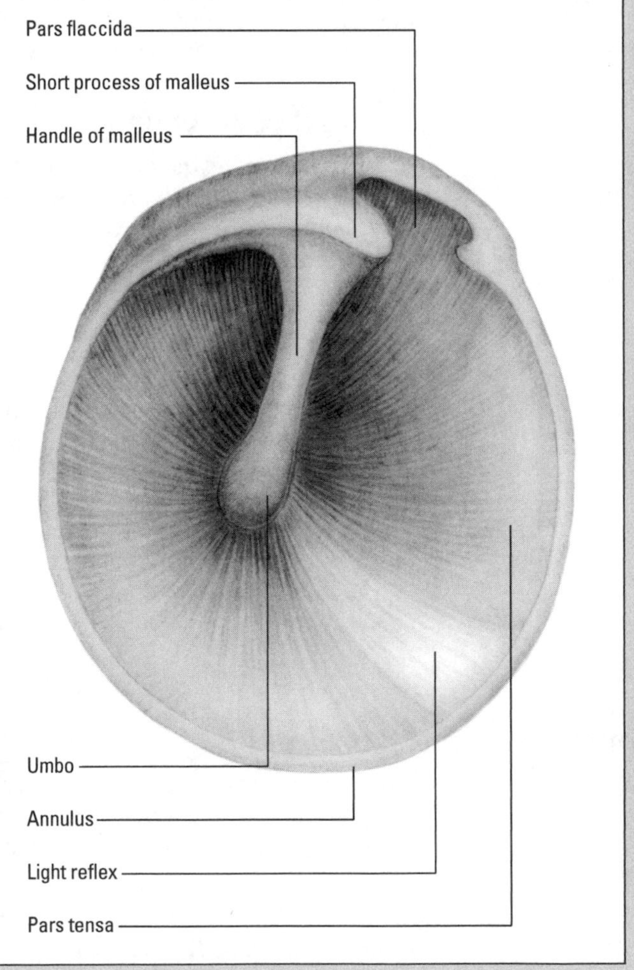

canal, check the canal for foreign bodies or discharge. (See *Using an otoscope.*)

Then palpate the tragus—the cartilaginous projection anterior to the external opening of the ear—and pull the auricle up. If this area is tender, don't insert the speculum. The patient could have otitis externa, and inserting the speculum could be painful.

Insert speculum A into ear B

To insert the speculum of the otoscope, tilt the patient's head away from you. Then grasp the superior posterior auricle with your thumb and index finger and pull it up and back to straighten the canal. Because everyone's ear canal is shaped differently, vary the angle of the speculum until you can see the tympanic membrane. If your patient is a child younger than age 3, pull the auricle down to get a good view of the membrane. Lean your hand holding the otoscope against the patient's head for steadiness.

Go gently into that good ear canal

Insert the speculum to about one-third its length when inspecting the canal. Be sure to insert it gently because the inner two-thirds of the canal are sensitive to pressure. Note the cerumen's color. (See *Cerumen variations.*) The elderly patient may have harder, drier cerumen because of rigid cilia in the ear canal. The external canal should be free from inflammation and scaling.

Blocked view

If your view of the tympanic membrane is obstructed by excessive cerumen, don't try to remove the cerumen with an instrument because you could cause the patient excessive pain. Instead, use ceruminolytic drops and warm water irrigation as ordered.

As the speculum turns

You may need to carefully rotate the speculum for a complete view of the tympanic membrane. The membrane should be pearl gray, glistening, and transparent. The annulus should be white and denser than the rest of the membrane. Inspect the membrane carefully for bulging, retraction, bleeding, lesions, and perforations, especially at the periphery. The elderly patient's eardrum may appear cloudy.

No lesions, drainage, nodules, or redness. Good!

"Timing" the light reflex?

Now, examine the membrane for the light reflex. The light reflex in the right ear should be between 4 and 6 o'clock; in the left ear, it should be between 6 and 8 o'clock. If the reflex is displaced or absent, the patient's tympanic membrane may be bulging, inflamed, or retracted.

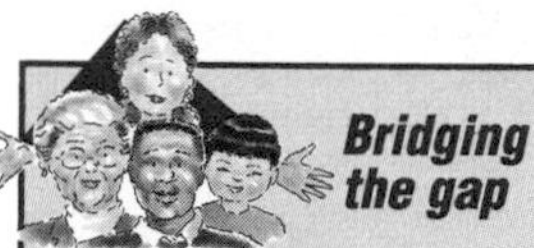

Cerumen variations

When examining your patient's ear canal, keep in mind that the presence of cerumen doesn't indicate poor hygiene. In fact, the appearance and type of cerumen is genetically determined. There are two types of cerumen:

- *Dry cerumen*—which is gray and flaky and is mostly found in Asians and Native Americans (including Eskimos).
- *Wet cerumen*—which has a dark brown, moist appearance and is commonly found in Blacks and Whites.

Finally, look for the bony landmarks. The malleus will appear as a dense, white streak at the 12 o'clock position. At the top of the light reflex, you'll find the umbo, the inferior point of the malleus.

Hearing acuity tests

The last part of an ear assessment involves testing the patient's hearing using Weber's test and the Rinne test. These tests assess conduction hearing loss, impaired sound transmission to the inner ear, sensorineural hearing loss, and impaired auditory nerve conduction or inner ear function. (See *Assessing hearing in young children.*)

Weber's test

Weber's test is performed when the patient reports diminished or lost hearing in one ear.

Choosing the right fork

This test uses a tuning fork to evaluate bone conduction. The tuning fork should be tuned to the frequency of normal human speech, 512 cycles/second. To perform Weber's test, strike the tuning fork lightly against your hand, and then place the fork on the patient's forehead at the midline or on the top of his head.

Do you hear what I hear?

If the patient hears the tone equally well in both ears, record this as a normal Weber's test. If he hears the tone better in one ear, record the result as right or left lateralization. If he hears the tone in his impaired ear, he has a conductive hearing loss. If he hears the tone in his unaffected ear, he has a sensorineural hearing loss.

Rinne test

Perform the Rinne test after Weber's test to compare air conduction of sound with bone conduction of sound. To administer this test, strike the tuning fork against your hand, and then place it over the patient's mastoid process. Ask him to tell you when the tone stops; note this time in seconds. Next, move the still-vibrating tuning fork to the ear's opening without touching the ear. Ask him to tell you when the tone stops. Note the time in seconds. (See *Positioning the tuning fork.*)

Air waves

The patient should hear the air-conducted tone for twice as long as he hears the bone-conducted tone. If he hears the bone-conducted tone as long as or longer than the air-conducted tone, conductive

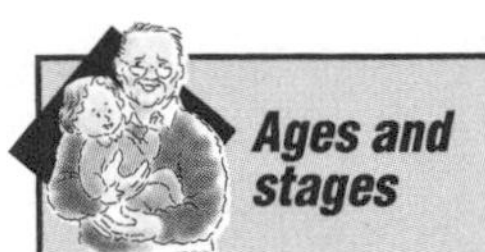

Ages and stages

Assessing hearing in young children

When assessing hearing in an infant or a young child, you can't use a tuning fork. Instead, for infants younger than age 6 months, test the startle reflex. Another option in neonates, infants, and young children is to have an audiologist test brain stem evoked response. Many states now require that all neonates undergo brain stem evoked response testing before they're discharged from the hospital.

Because hearing disorders in children may lead to speech, language, and learning problems, early identification and treatment is crucial. Undiagnosed hearing disorders can also cause some children to be incorrectly labeled as mentally challenged, brain damaged, or slow learners.

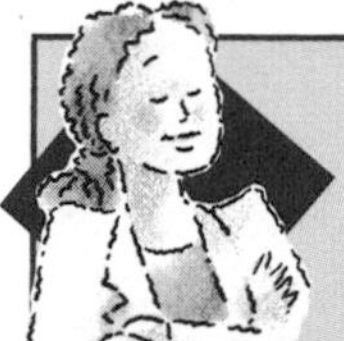

Peak technique

Positioning the tuning fork

These illustrations show how to hold a tuning fork to test a patient's hearing.

Weber's test
With the tuning fork vibrating lightly, position the tip on the patient's forehead at the midline, as shown below. Alternatively, place the tuning fork on the top of the patient's head.

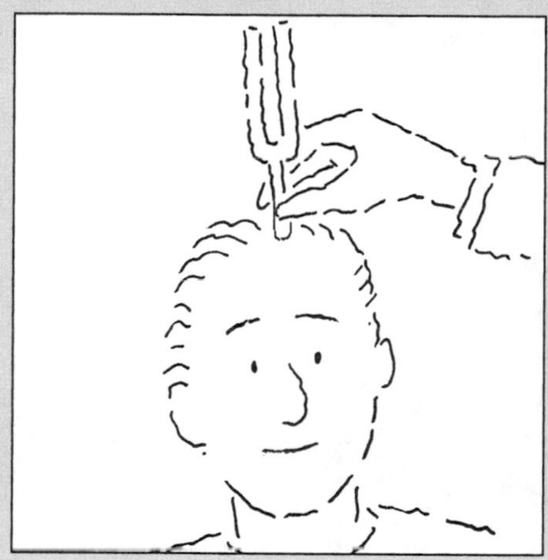

Rinne test
Strike the tuning fork against your hand, and then hold it behind the patient's ear, as shown below. When your patient tells you the tone has stopped, move the still-vibrating tuning fork to the opening of his ear.

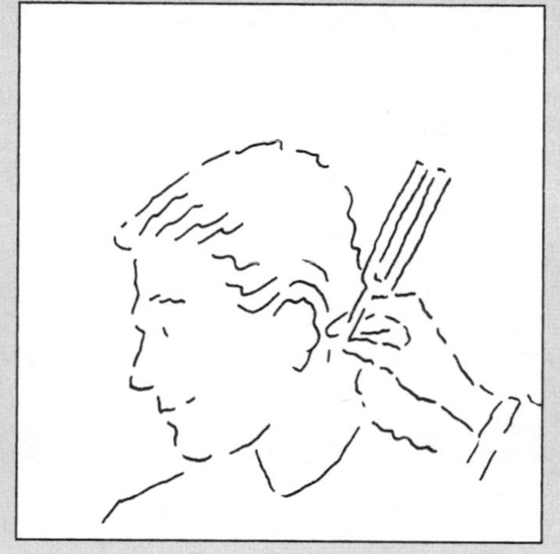

hearing loss is present. In sensorineural hearing loss, the air-conducted sound is heard longer than the bone-conducted sound.

Examining the nose and sinuses

A complete examination of the nose also includes checking the sinuses. To perform this examination, use the techniques of inspection and palpation.

Inspecting and palpating the nose

Begin by observing the patient's nose for position, symmetry, and color. Note variations, such as discoloration, swelling, or deformity. Variations in size and shape are largely caused by differences in cartilage and in the amount of fibroadipose tissue.

Peak technique

Inspecting the nostrils

The illustration below shows the proper placement of the nasal speculum during direct inspection and the structures you should be able to see during this examination.

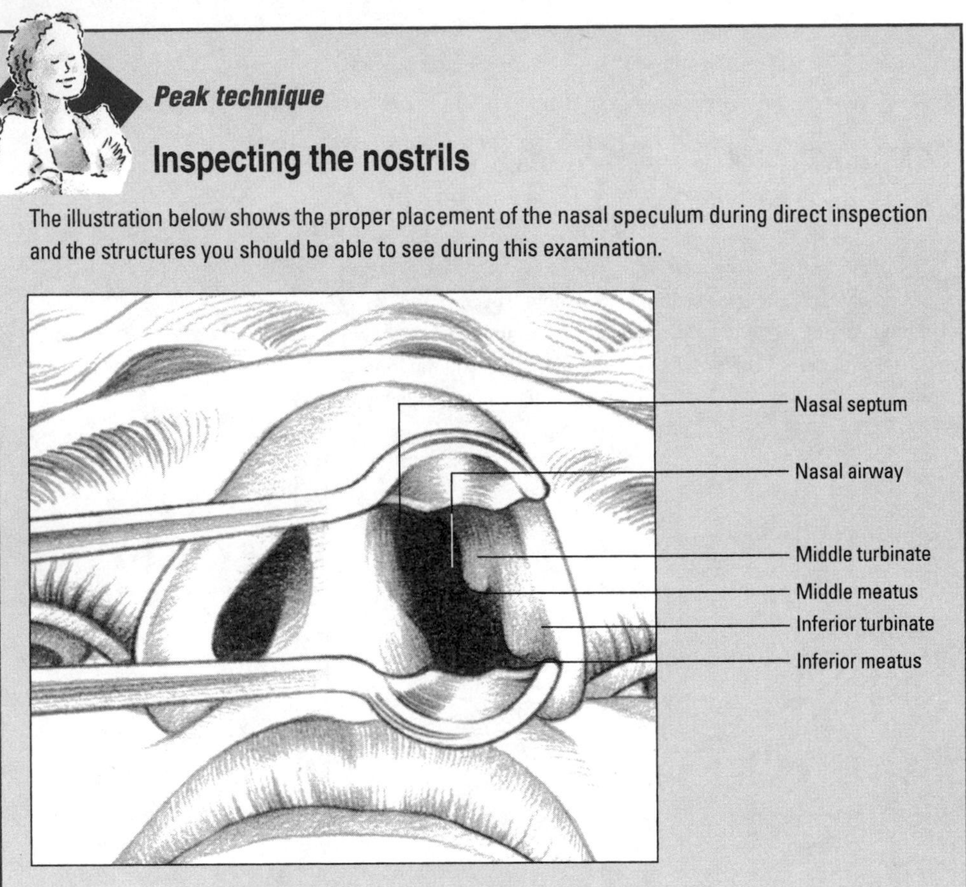

Observe for nasal discharge or flaring. If discharge is present, note the color, quantity, and consistency. If you notice flaring, observe for other signs of respiratory distress.

Name that smell...

To test nasal patency and olfactory nerve (cranial nerve I) function, ask the patient to block one nostril and inhale a familiar aromatic substance through the other nostril. Possible substances include soap, coffee, citrus, tobacco, or nutmeg. Ask him to identify the aroma. Then repeat the process with the other nostril, using a different aroma.

Turn up the patient's nose

Now, inspect the nasal cavity. Ask the patient to tilt his head back slightly, and then push the tip of his nose up. Use the light from the otoscope to illuminate his nasal cavities. Check for severe deviation or perforation of the nasal septum. Examine the vestibule and turbinates for redness, softness, swelling, and discharge.

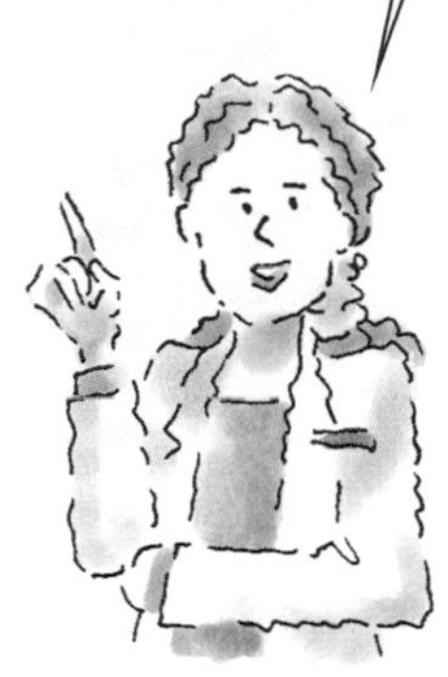

A light at the end of the speculum

Examine the nostrils by direct inspection, using a nasal speculum, a penlight or small flashlight, or an otoscope with a short, wide-tip attachment. Have the patient sit in front of you with his head tilted back. Put on gloves and insert the tip of the closed nasal speculum into one nostril to the point where the blade widens. Slowly open the speculum as wide as possible without causing discomfort. Shine the flashlight in the nostril to illuminate the area.

Observe the color and patency of the nostril, and check for exudate. The mucosa should be moist, pink to light red, and free from lesions and polyps. After inspecting one nostril, close the speculum, remove it, and inspect the other nostril. (See *Inspecting the nostrils.*)

Thumb his nose

Finally, palpate the patient's nose with your thumb and forefinger, assessing for pain, tenderness, swelling, and deformity.

Examining the sinuses

Next examine the sinuses. Remember, only the frontal and maxillary sinuses are accessible; you won't be able to palpate the ethmoidal and sphenoidal sinuses. However, if the frontal and maxillary sinuses are infected, you can assume that the other sinuses are, too.

Tell me if it hurts

Begin by checking for swelling around the eyes, especially over the sinus area. Then palpate the sinuses, checking for tenderness. (See *Palpating the maxillary sinuses*, page 136.) To palpate the frontal sinuses, place your thumbs above the patient's eyes just under the bony ridges of the upper orbits, and place your fingertips on his forehead. Apply gentle pressure. Next palpate the maxillary sinuses.

Shed some light on the subject

If the patient complains of tenderness during palpation of the sinuses, use transillumination to see if the sinuses are filled with fluid or pus. Transillumination can also help reveal tumors and obstructions. (See *Transilluminating the sinuses*, page 137.)

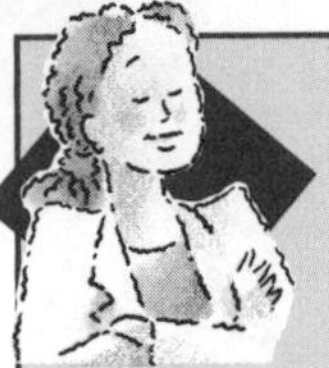

Peak technique

Palpating the maxillary sinuses

To palpate the maxillary sinuses, gently press your thumbs on each side of the nose just below the cheekbones, as shown. The illustration also shows the location of the frontal sinuses.

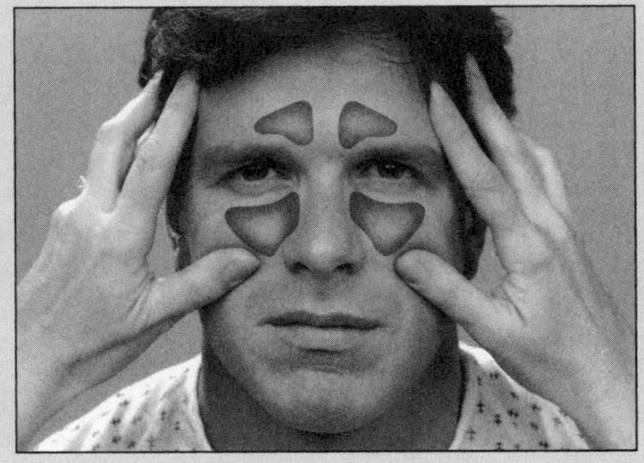

Examining the mouth, throat, and neck

Assessing the mouth and throat requires the techniques of inspection and palpation. Assessing the neck also involves auscultation.

Assessing the mouth and throat

First, inspect the patient's lips. They should be pink, moist, symmetrical, and without lesions. A bluish hue or flecked pigmentation is common in dark-skinned patients. Put on gloves and palpate the lips for lumps or surface abnormalities.

Mi casa, mucosa

Use a tongue blade and a bright light to inspect the oral mucosa. Have the patient open his mouth; then place the tongue blade on top of his tongue. The oral mucosa should be pink, smooth, moist, and free from lesions and unusual odors. Increased pigmentation is seen in dark-skinned patients.

Gums and then some

Next, observe the gingivae, or gums: They should be pink, moist, and have clearly defined margins at each tooth. They shouldn't be retracted. Inspect the teeth, noting their number, condition, and whether any are missing or crowded. If the patient is wearing dentures, ask him to remove them so you can inspect the gums underneath.

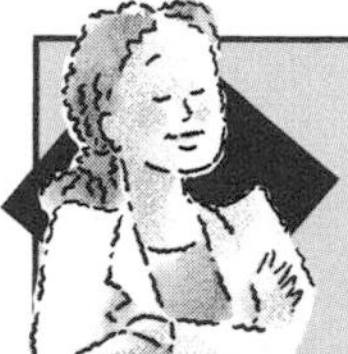

Peak technique

Transilluminating the sinuses

Transillumination of the sinuses helps detect sinus tumors and obstruction and requires only a penlight. Before you start, darken the room and have the patient close her eyes.

Frontal sinuses

Place the penlight on the supraorbital ring and direct the light upward to illuminate the frontal sinuses just above the eyebrow, as shown below.

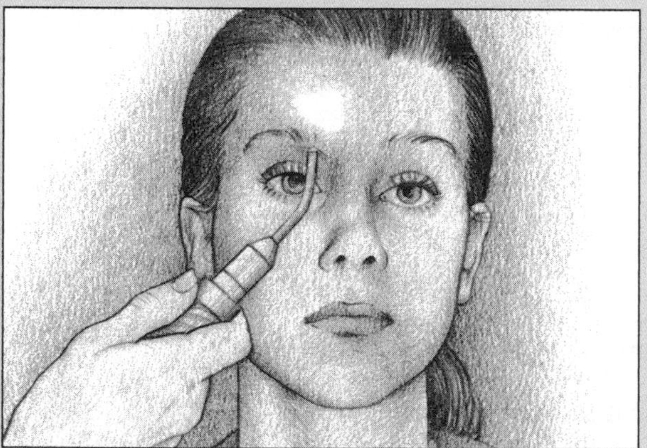

Maxillary sinuses

Place the penlight on the patient's cheekbone just below her eye and ask her to open her mouth, as shown below. The light should transilluminate easily and equally.

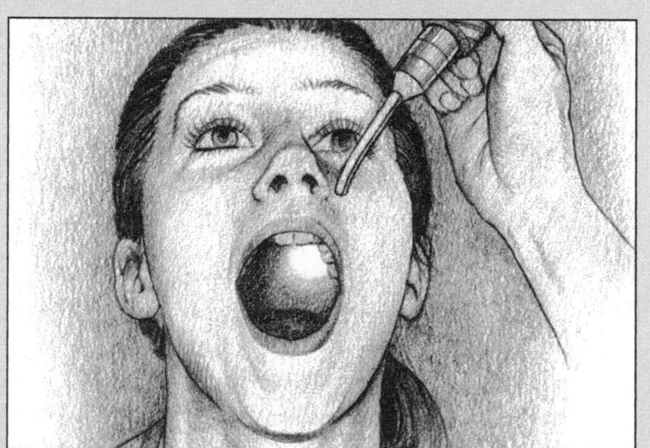

Give the tongue the once-over

Finally, inspect the tongue. It should be midline, moist, pink, and free from lesions. The posterior surface should be smooth, and the anterior surface should be slightly rough with small fissures. The tongue should move easily in all directions, and it should lie straight to the front at rest.

Ask the patient to raise the tip of his tongue and touch his palate directly behind his front teeth. Inspect the ventral surface of the tongue and the floor of the mouth. Next, wrap a piece of gauze around the tip of the tongue and move the tongue first to one side then the other to inspect the lateral borders. They should be smooth and even-textured. (See *Checking the surface.*)

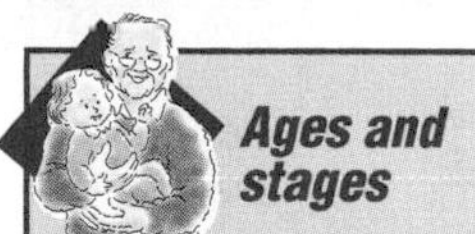

Ages and stages

Checking the surface

The elderly patient may have varicose veins on the ventral surface of the tongue. In addition, the area underneath the tongue is a common site for the development of oral cancers. This area must be assessed thoroughly.

Say "Ahhh"

Inspect the patient's oropharynx by asking him to open his mouth while you shine the penlight on the uvula and palate. You may need to insert a tongue blade into the mouth and depress the tongue. Place the tongue blade slightly off center to avoid eliciting the gag reflex. The uvula and oropharynx should be pink and moist, without inflammation or exudates. The tonsils should be pink and shouldn't be hypertrophied. Ask the patient to say "Ahhh." Observe for movement of the soft palate and uvula.

Gag order

Finally, palpate the lips, tongue, and oropharynx. Note lumps, lesions, ulcers, or edema of the lips or tongue. Assess the patient's gag reflex by gently touching the back of the pharynx with a cotton-tipped applicator or the tongue blade. This should produce a bilateral response.

Inspecting and palpating the neck

First, observe the patient's neck. It should be symmetrical, and the skin should be intact. Note any scars. No visible pulsations, masses, swelling, venous distention, or thyroid or lymph node enlargement should be present. Ask the patient to move his neck through the entire range of motion and to shrug his shoulders. Also ask him to swallow. Note rising of the larynx, trachea, or thyroid.

One lump or two?

Palpate the patient's neck to gather further data. Using the finger pads of both hands, bilaterally palpate the chain of lymph nodes under the patient's chin in the preauricular area; then proceed to the area under and behind the ears. (See *Locating lymph nodes.*) Assess the nodes for size, shape, mobility, consistency, temperature, and tenderness, comparing nodes on one side with those on the other.

By the throat

Palpate the trachea, which is normally located midline in the neck. Place your thumbs along each side of the trachea near the lower part of the neck. Assess whether the distance between the trachea's outer edge and the sternocleidomastoid muscle is equal on both sides.

Hard to swallow

To palpate the thyroid, stand behind the patient and put your hands around his neck, with the fingers of both hands over the lower trachea. Ask him to swallow as you feel the thyroid isthmus. The isthmus should rise with swallowing because it lies across the trachea, just below the cricoid cartilage.

Displace the thyroid to the right and then to the left, palpating both lobes for enlargement, nodules, tenderness, or a gritty sensation. (See *A close look at the thyroid gland*, page 140.) Lowering the patient's chin slightly and turning toward the side you're palpating helps relax the muscle and may facilitate assessment.

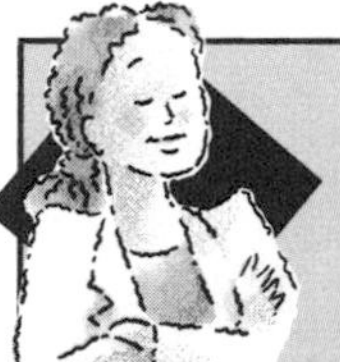

Peak technique

Locating lymph nodes

This illustration shows the location of the lymph nodes in the head and neck.

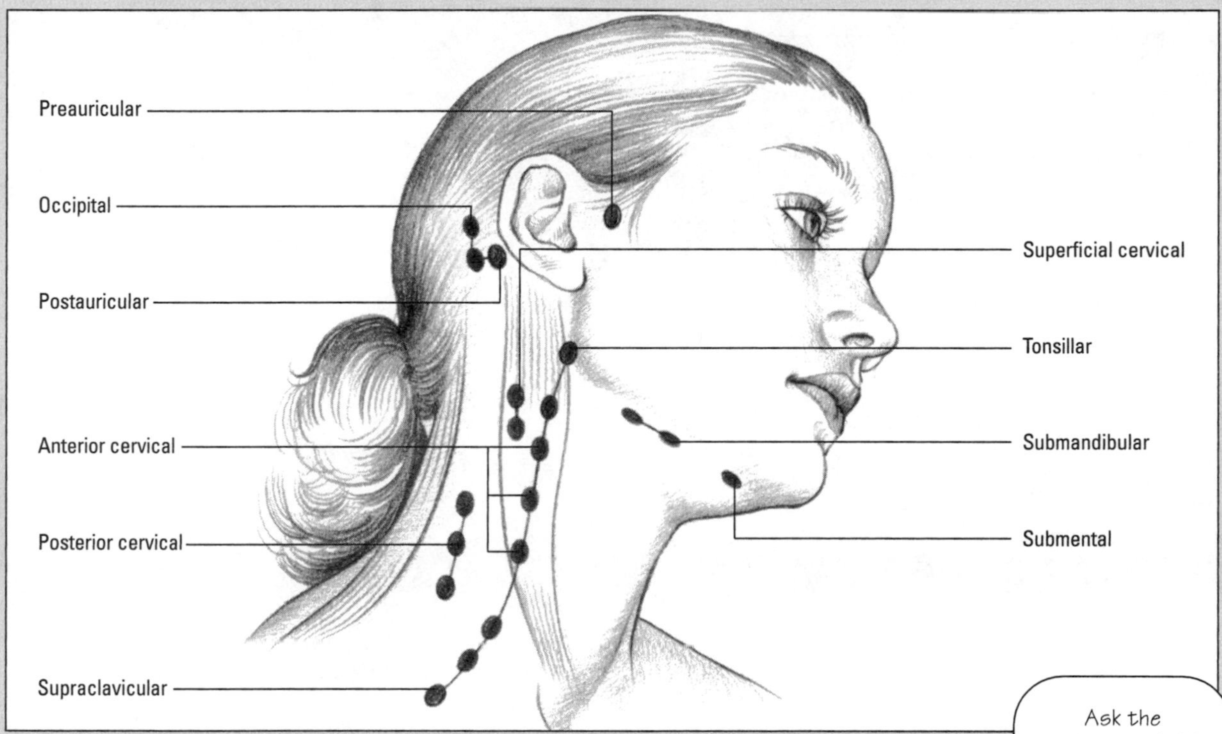
Preauricular
Occipital
Postauricular
Anterior cervical
Posterior cervical
Supraclavicular
Superficial cervical
Tonsillar
Submandibular
Submental

Auscultating the neck

Finally, auscultate the neck. Using light pressure on the bell of the stethoscope, listen over the carotid arteries. Ask the patient to hold his breath while you listen to prevent breath sounds from interfering with the sounds of circulation. Listen for bruits, which signal turbulent blood flow.

If you detect an enlarged thyroid gland, also auscultate the thyroid area with the bell. Check for a bruit or a soft rushing sound, which indicates a hypermetabolic state.

Ask the patient to hold his breath while you auscultate the neck.

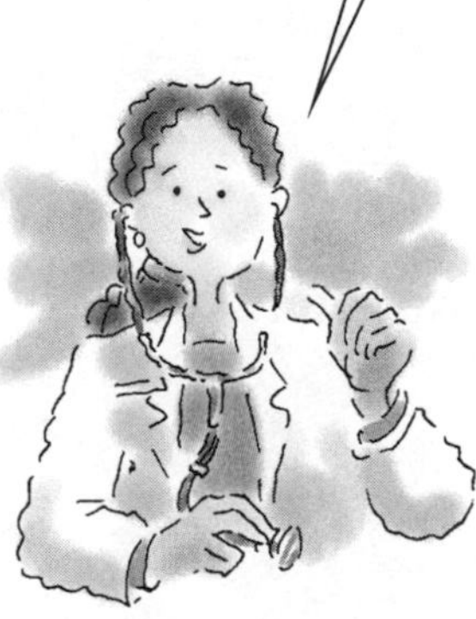

A close look at the thyroid gland

This illustration shows the structure and location of the thyroid gland.

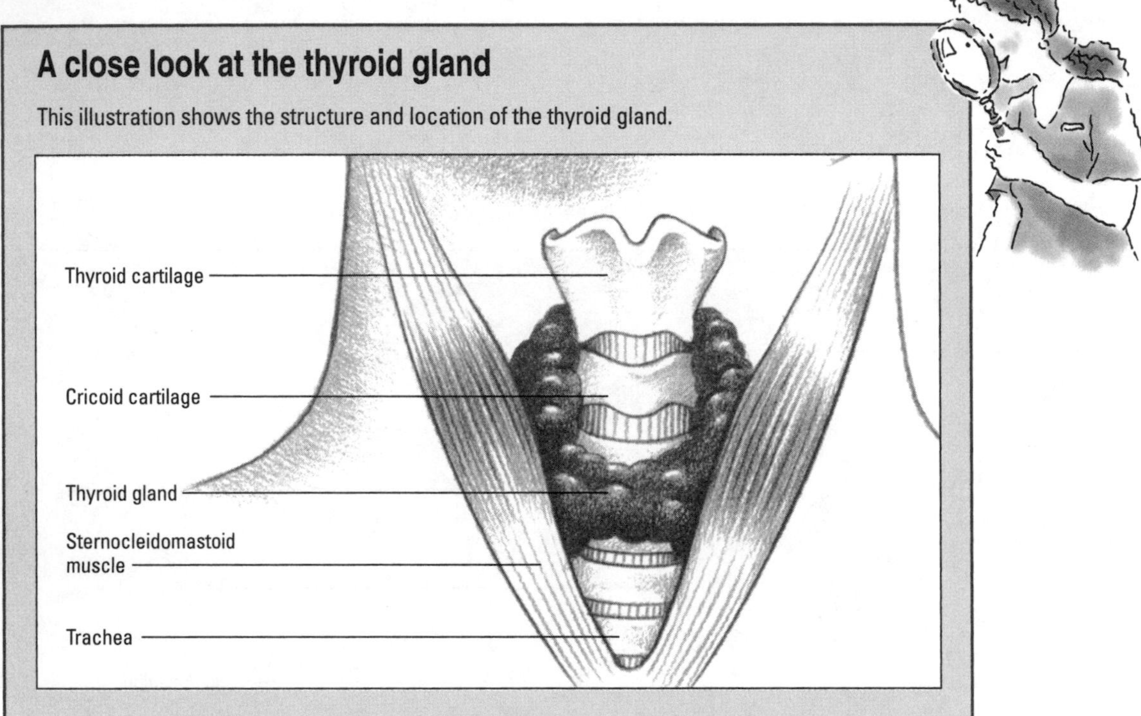

Abnormal findings

As you conclude your assessment, you'll need to record your findings and evaluate any abnormalities. (See *Ear, nose, and throat abnormalities.*)

Ear abnormalities

Common abnormalities you may find during an ear assessment include earache, hearing loss, and otorrhea.

Earache

Earaches usually result from disorders of the external and middle ear associated with infection, obstruction, or trauma.

An earful

Earaches range in severity from a feeling of fullness or blockage to deep, boring pain. At times, it may be difficult to determine the precise location of the earache. Earaches can be intermittent or continuous and may develop suddenly or gradually.

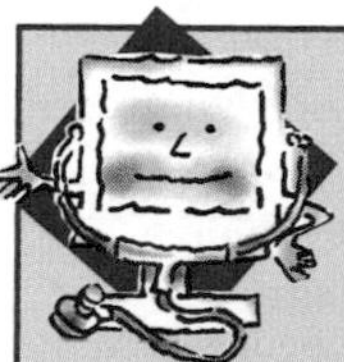

Interpretation station

Ear, nose, and throat abnormalities

The chart below shows common groups of findings for the signs and symptoms of the ear, nose, and throat, along with their probable causes.

Sign or symptom and findings	Probable cause
Dysphagia	
• Signs of respiratory distress, such as crowing and stridor • Phase 2 dysphagia with gagging and dysphonia	Airway obstruction
• Phase 2 and 3 dysphagia • Rapid weight loss • Steady chest pain • Cough with hemoptysis • Hoarseness • Sore throat • Hiccups	Esophageal cancer
• Painless, progressive dysphagia • Lead line on the gums • Metallic taste • Papilledema • Ocular palsy • Footdrop or wristdrop • Mental impairment or seizures	Lead poisoning
Earache	
• Sensation of blockage or fullness in the ear • Itching • Partial hearing loss • Possible dizziness	Cerumen impaction
***Earache** (continued)*	
• Mild to moderate ear pain that occurs with tragus manipulation • Low-grade fever • Sticky yellow or purulent ear discharge • Partial hearing loss • Feeling of blockage in the ear • Swelling of the tragus, external meatus, and external canal • Lymphadenopathy	Otitis externa
• Severe, deep throbbing pain • Hearing loss • High fever • Bulging, fiery red eardrum	Acute otitis media
Epistaxis	
• Ecchymoses • Petechiae • Bleeding from gums, mouth, and I.V. puncture sites • Menorrhagia • Signs of GI bleeding, such as melena and hematemesis	Coagulation disorders
• Unilateral or bilateral epistaxis • Nasal swelling • Periorbital ecchymoses and edema • Pain • Nasal deformity • Crepitation of the nasal bones	Nasal fracture

(continued)

Ear, nose, and throat abnormalities *(continued)*

Sign or symptom and findings	Probable cause
Epistaxis *(continued)*	
• Oozing epistaxis • Dry cough • Abrupt onset of chills and high fever • "Rose-spot" rash • Vomiting • Profound fatigue • Anorexia	Typhoid fever
Nasal obstruction	
• Watery nasal discharge • Sneezing • Temporary loss of smell and taste • Sore throat • Malaise • Arthralgia • Mild headache	Common cold
• Anosmia • Clear, watery nasal discharge • History of allergies, chronic sinusitis, trauma, cystic fibrosis, or asthma • Translucent, pear-shaped polyps that are unilateral or bilateral	Nasal polyps
• Thick, purulent drainage • Severe pain over the sinuses • Fever • Inflamed nasal mucosa with purulent mucus	Sinusitis
Throat pain	
• Throat pain that occurs seasonally or year-round • Nasal congestion with a thin nasal discharge and postnasal drip • Paroxysmal sneezing • Decreased sense of smell • Frontal or temporal headache • Pale and glistening nasal mucosa with edematous nasal turbinates • Watery eyes	Allergic rhinitis
• Mild to severe hoarseness • Temporary loss of voice • Malaise • Low-grade fever • Dysphagia • Dry cough • Tender, enlarged cervical lymph nodes	Laryngitis
• Mild to severe sore throat • Pain may radiate to the ears • Dysphagia • Headache • Malaise • Fever with chills • Tender cervical lymphadenopathy	Tonsillitis, acute

Hearing loss

Several factors can interfere with the ear's ability to conduct sound waves. Cerumen, a foreign body, or a polyp may be obstructing the ear canal. Otitis media may have thickened the fluid in the middle ear, which interferes with the vibrations that transmit sound. Otosclerosis, a hardening of the bones in the middle ear, also interferes with the transmission of sound vibrations. Trauma can disrupt the middle ear's bony chain.

Hear today, gone tomorrow

Sensorineural hearing loss also has several causes. The most common cause is loss of hair cells in the organ of Corti. In elderly people, presbycusis, or progressive hearing loss, results from atrophy of the organ of Corti and the auditory nerve. Hearing loss can also result from trauma to the hair cells caused by loud noise or ototoxicity. (See *Hearing loss*.)

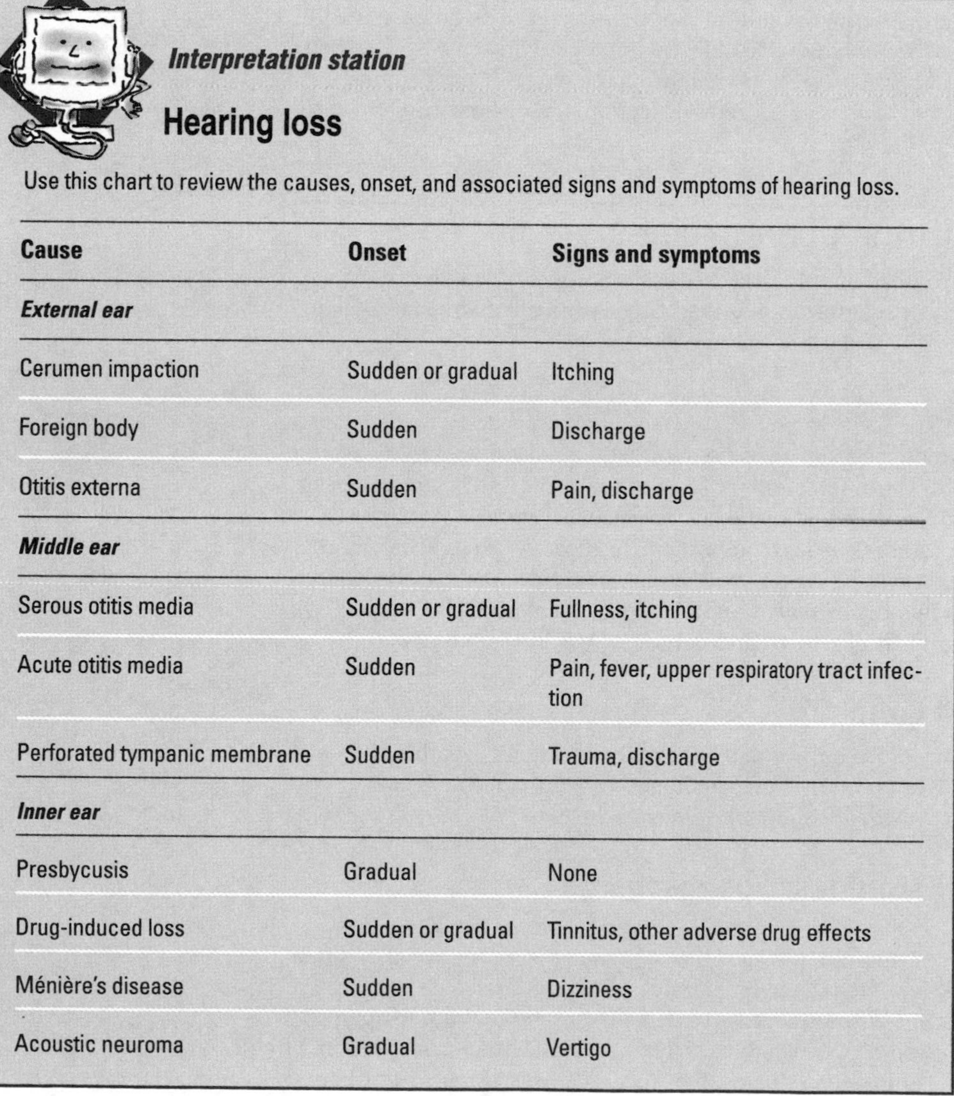

Interpretation station

Hearing loss

Use this chart to review the causes, onset, and associated signs and symptoms of hearing loss.

Cause	Onset	Signs and symptoms
External ear		
Cerumen impaction	Sudden or gradual	Itching
Foreign body	Sudden	Discharge
Otitis externa	Sudden	Pain, discharge
Middle ear		
Serous otitis media	Sudden or gradual	Fullness, itching
Acute otitis media	Sudden	Pain, fever, upper respiratory tract infection
Perforated tympanic membrane	Sudden	Trauma, discharge
Inner ear		
Presbycusis	Gradual	None
Drug-induced loss	Sudden or gradual	Tinnitus, other adverse drug effects
Ménière's disease	Sudden	Dizziness
Acoustic neuroma	Gradual	Vertigo

Now hear this!

A toxic reaction to a drug can cause a rapid loss of hearing. If hearing loss is detected, the medication must be discontinued immediately. Drugs that may affect hearing include aspirin, aminoglycosides, loop diuretics, and several chemotherapeutic agents, including cisplatin.

Such drugs as aspirin, aminoglycosides, loop diuretics, and certain chemotherapeutic agents may cause rapid hearing loss.

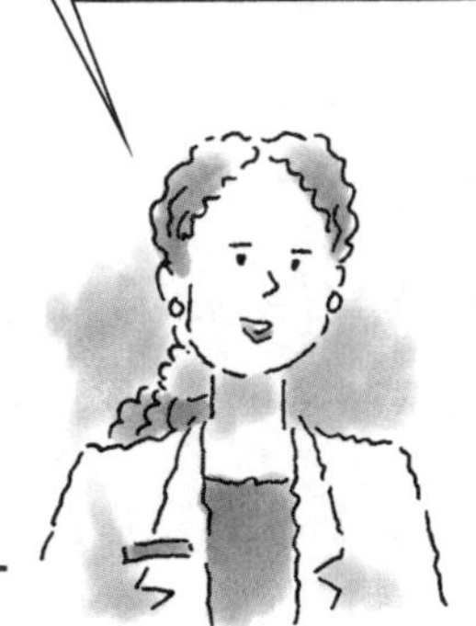

Otorrhea

Otorrhea—or drainage from the ear—may be bloody (otorrhagia), purulent, clear, or serosanguineous. Otorrhea may occur alone or with other symptoms such as ear pain. Its onset, duration, and severity provide clues to the underlying cause. Otorrhea may result from disorders that affect the external ear canal or the middle ear, including allergies, infection, neoplasms, trauma, and collagen disease.

Nose, mouth, and throat abnormalities

During a nose, mouth, and throat assessment, you may detect epistaxis, nasal flaring, nasal stuffiness and discharge, nasal pain, pharyngitis, and peritonsillar abscess.

Epistaxis

A common sign, epistaxis (nosebleed) can occur spontaneously or be induced from the front or back of the nose. A rich supply of fragile blood vessels makes the nose particularly vulnerable to bleeding. Dry, irritated mucous membranes bleed easily; they're also more susceptible to infection, which may trigger epistaxis. Additional causes include trauma; septal deviation; hematologic, coagulation, renal, and GI disorders; and certain drugs and treatments.

Nasal flaring

Some nasal flaring normally occurs during quiet breathing in adults and children. However, marked, regular nasal flaring in an adult may signal respiratory distress.

Nasal stuffiness and discharge

Obstruction of the nasal mucous membranes along with a discharge of thin mucus can signal systemic disorders, nasal or sinus disorders such as a deviated septum, trauma such as a basilar skull or nasal fracture, excessive use of vasoconstricting nose drops or sprays, or allergies or exposure to irritants, such as dust, tobacco smoke, and fumes. Nasal drainage accompanied by sinus tenderness and fever suggests acute sinusitis, which usually involves the frontal or maxillary sinuses. Thick, white, yellow, or greenish drainage suggests an infection.

Take a closer look

Be sure to evaluate clear, thin drainage closely. It may simply indicate rhinitis, or it may be cerebrospinal fluid leaking from a basilar skull fracture or other defect.

Dysphagia

Dysphagia — difficulty swallowing — is the most common symptom of esophageal disorders. However, it may also result from oropharyngeal, respiratory, neurologic, and collagen disorders, or from the effects of toxins and treatments. Dysphagia increases the risk of choking and aspiration.

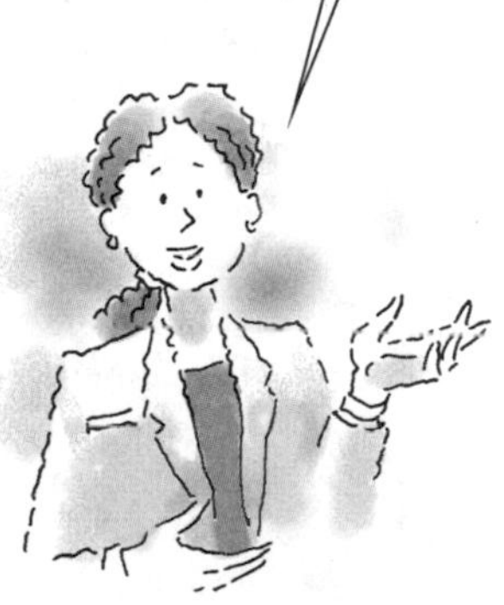

Throat pain

Commonly know as a *sore throat*, throat pain refers to discomfort in any part of the pharynx. This common symptom ranges from a sensation of scratchiness to severe pain. Throat pain may result from infection, trauma, allergy, cancer, or a systemic disorder. It may also follow surgery and endotracheal intubation. Additional causes include mouth breathing, alcohol consumption, inhaling smoke or chemicals such as ammonia, and vocal strain.

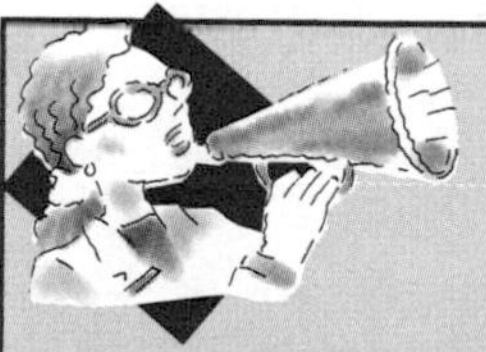

That's a wrap!

Ears, nose, and throat review

Health history

- Ask about common ear complaints, such as hearing loss, tinnitus, pain, and dizziness.
- Discuss past medical history, including allergies.
- Ask about common nose complaints, such as nasal stuffiness, nasal discharge, and nosebleed.
- Ask about colds, headaches, and sinus problems.
- Ask about common throat complaints, such as bleeding or sore gums, sore throat, and tooth problems.
- Ask the patient whether he smokes or uses other types of tobacco.
- Ask about neck problems, such as neck pain, swelling, or trouble moving the neck.

Ear

External ear

- Consists mainly of elastic cartilage.
- Collects sounds and transmits them to the middle ear.

Middle ear

- Separated from the external ear by the tympanic membrane
- Contains three small bones: the malleus, the incus, and the stapes
- Connects to the nasopharynx via the eustachian tube
- Transmits sound vibrations to the inner ear, protects the auditory apparatus, and equalizes air pressure on both sides of the tympanic membrane

(continued)

Ears, nose, and throat review *(continued)*

Inner ear

- Consists of closed, fluid-filled spaces
- Contains the vestibule and semicircular canals that help to maintain equilibrium, and the cochlea, the organ of hearing

Assessment

- Observe the ears for position and symmetry.
- Inspect the external ear for lesions, drainage, nodules, or redness.
- Inspect and palpate the mastoid area behind each auricle.
- Perform an otoscopic examination: examine the external canal, noting the presence and color of cerumen, and then advance the otoscope to view the tympanic membrane.
- Use Weber's test to evaluate a patient with diminished or lost hearing in one ear.
- Use the Rinne test to compare air conduction of sound with bone conduction of sound.

Abnormal findings

- Earache—severity ranges from a feeling of fullness or blockage to deep, boring pain
- Hearing loss—can be conductive or sensorineural
- Otorrhea—drainage from the ear

Nose

- Acts as sensory organ of smell
- Filters, warms, and humidifies inhaled air
- Linked internally to four pairs of paranasal sinuses: maxillary (on the cheeks below the eyes), frontal (above the eyebrows), and ethmoidal and sphenoidal (behind the eyes and nose)

Assessment

- Observe the nose for position, symmetry, and color. Note nasal flaring or discharge.
- Test nasal patency and the olfactory nerve (cranial nerve I) by having the patient obstruct one nostril and identify a smell with the other.
- Inspect the nasal cavity using the light from the otoscope, checking the vestibule, turbinates, and nostrils.
- Palpate the nose for pain, tenderness, swelling, and deformity.
- Examine the frontal and maxillary sinuses (the only sinuses that are accessible for examination).
- Check for swelling around the eyes.
- Palpate the sinuses. Use transillumination, if necessary, to help reveal obstructions and tumors.

Abnormal findings

- Epistaxis—nosebleed; a common sign
- Nasal flaring—may be a sign of respiratory distress
- Nasal stuffiness and discharge—obstruction of the nasal mucous membranes along with a discharge of thin mucus

Throat and neck

- Consists of nasopharynx, oropharynx, and laryngopharynx
- Contains cervical vertebrae, the major neck and shoulder muscles, and their ligaments
- Contains trachea, thyroid gland, and chains of lymph nodes

Assessment

- Inspect the lips.
- Use a tongue blade and a bright light to inspect the oral mucosa, gingivae, gums, and teeth.
- Inspect the tongue and note the patient's ability to move it in all directions. Also inspect underneath the tongue.
- Inspect and palpate the neck.
- Assess lymph nodes.
- Palpate the trachea and thyroid gland.
- Auscultate the neck by listening over the carotid arteries and over the thyroid gland (if it's enlarged).

Abnormal findings

- Dysphagia—difficulty swallowing
- Throat pain—discomfort in any part of the pharynx; may range from a scratchy sensation to severe pain

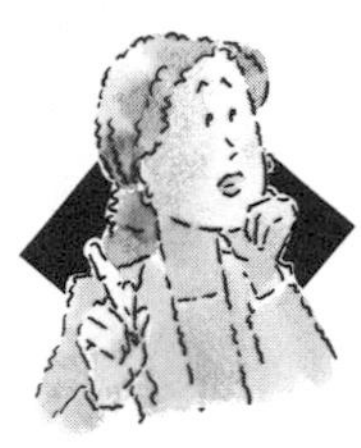

Quick quiz

1. Before inserting the otoscope into a patient's ear, the nurse should palpate the:
- A. helix.
- B. earlobe.
- C. lymph nodes.
- D. tragus.

Answer: D. Before inserting the otoscope, palpate the tragus to make sure it isn't tender. A tender tragus signals otitis externa.

2. During an otoscopic examination, the nurse should pull the superior posterior auricle of an adult patient's ear:
- A. up and back.
- B. up and forward.
- C. down and back.
- D. straight back.

Answer: A. In the adult patient, the superior posterior auricle should be pulled up and back to straighten the ear canal.

3. To assess the frontal sinuses, the nurse should palpate:
- A. the forehead.
- B. below the cheekbones.
- C. over the temporal areas.
- D. below the ears.

Answer: A. The frontal sinuses are located in the forehead, the site of palpation for those structures.

4. A cerumen impaction may contribute to a form of hearing loss called:
- A. central hearing loss.
- B. conductive hearing loss.
- C. sensorineural hearing loss.
- D. lateral hearing loss.

Answer: B. Conductive hearing loss occurs from abnormal function of the external or middle ear, resulting in impaired sound transmission.

5. The patient's ability to identify a particular aroma depends on proper functioning of cranial nerve:
- A. I.
- B. II.
- C. IV.
- D. VI.

Answer: A. Nasal patency and the olfactory nerve (cranial nerve I) are tested by having the patient identify an aroma.

6. Clear, thin nasal drainage may indicate:
A. infection.
B. cerebrospinal fluid leak.
C. epistaxis.
D. the presence of a foreign object.

Answer: B. Clear, thin nasal drainage may indicate a cerebrospinal fluid leak; therefore, you should evaluate this finding closely.

Scoring

☆☆☆ If you answered all six questions correctly, fantastic! We wouldn't blame you if you have a lump of pride in your throat.

☆☆ If you answered four or five questions correctly, way to go! We heard that you've been studying, and it must be true.

☆ If you answered fewer than four questions correctly, don't sniffle! Just set your eyes on the prize and move to the next chapter.

Respiratory system

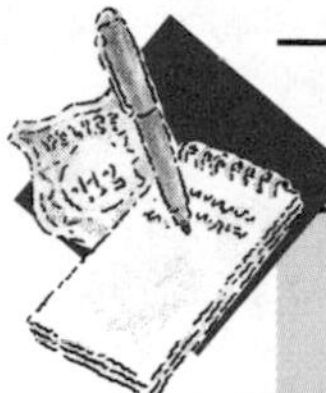

Just the facts

In this chapter, you'll learn:

- anatomy and physiology of the respiratory system
- methods for assessing the respiratory system
- abnormal respiratory system findings and their causes.

A look at the respiratory system

The respiratory system includes the airways, lungs, bony thorax, respiratory muscles, and central nervous system (CNS). (See *A close look at the respiratory system*, page 150.) They work together to deliver oxygen to the bloodstream and remove excess carbon dioxide from the body. Knowing the basic structures and functions of the respiratory system will help you perform a comprehensive respiratory assessment and recognize any abnormalities.

Airways and lungs

The airways are divided into the upper and lower airways. The upper airways include the nasopharynx (nose), oropharynx (mouth), laryngopharynx, and larynx. Their purpose is to warm, filter, and humidify inhaled air. They also help to make sound and send air to the lower airways.

Flapped for your protection

The epiglottis is a flap of tissue that closes over the top of the larynx when the patient swallows. The epiglottis protects the patient from aspirating food or fluid into the lower airways.

A close look at the respiratory system

The major structures of the upper and lower airways are illustrated below. The alveolus, or acinus, is shown in the inset.

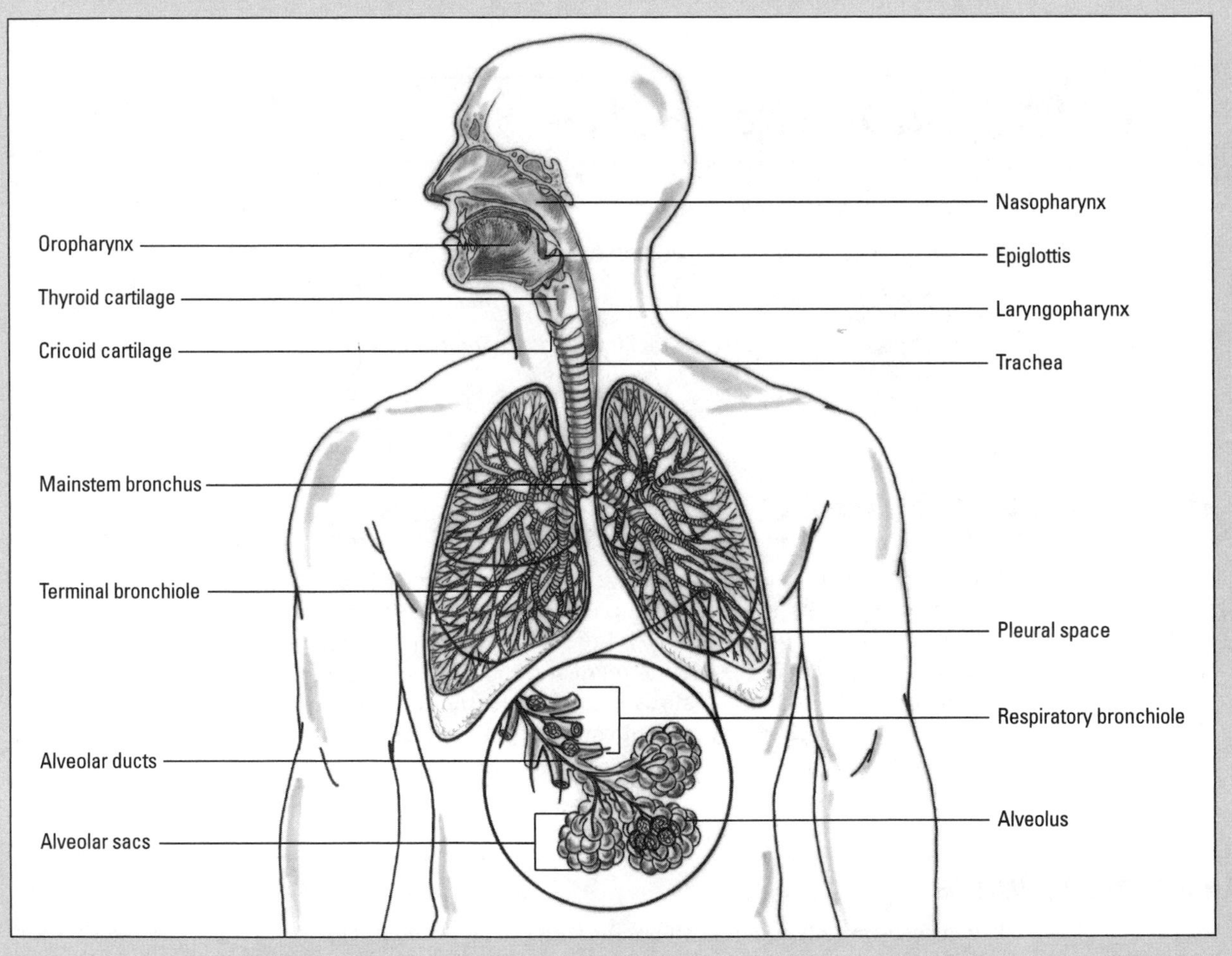

Vocal point

The larynx is located at the top of the trachea and houses the vocal cords. It's the transition point between the upper and lower airways.

The lowdown on the lower airways

The lower airways begin with the trachea, which then divides into the right and left mainstem bronchi. The mainstem bronchi divide into the lobar bronchi, which are lined with mucus-producing ciliated epithelium, one of the lungs' major defense systems.

The lobar bronchi then divide into secondary bronchi, tertiary bronchi, terminal bronchioles, respiratory bronchioles, alveolar ducts and, finally, into the alveoli, the gas-exchange units of the lungs. An adult's lungs typically contain about 300 million alveoli.

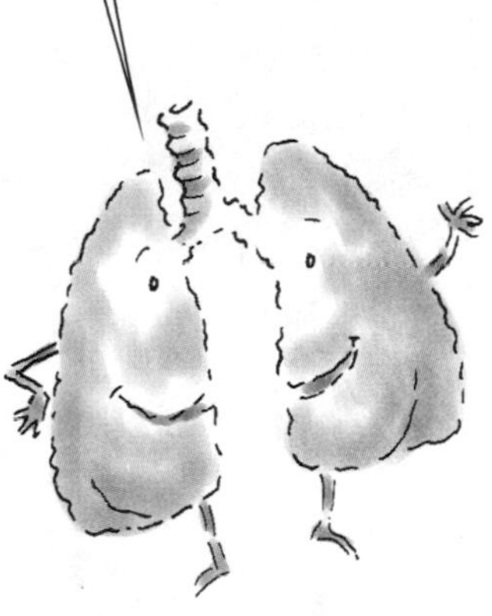

Lungs and lobes

Each lung is wrapped in a lining called the *visceral pleura.* The right lung is larger and has three lobes: upper, middle, and lower. The left lung is smaller and has only an upper and a lower lobe.

Smooth moves

The lungs share space in the thoracic cavity with the heart and great vessels, the trachea, the esophagus, and the bronchi. All areas of the thoracic cavity that come in contact with the lungs are lined with parietal pleura.

A small amount of fluid fills the area between the two layers of the pleura. This pleural fluid allows the layers to slide smoothly over each other as the chest expands and contracts. The parietal pleura also contain nerve endings that transmit pain signals when inflammation occurs.

Thorax

The bony thorax includes the clavicles, sternum, scapula, 12 sets of ribs, and 12 thoracic vertebrae. You can use specific parts of the thorax, along with some imaginary vertical lines drawn on the chest, to help describe the locations of your findings. (See *Respiratory assessment landmarks*, page 152.)

Rack of ribs

Ribs consist of bone and cartilage and allow the chest to expand and contract during each breath. All ribs attach to the thoracic vertebrae. The first seven ribs also attach directly to the sternum. The eighth, ninth, and tenth ribs attach to the cartilage of the preceding rib. The eleventh and twelfth ribs are called *floating ribs* because they don't attach to anything in the anterior thorax.

Respiratory muscles

The diaphragm and the external intercostal muscles are the primary muscles used in breathing. They contract when the patient inhales and relax when the patient exhales.

Respiratory assessment landmarks

The illustrations below show common landmarks used in respiratory assessment.

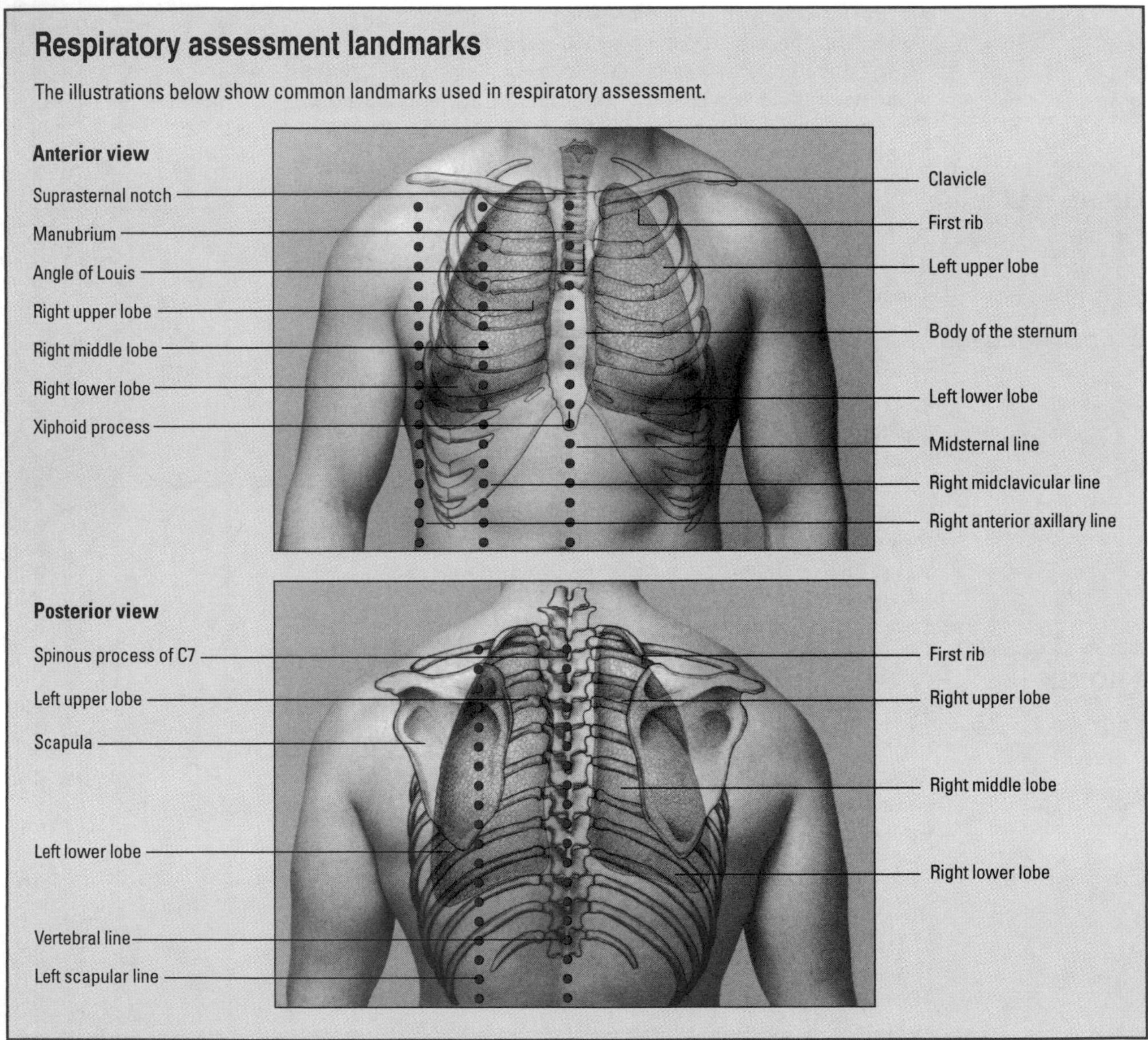

Message in a nerve

The respiratory center in the medulla initiates each breath by sending messages to the primary respiratory muscles over the phrenic nerve. Impulses from the phrenic nerve adjust the rate and depth of breathing, depending on the carbon dioxide and pH levels in the cerebrospinal fluid. (See *A close look at the mechanics of breathing.*)

A close look at the mechanics of breathing

These illustrations show how mechanical forces, such as the movement of the diaphragm and intercostal muscles, produce a breath. A plus sign (+) indicates positive pressure, and a minus sign (–) indicates negative pressure.

At rest

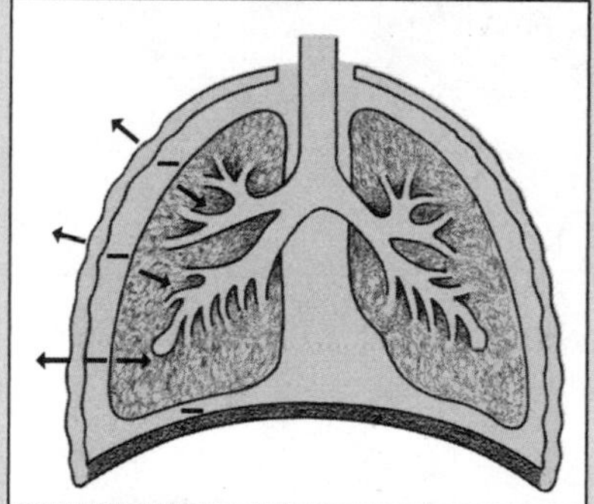

- Inspiratory muscles relax.
- Atmospheric pressure is maintained in the tracheobronchial tree.
- No air movement occurs.

Inhalation

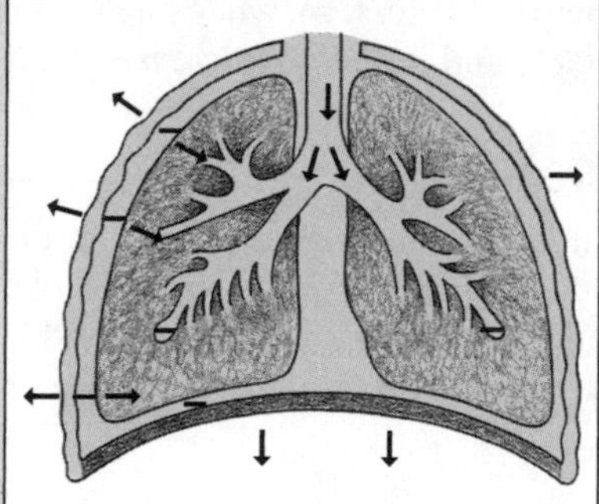

- Inspiratory muscles contract.
- The diaphragm descends and flattens.
- Negative alveolar pressure is maintained.
- Air moves into the lungs

Exhalation

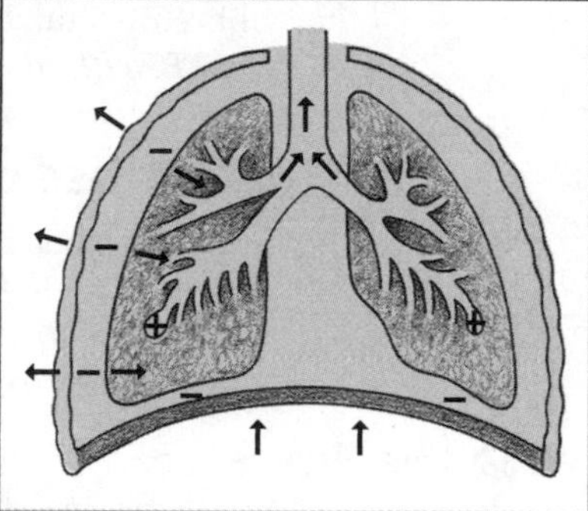

- Inspiratory muscles relax, causing lungs to recoil to their resting size and position.
- The diaphragm ascends, returning to its resting position.
- Positive alveolar pressure is maintained.
- Air moves out of the lungs

Accessory to breathing

Other muscles assist in breathing. Accessory inspiratory muscles include the trapezius, the sternocleidomastoid, and the scalenes, which combine to elevate the scapula, clavicle, sternum, and upper ribs. That elevation expands the front-to-back diameter of the chest when use of the diaphragm and intercostal muscles isn't effective.

Expiration occurs when the diaphragm and external intercostal muscles relax. If the patient has an airway obstruction, he may also use the abdominal muscles and internal intercostal muscles to exhale.

Obtaining a health history

When obtaining the health history of a patient with a respiratory disorder, first ask questions pertinent to the respiratory system.

Then broaden your assessment to include questions about other health issues.

Questions about the respiratory system

A patient with a respiratory disorder may complain of shortness of breath, cough, sputum production, wheezing, and chest pain. (See *Breathtaking facts* and *Listen and learn, then teach.*)

Shortness of breath

You can gain a history of the patient's shortness of breath by using several scales. Ask the patient to rate his usual level of dyspnea on a scale of 0 to 10, in which 0 means no dyspnea and 10 means the worst he has experienced. Then ask him to rate the level that day.

Making the grade

Other scales grade dyspnea as it relates to activity. In addition to using one of the severity scales, you might also ask these questions: What do you do to relieve the dyspnea? How well does it work? (See *Grading dyspnea.*)

Orthopnea

A patient with orthopnea (shortness of breath when lying down) tends to sleep with his upper body elevated.

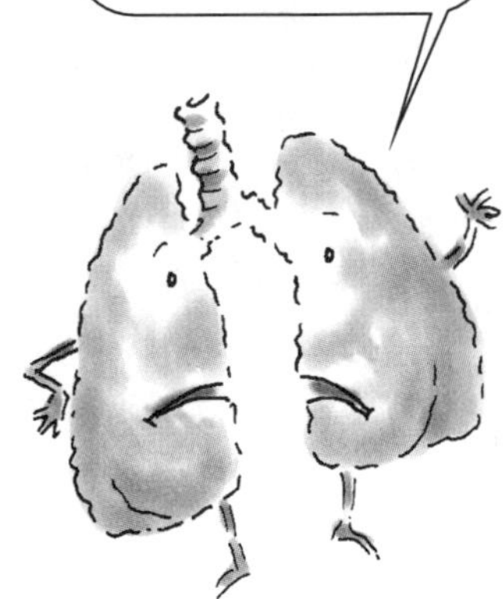

Breathtaking facts

Cough it up

Coughing clears unwanted material from the tracheobronchial tree. Sputum from the bronchial tubes traps foreign matter and protects the lungs from damage.

Pain sites

The lungs themselves don't contain pain receptors, but chest pain may be caused by inflammation of the pleura or the costochondral joints at the midclavicular line or at the edge of the sternum.

How much oxygen?

Patients with chronically high partial pressure of arterial carbon dioxide ($Paco_2$), such as those with chronic obstructive pulmonary disease or a neuromuscular disease, may be stimulated to breathe by a low oxygen level (the hypoxic drive) rather than by a slightly high $Paco_2$ level, which is normal. For such patients, supplemental oxygen therapy should be provided cautiously because it may depress the stimulus to breathe, further increasing $Paco_2$.

Listen and learn, *then* teach

Listening to what your patient says about his respiratory problems will help you know when he needs patient education. These typical responses indicate that the patient needs to know more about self-care techniques:

"Whenever I feel breathless, I just take a shot of my inhaler." This patient needs to know more about proper use of an inhaler and when to call the doctor.

"If I feel all congested, I just smoke a cigarette, and then I can cough up that phlegm!" This patient needs to know about the dangers of cigarette smoking.

"None of the other guys wear a mask when we're working." This patient needs to know the importance of wearing an appropriate safety mask when working around heavy dust and particles in the air, such as sawdust or powders.

Grading dyspnea

To assess dyspnea as objectively as possible, ask your patient to briefly describe how various activities affect his breathing. Then document his response using this grading system:

Grade 0: not troubled by breathlessness except with strenuous exercise

Grade 1: troubled by shortness of breath when hurrying on a level path or walking up a slight hill

Grade 2: walks more slowly on a level path than people of the same age because of breathlessness or has to stop to breathe when walking on a level path at his own pace

Grade 3: stops to breathe after walking about 100 yards (91 m) on a level path

Grade 4: too breathless to leave the house or breathless when dressing or undressing

Need a lift?

Ask the patient how many pillows he uses. The answer describes the severity of orthopnea. For instance, a patient who uses three pillows can be said to have "three-pillow orthopnea."

Cough

Ask the patient with a cough these questions: Is the cough productive? If the cough is a chronic problem, has it changed recently? If so, how? What makes the cough better? What makes it worse?

Sputum

When a patient produces sputum, ask him to estimate the amount produced in teaspoons or some other common measurement.

Now that you've brought it up...

Also ask him these questions: At what time of day do you cough most often? What's the color and consistency of the sputum? If sputum is a chronic problem, has it changed recently? If so, how? Do you cough up blood (hemoptysis)? If so, how much and how often?

Wheezing

If a patient wheezes, ask these questions: When does wheezing occur? What makes you wheeze? Do you wheeze loudly enough for others to hear it? What helps stop your wheezing?

Chest pain

If the patient has chest pain, ask him these questions: Where's the pain? What does it feel like? Is it sharp, stabbing, burning, or aching? Does it move to another area? How long does it last? What causes it to occur? What makes it better?

Chest pain associated with a respiratory problem usually results from pneumonia, pulmonary embolism, or pleural inflammation. Coughing or fractures can also cause musculoskeletal chest pain.

Questions about general health

Remember to look at the patient's medical and family history, being particularly watchful for a smoking habit, allergies, previous operations, and respiratory diseases, such as pneumonia and tuberculosis.

Also, ask about environmental exposure to irritants such as asbestos. People who work in mining, construction, or chemical manufacturing are commonly exposed to environmental irritants.

Assessing the respiratory system

Any patient can develop a respiratory disorder. By using a systematic assessment, you'll be able to detect subtle or obvious respiratory changes. The depth of your assessment will depend on several factors, including the patient's primary health problem and his risk of developing respiratory complications.

A physical examination of the respiratory system follows four steps: inspection, palpation, percussion, and auscultation. Before you begin, make sure the room is well lit and warm.

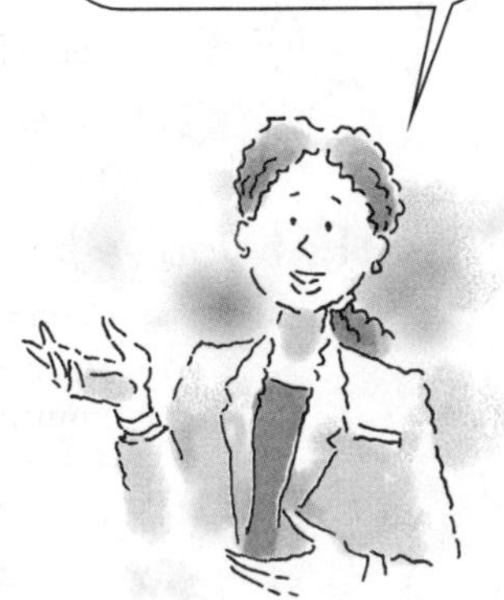

First impressions

Make a few observations about the patient as soon as you enter the room. Note how the patient is seated, which will most likely be the position most comfortable for him. Take note of his level of awareness and general appearance. Does he appear relaxed? Anxious? Uncomfortable? Is he having trouble breathing? You'll include these observations in your final assessment.

Inspecting the chest

Introduce yourself and explain why you're there. Help the patient into an upright position. The patient should be undressed from the waist up or clothed in an examination gown that allows you access to his chest.

Back, then front

Examine the back of the chest first, using inspection, palpation, percussion, and auscultation. Always compare one side with the other. Then examine the front of the chest using the same sequence. The patient can lie back when you examine the front of the chest if that's more comfortable for him.

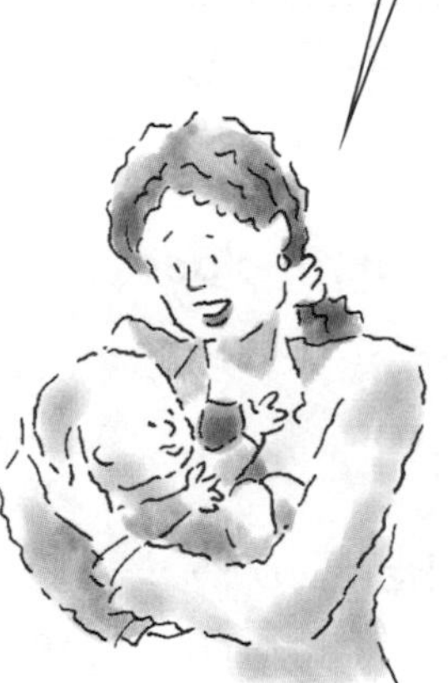

Beauty in symmetry

Note masses or scars that indicate trauma or surgery. Look for chest wall symmetry. Both sides of chest should be equal at rest and expand equally as the patient inhales. The diameter of the chest, from front to back, should be about half the width of the chest.

A new angle

Also, look at the angle between the ribs and the sternum at the point immediately above the xiphoid process. This angle—the costal angle—should be less than 90 degrees in an adult. The angle will be larger if the chest wall is chronically expanded because of an enlargement of the intercostal muscles, as can happen with chronic obstructive pulmonary disease (COPD).

Every breath you take

To find the patient's respiratory rate, count for a full minute—longer if you note abnormalities. Don't tell him what you're doing or he might alter his natural breathing pattern. One trick is to count respirations while the patient thinks you're taking his pulse or listening to his heart.

Adults normally breathe at a rate of 12 to 20 breaths/minute. An infant's breathing rate may reach about 40 breaths/minute. The respiratory pattern should be even, coordinated, and regular, with occasional sighs. The ratio of inspiration to expiration (I:E) is about 1:2. (See *Types of breathing*.)

> **Types of breathing**
>
> Men, children, and infants usually use abdominal, or diaphragmatic, breathing. Athletes and singers do as well. Most women, however, usually use chest, or intercostal, breathing.

Raising a red flag

Watch for paradoxical, or uneven, movement of the chest wall. Paradoxical movement may appear as an abnormal collapse of part of the chest wall when the patient inhales or an abnormal expansion when the patient exhales. In either case, this uneven movement indicates a loss of normal chest wall function.

Muscles in motion

When the patient inhales, his diaphragm should descend and the intercostal muscles should contract. This dual motion causes the abdomen to push out and the lower ribs to expand laterally. When the patient exhales, his abdomen and ribs return to their resting position. The upper chest shouldn't move much.

Helping more than they should

Accessory muscles may hypertrophy, indicating frequent use. Frequent use of accessory muscles may be normal in some athletes, but for other patients it indicates a respiratory problem, particularly when the patient purses his lips and flares his nostrils when breathing.

Inspecting related structures

Inspection of the skin, tongue, mouth, fingers, and nail beds also may provide information about respiratory status.

Colorful clues

Skin color varies considerably among patients, but in all cases patients with a bluish tint to their skin and mucous membranes are considered cyanotic. Cyanosis, which occurs when oxygenation to the tissues is poor, is a late sign of hypoxemia.

Blue is a great color for the eyes, but not the nail beds!

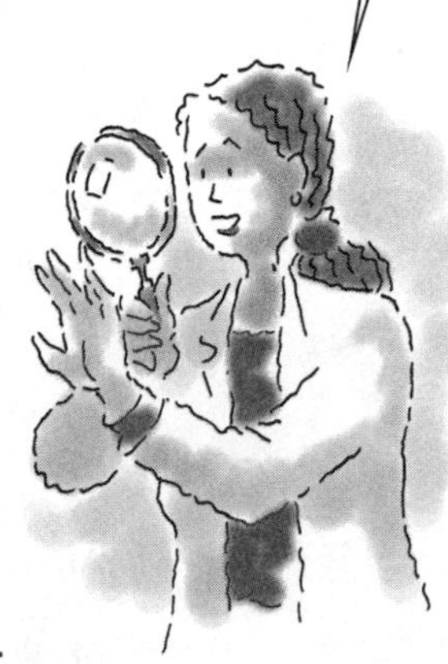

Where to look

The most reliable place to check for cyanosis is the tongue and mucous membranes of the mouth. A chilled patient may have cyanotic nail beds, nose, or ears, indicating low blood flow to those areas but not necessarily to major organs.

Join the club

When you check the fingers, look for clubbing, a possible sign of long-term hypoxia. A fingernail normally enters the skin at an angle of less than 180 degrees. When clubbing occurs, the angle is greater than or equal to 180 degrees.

Palpating the chest

Palpation of the chest provides important information about the respiratory system and the processes involved in breathing. (See *Palpating the chest.*)

Here's what to look for when palpating the chest.

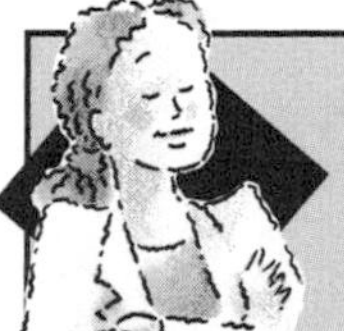

Peak technique

Palpating the chest

To palpate the chest, place the palm of your hand (or hands) lightly over the thorax, as shown. Palpate for tenderness, alignment, bulging, and retractions of the chest and intercostal spaces. Assess the patient for crepitus, especially around drainage sites. Repeat this procedure on the patient's back.

Next, use the pads of your fingers, as shown, to palpate the front and back of the thorax. Pass your fingers over the ribs and any scars, lumps, lesions, or ulcerations. Note the skin temperature, turgor, and moisture. Also note tenderness and bony or subcutaneous crepitus. The muscles should feel firm and smooth.

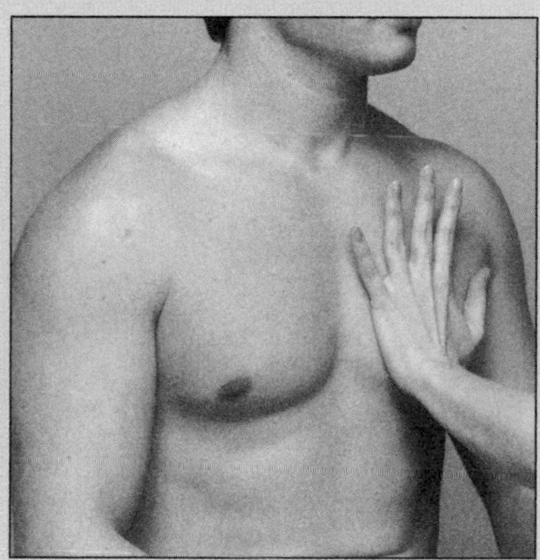

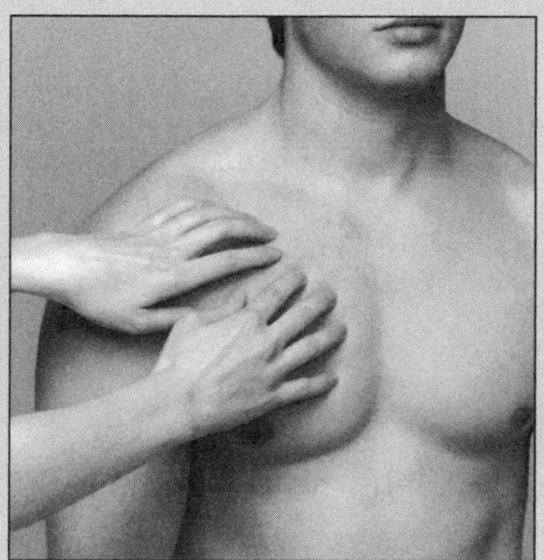

Snap, crackle, pop

The chest wall should feel smooth, warm, and dry. Crepitus indicates subcutaneous air in the chest, an abnormal condition. Crepitus feels like puffed-rice cereal crackling under the skin and indicates that air is leaking from the airways or lungs.

If a patient has a chest tube, you may find a small amount of subcutaneous air around the insertion site. If the patient has no chest tube or the area of crepitus is getting larger, alert the doctor immediately.

Tender touch

Gentle palpation shouldn't cause the patient pain. If the patient complains of chest pain, try to find a painful area on the chest wall. Painful costochondral joints are typically located at the midclavicular line or next to the sternum. Rib or vertebral fractures will be quite painful over the fracture, although pain may radiate around the chest as well. Pain may also be caused by sore muscles as a result of protracted coughing. A collapsed lung may also cause pain.

Vibratin' fremitus

Palpate for tactile fremitus, palpable vibrations caused by the transmission of air through the bronchopulmonary system. Fremitus is decreased over areas where pleural fluid collects, at times when the patient speaks softly, and within pneumothorax, atelectasis, and emphysema. Fremitus is increased normally over the large bronchial tubes and abnormally over areas in which alveoli are filled with fluid or exudate, as happens in pneumonia. (See *Checking for tactile fremitus.*)

Equal measure

To evaluate the patient's chest wall symmetry and expansion, place your hands on the front of the chest wall with your thumbs

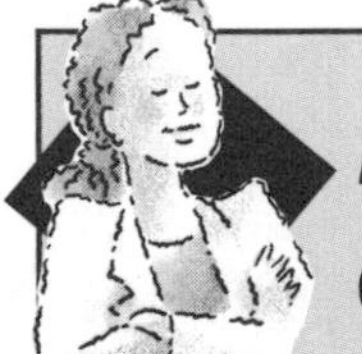

Peak technique

Checking for tactile fremitus

When you check the back of the thorax for tactile fremitus, ask the patient to fold his arms across his chest. This movement shifts the scapulae out of the way.

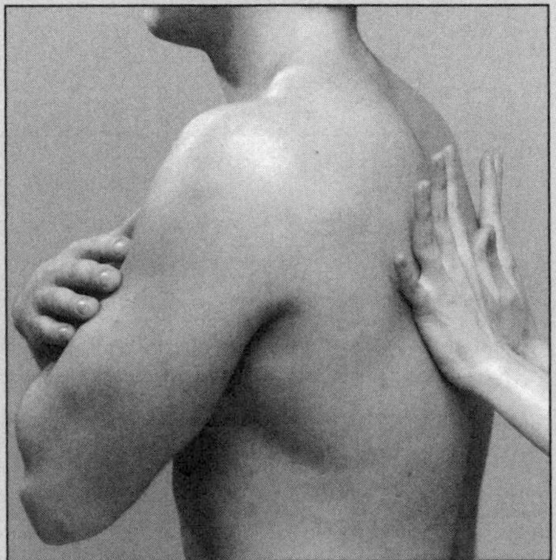

What to do

Check for tactile fremitus by lightly placing your open palms on both sides of the patient's back, as shown, without touching his back with your fingers. Ask the patient to repeat the phrase "ninety-nine" loud enough to produce palpable vibrations. Then palpate the front of the chest using the same hand positions.

What the results mean

Vibrations that feel more intense on one side than the other indicate tissue consolidation on that side. Less intense vibrations may indicate emphysema, pneumothorax, or pleural effusion. Faint or no vibrations in the upper posterior thorax may indicate bronchial obstruction or a fluid-filled pleural space.

touching each other at the second intercostal space. As the patient inhales deeply, watch your thumbs. They should separate simultaneously and equally to a distance several centimeters away from the sternum.

Repeat the measurement at the fifth intercostal space. The same measurement may be made on the back of the chest near the tenth rib.

There's no need for drums. The only percussion instruments you need in a respiratory assessment are your hands.

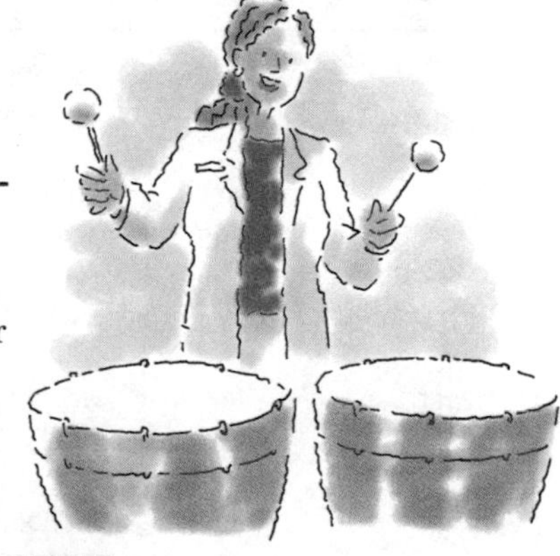

Warning signs

The patient's chest may expand asymmetrically if he has pleural effusion, atelectasis, pneumonia, or pneumothorax. Chest expansion may be decreased at the level of the diaphragm if the patient has emphysema, respiratory depression, diaphragm paralysis, atelectasis, obesity, or ascites.

Percussing the chest

You'll percuss the chest to find the boundaries of the lungs, to determine whether the lungs are filled with air or fluid or solid material, and to evaluate the distance the diaphragm travels between the patient's inhalation and exhalation. (See *Percussing the chest.*)

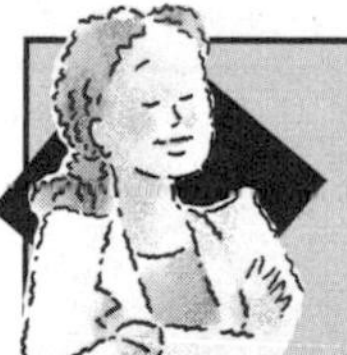

Peak technique

Percussing the chest

To percuss the chest, hyperextend the middle finger of your left hand if you're right-handed or the middle finger of your right hand if you're left-handed. Place your hand firmly on the patient's chest. Use the tip of the middle finger of your dominant hand—your right hand if you're right-handed, left hand if you're left-handed—to tap on the middle finger of your other hand just below the distal joint (as shown).

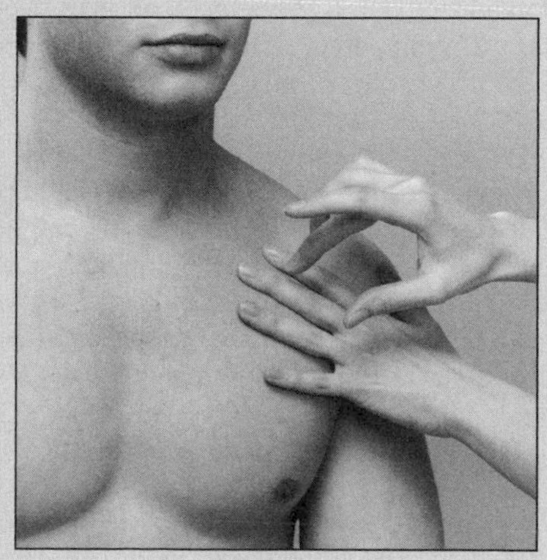

The movement should come from the wrist of your dominant hand, not your elbow or upper arm. Keep the fingernail you use for tapping short so you won't hurt yourself. Follow the standard percussion sequence over the front and back chest walls.

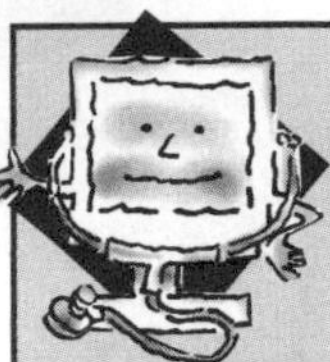

Interpretation station

Percussion sounds

Use this chart to help you become more comfortable with percussion and to interpret percussion sounds quickly. Learn the different percussion sounds by practicing on yourself, your patients, and other people willing to help.

Sound	Description	Clinical significance
Flat	Short, soft, high-pitched, extremely dull, found over the thigh	Consolidation, as in atelectasis and extensive pleural effusion
Dull	Medium in intensity and pitch, moderate length, thudlike, found over the liver	Solid area, as in lobar pneumonia
Resonant	Long, loud, low-pitched, hollow	Normal lung tissue; bronchitis
Hyperresonant	Very loud, lower-pitched, found over the stomach	Hyperinflated lung, as in emphysema or pneumothorax
Tympanic	Loud, high-pitched, moderate length, musical, drumlike, found over a puffed-out cheek	Air collection, as in a gastric air bubble, air in the intestines, or a large pneumothorax

Different sites, different sounds

Percussion allows you to assess structures as deep as 3″ (7.6 cm). You'll hear different percussion sounds in different areas of the chest. (See *Percussion sounds.*)

Tainted by treatments

You may also hear different sounds after certain treatments. For example, if your patient has atelectasis and you percuss his chest before chest physiotherapy, you'll hear a high-pitched, dull, soft sound. After physiotherapy, you should hear a low-pitched, hollow sound. In all cases, make sure you use other assessment techniques to confirm percussion findings. (*Double-check percussion findings.*)

Ringing with resonance

You'll hear resonant sounds over normal lung tissue, which you should find over most of the chest. In the left front chest from the third or fourth intercostal space at the sternum to the third or

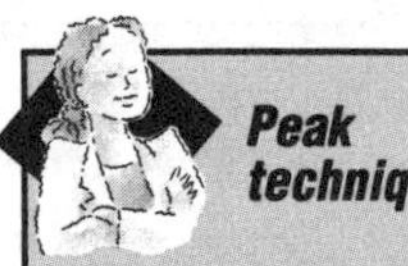

Peak technique

Double-check percussion findings

Use other assessment findings to verify the results of respiratory percussion. For example, if you hear low-pitched, loud, booming sounds when you percuss the chest of a patient with chronic obstructive pulmonary disease, an X-ray can be used to confirm emphysema.

Percussion sequences

Follow these percussion sequences to distinguish between normal and abnormal sounds in the patient's lungs. Remember to compare sound variations from one side with the other as you proceed. Carefully describe abnormal sounds you hear and include their locations. You'll follow the same sequences for auscultation.

Anterior

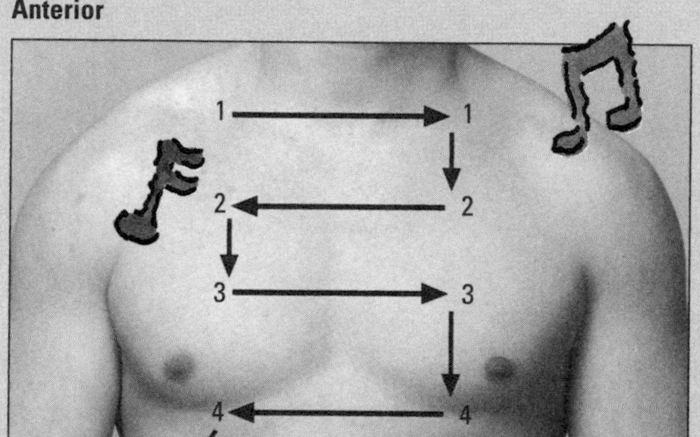

Posterior

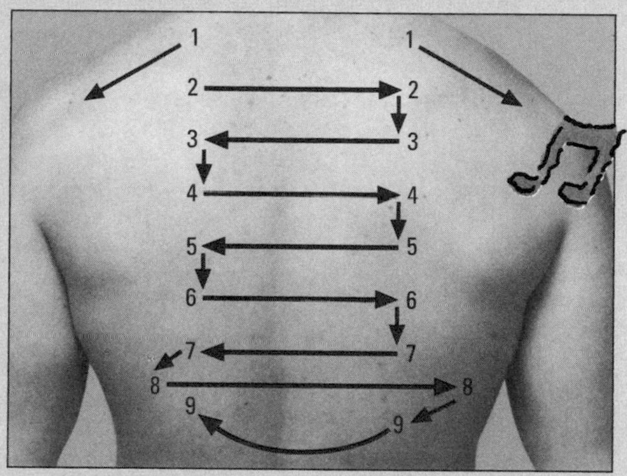

fourth intercostal space at the midclavicular line, you should hear a dull sound. Percussion is dull there because that's the space occupied by the heart. Resonance resumes at the sixth intercostal space. The sequence of sounds in the back is slightly different. (See *Percussion sequences*.)

Sounds serious

When you hear hyperresonance during percussion, it means you've found an area of increased air in the lung or pleural space. Expect hyperresonance with pneumothorax, acute asthma, bullous emphysema (large holes in the lungs from alveolar destruction), or gastric distention that pushes up on the diaphragm.

When you hear abnormal dullness, it means you've found areas of decreased air in the lungs. Expect abnormal dullness in the presence of pleural fluid, consolidation, atelectasis, or a tumor.

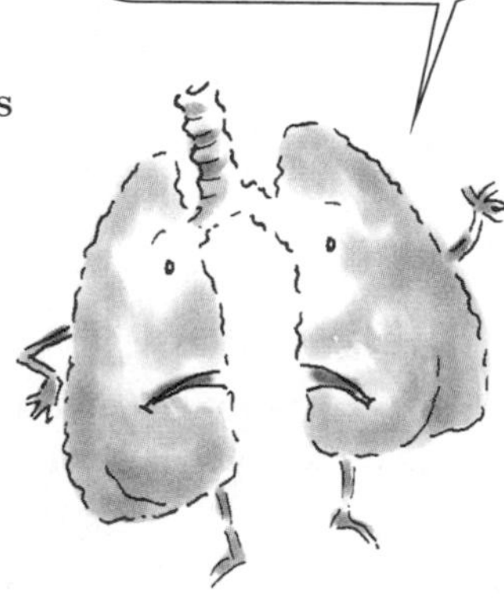

On the move

Percussion also allows you to assess how much the diaphragm moves during inspiration and expiration. The normal diaphragm descends 1¼″ to 2″ (3 to 5 cm) when the patient inhales. The diaphragm doesn't move as far in a patient with emphysema, respi-

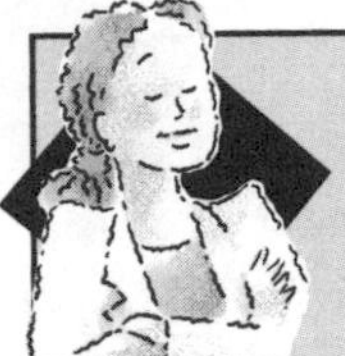

Peak technique

Measuring diaphragm movement

You can measure how much the diaphragm moves by asking the patient to exhale. Percuss the back on one side to locate the upper edge of the diaphragm, the point at which normal lung resonance changes to dullness. Use a pen to mark the spot indicating the position of the diaphragm at full expiration on that side of the back.

Then ask the patient to inhale as deeply as possible. Percuss the back when the patient has breathed in fully until you locate the diaphragm. Use the pen to mark this spot as well. Repeat on the opposite side of the back.

Measure

Use a ruler or tape measure to determine the distance between the marks. The distance, normally 1¼″ to 2″ (3 to 5 cm), should be equal on both the right and left sides.

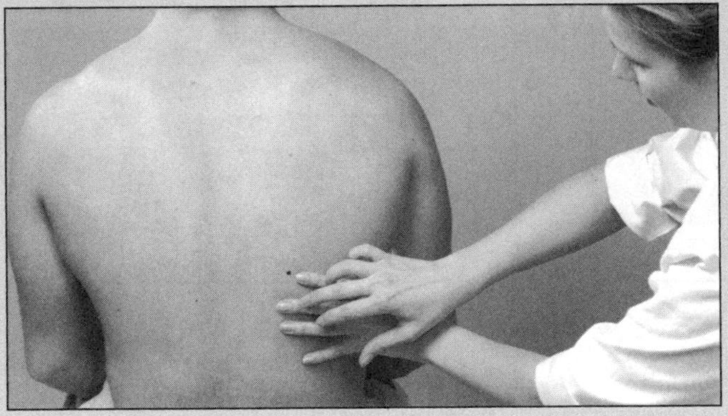

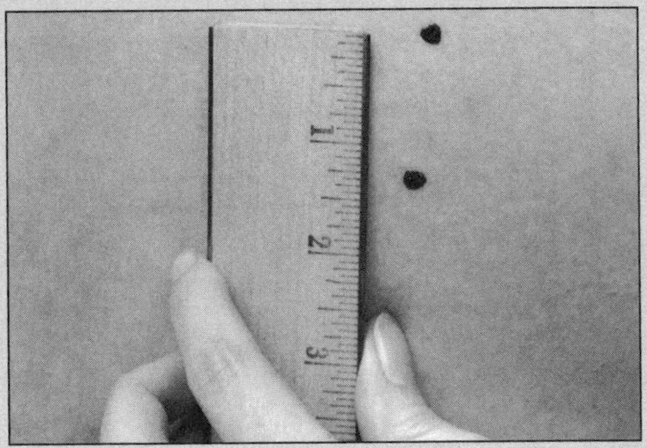

ratory depression, diaphragm paralysis, atelectasis, obesity, or ascites. (See *Measuring diaphragm movement.*)

When auscultating the chest, have the patient breathe through his mouth; nose breathing alters the pitch of breath sounds.

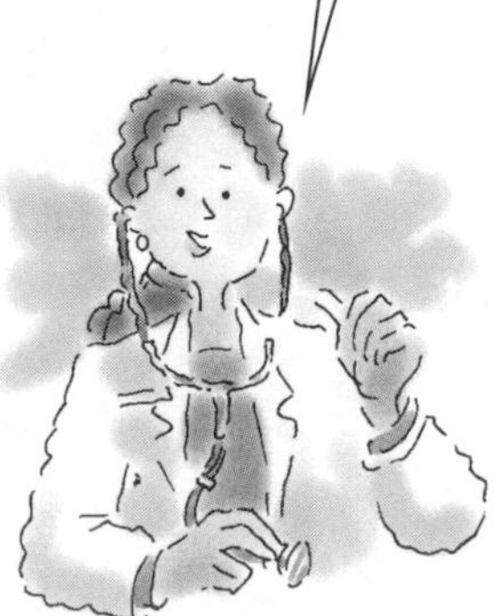

Auscultating the chest

As air moves through the bronchi, it creates sound waves that travel to the chest wall. The sounds produced by breathing change as air moves from larger airways to smaller airways. Sounds also change if they pass through fluid, mucus, or narrowed airways.

Auscultation of these sounds helps you to determine the condition of the alveoli and surrounding pleura.

Familiar sites

Auscultation sites are the same as percussion sites. Listen to a full inspiration and a full expiration at each site, using the diaphragm of the stethoscope. Ask the patient to breathe through his mouth;

nose breathing alters the pitch of breath sounds. If the patient has abundant chest hair, mat it down with a damp washcloth so the hair doesn't make sounds like crackles.

Be firm

To auscultate for breath sounds, you'll press the stethoscope firmly against the skin. Remember that if you listen through clothing or dry chest hair, you may hear unusual and deceptive sounds.

Sounds perfectly normal!

You'll hear four types of breath sounds over normal lungs:

- tracheal (heard when a patient inhales or exhales)
- bronchial (heard loudest when the patient exhales; discontinuous)
- bronchovesicular (heard when the patient inhales or exhales; continuous)
- vesicular (are prolonged during inhalation and shortened during exhalation).

(See *Qualities of normal breath sounds.*)

The type of sound you hear depends on where you listen. (See *Locations of normal breath sounds.*)

Qualities of normal breath sounds

Breath sound	Quality	Inspiration-expiration (I:E) ratio	Location
Tracheal	Harsh, high-pitched	I = E	Above supraclavicular notch
Bronchial	Loud, high-pitched	I < E	Just above clavicles on each side of the sternum, between scapulae, over the manubrium
Bronchovesicular	Medium in loudness and pitch	I = E	Next to sternum, between scapulae
Vesicular	Soft, low-pitched	I > E	Remainder of lungs

Locations of normal breath sounds

These photographs show the normal locations of different types of breath sounds.

Anterior thorax

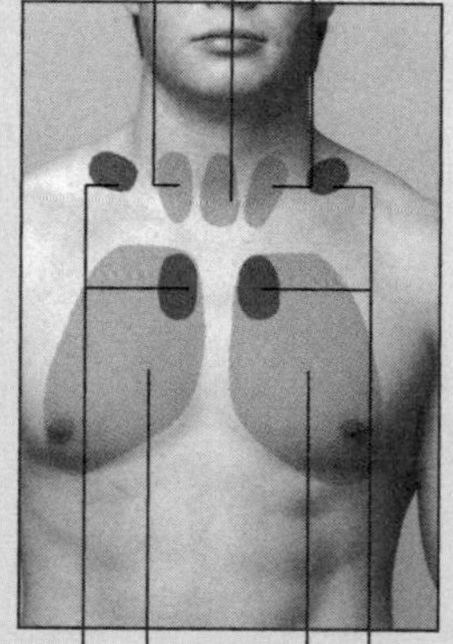

Posterior thorax

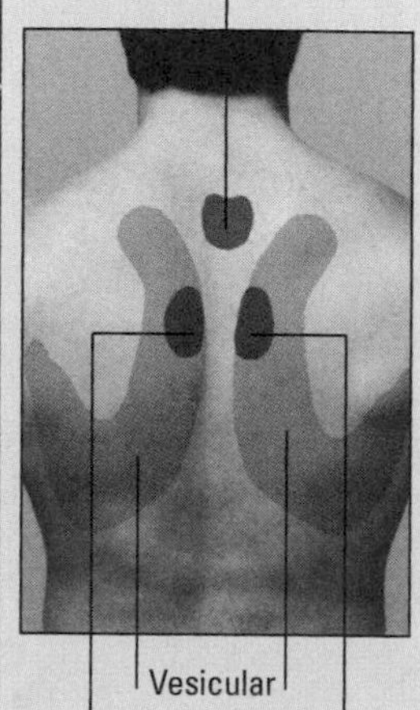

In a class by itself

Classify each sound according to its intensity, location, pitch, duration, and characteristic. Note whether the sound occurs when the patient inhales, exhales, or both.

Sounds of silence

If you hear diminished but normal breath sounds in both lungs, the patient may have emphysema, atelectasis, severe bronchospasm, or shallow breathing. If you hear breath sounds in one lung only, the patient may have pleural effusion, pneumothorax, a tumor, or mucus plugs in the airways. In such cases, the doctor may order pulmonary function tests (PFTs) to further assess the patient's condition. (See *PFT results*.)

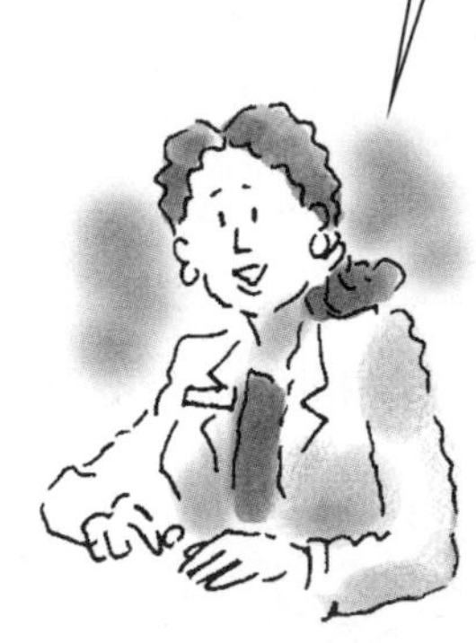

Voicing complaints

Also check the patient for vocal fremitus — voice sounds resulting from chest vibrations that occur as the patient speaks. Abnormal transmission of voice sounds — the most common of which are bronchophony, egophony, and whispered pectoriloquy — may occur over consolidated areas. (See *Assessing vocal fremitus*, page 168.)

Sound check

To test for bronchophony, ask the patient to say "ninety-nine" or "blue moon." Over normal lung tissue, the words sound muffled. Over consolidated areas, the words sound unusually loud. To test for egophony, ask the patient to say "E." Over normal lung tissue, the sound is muffled. Over consolidated lung tissue, it will sound like the letter *a*. To test for whispered pectoriloquy, ask the patient to whisper "1, 2, 3." Over normal lung tissue, the numbers will be almost indistinguishable. Over consolidated lung tissue, the numbers will be loud and clear.

The next step

A patient with abnormal findings during a respiratory assessment may be further evaluated using such diagnostic tests as arterial blood gas analysis and PFTs.

Abnormal findings

Your assessment of the chest may reveal several abnormalities of the chest wall and lungs. In this section, we'll look at chest-wall abnormalities, abnormal respiratory patterns, and abnormal breath sounds. (See *Respiratory abnormalities*, pages 169 and 170.)

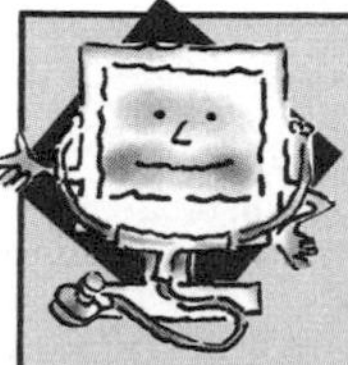

Interpretation station

PFT results

You may need to interpret results of pulmonary function tests (PFTs) in your assessment of a patient's respiratory status. Use the chart below as a guide to common PFTs.

Restrictive and obstructive

The chart mentions restrictive and obstructive defects. A restrictive defect is one in which a person can't inhale a normal amount of air. It may occur with chest-wall deformities, neuromuscular diseases, or acute respiratory tract infections.

An obstructive defect is one in which something obstructs the flow of air into or out of the lungs. It may occur with a disease such as asthma, chronic bronchitis, emphysema, or cystic fibrosis.

Test	Implications
Tidal volume (V_T): amount of air inhaled or exhaled during normal breathing	Decreased V_T may indicate restrictive disease and requires further tests, such as full pulmonary function studies or chest X-rays.
Minute volume (MV): amount of air breathed per minute	Normal MV can occur in emphysema. Decreased MV may indicate other abnormalities such as pulmonary edema.
Inspiratory reserve volume (IRV): amount of air inhaled after normal inspiration	Abnormal IRV alone doesn't indicate respiratory dysfunction. IRV decreases during normal exercise.
Expiratory reserve volume (ERV): amount of air that can be exhaled after normal expiration	ERV varies, even in healthy people.
Vital capacity (VC): amount of air that can be exhaled after maximum inspiration	Normal or increased VC with decreased flow rates may indicate reduction in functional pulmonary tissue. Decreased VC with normal or increased flow rates may indicate decreased respiratory effort, decreased thoracic expansion, or limited movement of the diaphragm.
Inspiratory capacity (IC): amount of air that can be inhaled after normal expiration	Decreased IC indicates restrictive disease.
Forced vital capacity (FVC): amount of air that can be exhaled after maximum inspiration	Decreased FVC indicates flow resistance in the respiratory system from obstructive disease, such as chronic bronchitis, emphysema, and asthma.
Forced expiratory volume (FEV): volume of air exhaled in the first (FEV_1), second (FEV_2), or third (FEV_3) FVC maneuver	Decreased FEV_1 and increased FEV_2 and FEV_3 may indicate obstructive disease. Decreased or normal FEV_1 may indicate restrictive disease.

Assessing vocal fremitus

To assess for vocal fremitus, ask the patient to repeat the words below while you listen. Auscultate over an area where you heard abnormally located bronchial breath sounds to check for abnormal voice sounds.

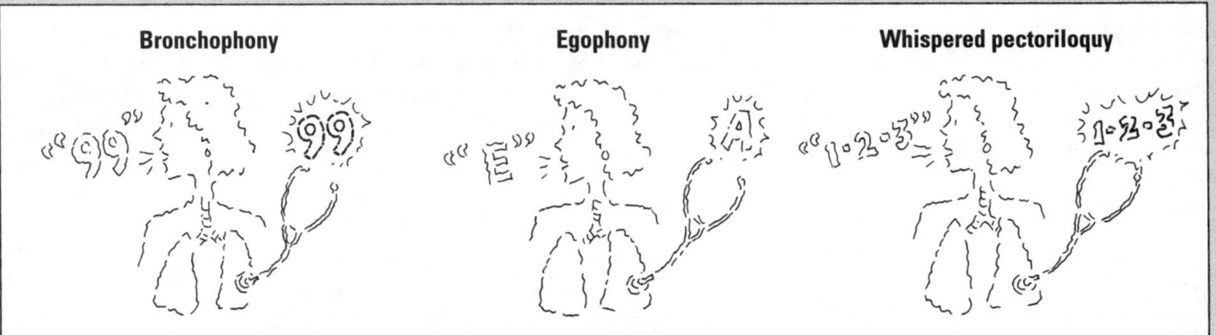

Chest-wall abnormalities

Chest-wall abnormalities may be congenital or acquired. As you examine a patient for chest-wall abnormalities, keep in mind that a patient with a deformity of the chest wall might have completely normal lungs and that the lungs might be cramped within the chest. The patient might have a smaller-than-normal lung capacity and limited exercise tolerance, and he may more easily develop respiratory failure from a respiratory tract infection. (See *Chest deformities*, page 171.)

I may be normal, but a chest-wall abnormality may affect how I work.

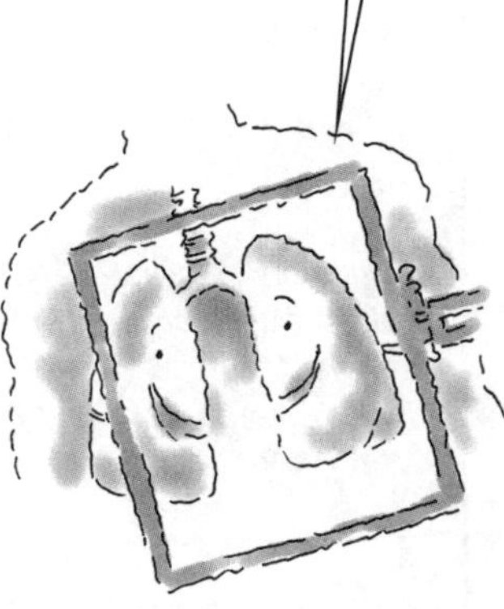

Barrel chest

A barrel chest looks like its name implies: The chest is abnormally round and bulging, with a greater-than-normal front-to-back diameter. Barrel chest may be normal in infants and elderly patients. In other patients, barrel chest occurs as a result of COPD.

Calling for backup

In patients with COPD, barrel chest indicates that the lungs have lost their elasticity and that the diaphragm is flattened. You'll note that this patient typically uses accessory muscles when he inhales and easily becomes breathless. You'll also note kyphosis of the thoracic spine, ribs that run horizontally rather than tangentially, and a prominent sternal angle.

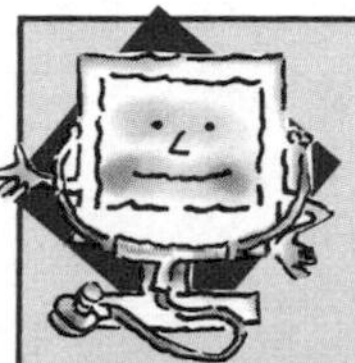

Interpretation station

Respiratory abnormalities

The chart below shows common respiratory complaints, their accompanying signs and symptoms, and their probable causes.

Sign or symptom and findings	Probable cause
Cough	
• Nonproductive cough • Pleuritic chest pain • Dyspnea • Tachypnea • Anxiety • Decreased vocal fremitus • Tracheal deviation toward the affected side	Atelectasis
• Productive cough with small amounts of purulent (or mucopurulent), blood-streaked sputum or large amounts of frothy sputum • Dyspnea • Anorexia • Fatigue • Weight loss • Wheezing • Clubbing	Lung cancer
• Nonproductive cough • Dyspnea • Pleuritic chest pain • Decreased chest motion • Pleural friction rub • Tachypnea • Tachycardia • Flatness on percussion • Egophony	Pleural effusion

Sign or symptom and findings	Probable cause
Dyspnea	
• Acute dyspnea • Tachypnea • Crackles and rhonchi in both lung fields • Intercostal and suprasternal retractions • Restlessness • Anxiety • Tachycardia	Acute respiratory distress syndrome
• Progressive exertional dyspnea • A history of smoking • Barrel chest • Accessory muscle hypertrophy • Diminished breath sounds • Pursed-lip breathing • Prolonged expiration • Anorexia • Weight loss	Emphysema
• Acute dyspnea • Pleuritic chest pain • Tachycardia • Decreased breath sounds • Low-grade fever • Dullness on percussion • Cool, clammy skin	Pulmonary embolism

(continued)

Respiratory abnormalities *(continued)*

Sign or symptom and findings	Probable cause
Hemoptysis	
• Sputum ranging in color from pink to dark brown • Productive cough • Dyspnea • Chest pain • Crackles on auscultation • Chills • Fever	Pneumonia
• Frothy, blood-tinged, pink sputum • Severe dyspnea • Orthopnea • Gasping • Diffuse crackles • Cold, clammy skin • Anxiety	Pulmonary edema
• Blood-streaked or blood-tinged sputum • Chronic productive cough • Fine crackles after coughing • Dyspnea • Dullness to percussion • Increased tactile fremitus	Pulmonary tuberculosis
Wheezing	
• Sudden onset of wheezing • Stridor • Dry, paroxysmal cough • Gagging • Hoarseness • Decreased breath sounds • Dyspnea • Cyanosis	Aspiration of a foreign body
• Audible wheezing on expiration • Prolonged expiration • Apprehension • Intercostal and supraclavicular retractions • Rhonchi • Nasal flaring • Tachypnea	Asthma
• Wheezing • Coarse crackles • Hacking cough that later becomes productive • Dyspnea • Barrel chest • Clubbing • Edema • Weight gain	Chronic bronchitis

Pigeon chest

A patient with pigeon chest, or pectus carinatum, has a chest with a sternum that protrudes beyond the front of the abdomen. The displaced sternum increases the front-to-back diameter of the chest.

Funnel chest

A patient with funnel chest, or pectus excavatum, has a funnel-shaped depression on all or part of the sternum. The shape of the

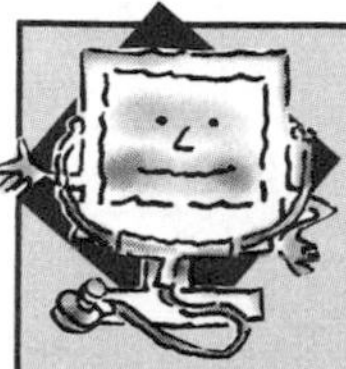

Interpretation station

Chest deformities

As you inspect the patient's chest, note deviations in size and shape. The illustrations here show a normal adult chest and four common chest deformities.

Normal adult chest

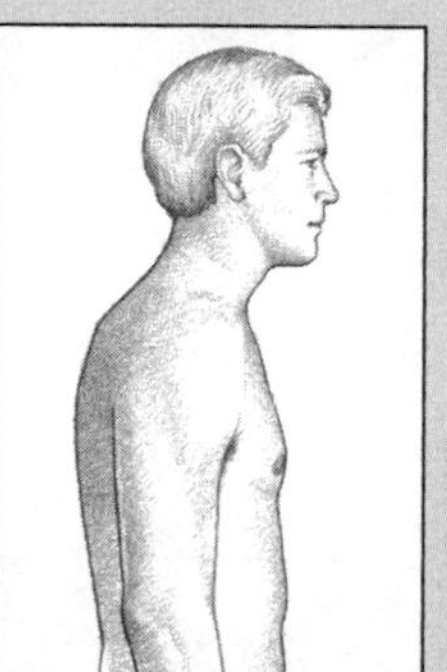

Barrel chest

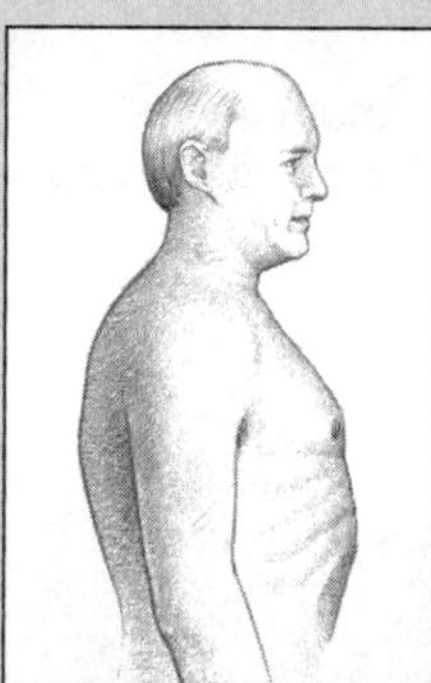

Increased anteroposterior diameter

Funnel chest

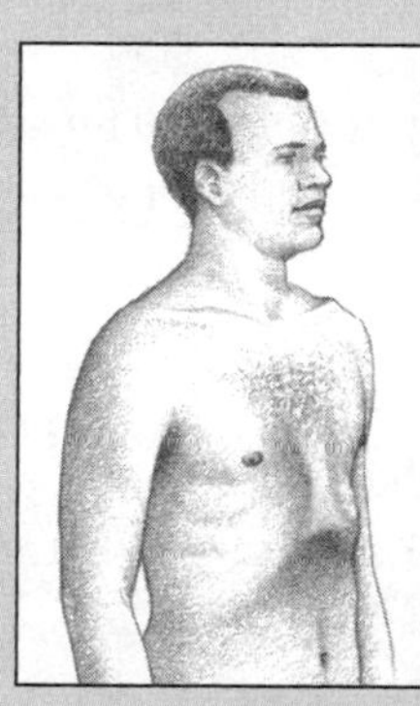

Depressed lower sternum

Pigeon chest

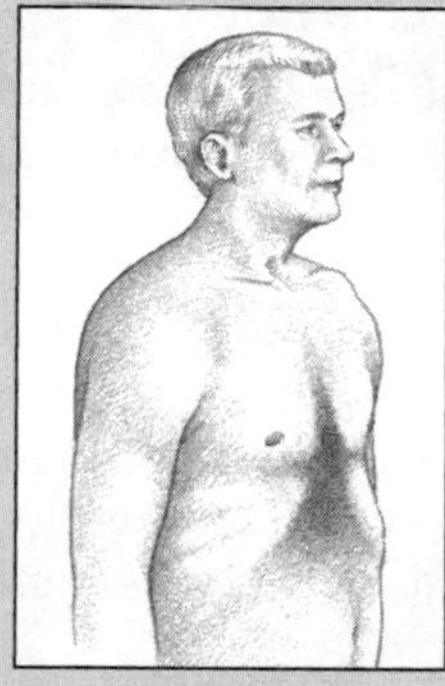

Anteriorly displaced sternum

Thoracic kyphoscoliosis

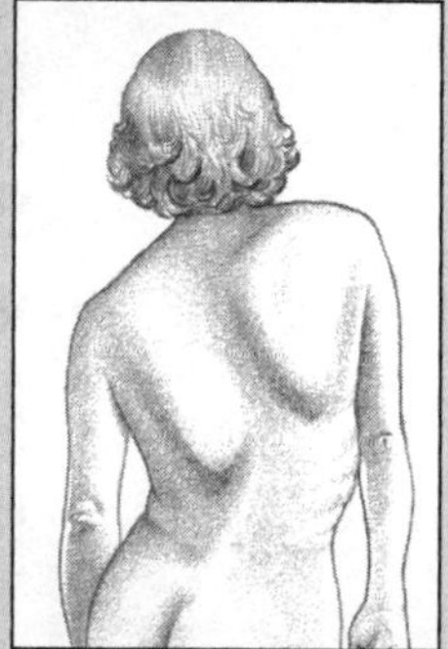

Raised shoulder and scapula, thoracic convexity, and flared interspaces

chest may interfere with respiratory and cardiac function. Compression of the heart and great vessels may cause murmurs.

Thoracic kyphoscoliosis

In thoracic kyphoscoliosis, the patient's spine curves to one side and the vertebrae are rotated. Because the rotation distorts lung tissues, it may be more difficult to assess respiratory status.

Abnormal respiratory patterns

Identifying abnormal respiratory patterns can help you assess more completely a patient's respiratory status and his overall condition. (See *Abnormal respiratory patterns*, page 173.)

Tachypnea

Tachypnea is a respiratory rate greater than 20 breaths/minute with shallow breathing. It's commonly seen in patients with restrictive lung disease, pain, sepsis, obesity, and anxiety.

Hot and bothered

Fever may be another cause of tachypnea. The respiratory rate may increase by 4 breaths/minute for every 1° F (0.6° C) rise in body temperature.

Bradypnea

Bradypnea is a respiratory rate below 10 breaths/minute and is typically noted just before a period of apnea or full respiratory arrest.

Feeling depressed

Patients with bradypnea might have CNS depression as a result of excessive sedation, tissue damage, or diabetic coma, which all depress the brain's respiratory control center. (The respiratory rate normally decreases during sleep.)

Apnea

Apnea is the absence of breathing. Periods of apnea may be short and occur sporadically during Cheyne-Stokes respirations, Biot's respirations, or other abnormal respiratory patterns. This condition may be life-threatening if periods of apnea last long enough.

Hyperpnea

Characterized by deep, rapid breathing, hyperpnea occurs in patients who exercise or who have anxiety, pain, or metabolic acidosis. In a comatose patient, hyperpnea may indicate hypoxia or hypoglycemia.

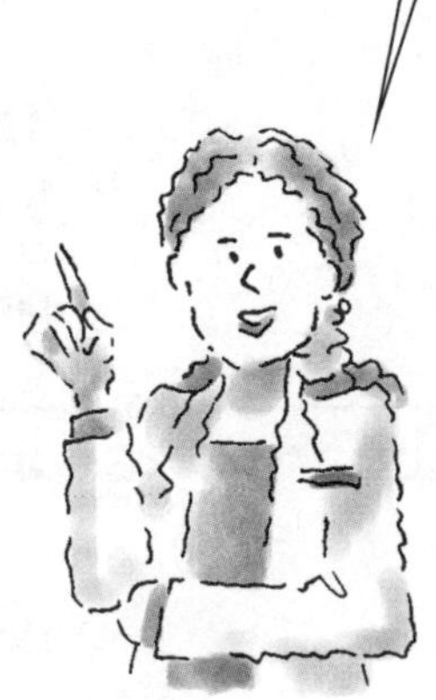

You need to do more than just count your patient's respiratory rate. Assessing his pattern of breathing can provide valuable clues about his respiratory status and overall health.

Kussmaul's respirations

Kussmaul's respirations are rapid, deep, sighing breaths that occur in patients with metabolic acidosis, especially when associated with diabetic ketoacidosis.

Cheyne-Stokes respirations

Cheyne-Stokes respirations have a regular pattern of variations in the rate and depth of breathing. Deep breaths alternate with short periods of apnea. This respiratory pattern occurs in patients with

Interpretation station

Abnormal respiratory patterns

Here are typical characteristics of the most common abnormal respiratory patterns.

Tachypnea
Shallow breathing with increased respiratory rate

Bradypnea
Decreased rate but regular breathing

Apnea
Absence of breathing; may be periodic

Hyperpnea
Deep, fast breathing

Kussmaul's respirations
Rapid, deep breathing without pauses; in adults, more than 20 breaths/minute; breathing usually sounds labored with deep breaths that resemble sighs

Cheyne-Stokes respirations
Breaths that gradually become faster and deeper than normal, then slower, during a 30- to 170-second period; alternates with 20- to 60-second periods of apnea

Biot's respirations
Rapid, deep breathing with abrupt pauses between each breath; equal depth to each breath

heart failure, kidney failure, or CNS damage. However, Cheyne-Stokes respirations may be normal during sleep in children and elderly patients.

Biot's respirations

Biot's respirations involve rapid, deep breaths that alternate with abrupt periods of apnea. Biot's respirations are an ominous sign of severe CNS damage.

Abnormal breath sounds

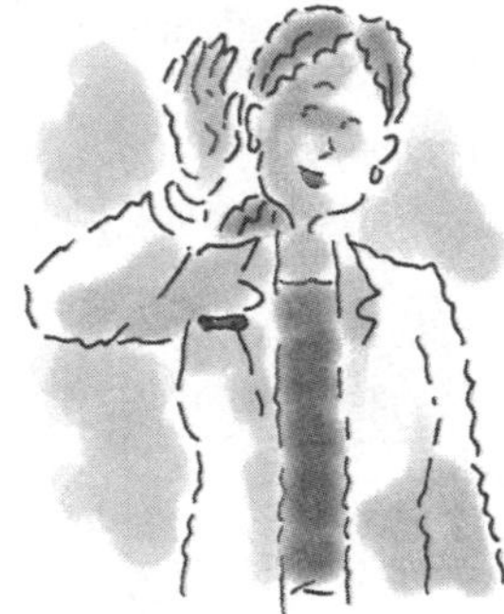

If you hear a sound in an area other than where you would expect to hear it, consider the sound abnormal. For example, if you hear bronchial or bronchovesicular breath sounds in an area where you would normally hear vesicular breath sounds, then the alveoli and small bronchioles in that area might be filled with fluid or exudate, as occurs in pneumonia and atelectasis. You won't hear vesicular sounds in those areas because no air is moving through the small airways.

Keep in mind that solid tissue transmits sound better than air or fluid. Therefore, breath sounds (as well as spoken or whispered words) will be louder than normal over areas of consolidation.

On the other hand, if pus, fluid, or air fills the pleural space, breath sounds will be quieter than normal. If a foreign body or secretions obstruct a bronchus, breath sounds will be diminished or absent over lung tissue located distal to the obstruction.

Troublemakers

Other breath sounds, called *adventitious sounds*, are abnormal no matter where you hear them in the lungs. Those sounds include fine and coarse crackles, wheezes, rhonchi, stridor, and pleural friction rub.

Crackles

Crackles are intermittent, nonmusical, brief crackling sounds that are caused by collapsed or fluid-filled alveoli popping open. Heard primarily when the patient inhales, crackles are classified as ei-

Types of crackles

Here's how to differentiate fine crackles from coarse crackles, a critical distinction when assessing the lungs.

Fine crackles

These characteristics distinguish fine crackles:
- occur when the patient stops inhaling
- are usually heard in lung bases
- sound like a piece of hair being rubbed between the fingers or like Velcro being pulled apart
- are unaffected by coughing
- occur in restrictive diseases, such as pulmonary fibrosis, asbestosis, silicosis, atelectasis, heart failure, and pneumonia.

Coarse crackles

These characteristics distinguish coarse crackles:
- occur when the patient starts to inhale; may be present when the patient exhales
- may be heard through the lungs and even at the mouth
- sound more like bubbling or gurgling, as air moves through secretions in larger airways
- usually clear or diminish after coughing
- occur in chronic obstructive pulmonary disease, bronchiectasis, pulmonary edema, and with severely ill patients who can't cough; also called the "death rattle."

ther fine or coarse and usually don't clear with coughing. If crackles do clear with coughing, secretions most likely caused them. (See *Types of crackles.*)

Wheezes

Wheezes are high-pitched sounds heard first when a patient exhales. (See *When wheezing stops.*) The sounds occur when airflow is blocked. As severity of the block increases, wheezes may also be heard when the patient inhales. The sound of a wheeze doesn't change with coughing. Patients may wheeze as a result of asthma, infection, heart failure, or airway obstruction from a tumor or foreign body. (See *Signs and symptoms of upper airway obstruction.*)

Rhonchi

Rhonchi are low-pitched, snoring, rattling sounds that occur primarily during exhalation, although they may also be heard on inhalation. Rhonchi usually change or disappear with coughing. The sounds occur when fluid partially blocks the large airways.

Stridor

Stridor is a loud, high-pitched crowing sound that's heard, usually without a stethoscope, during inspiration. Stridor, which is caused by an obstruction in the upper airway, requires immediate attention.

Pleural friction rub

Pleural friction rub is a low-pitched, grating, rubbing sound heard when the patient inhales and exhales. Pleural inflammation causes the two layers of pleura to rub together. The patient may complain of pain in areas where the rub is heard.

When wheezing stops

If you no longer hear wheezing in a patient having an acute asthma attack, the attack may be far from over. When bronchospasm and mucosal swelling become severe, little air can move through the airways. As a result, you won't hear wheezing.

If all other assessment criteria—labored breathing, prolonged expiratory time, and accessory muscle use—point to acute bronchial obstruction, act to maintain the patient's airway and give oxygen as ordered. The patient may begin to wheeze again when the airways open.

Signs and symptoms of upper airway obstruction

If a patient can't maintain a patent airway, he may end up in respiratory arrest. Refer to this list of potential signs and symptoms when assessing a patient for partial or complete airway obstruction.

- Anxiety
- Dyspnea
- Stridor
- Wheezing
- Decreased or absent breath sounds
- Use of accessory muscles
- Seesaw movement between chest and abdomen
- Inability to speak (complete obstruction)
- Cyanosis

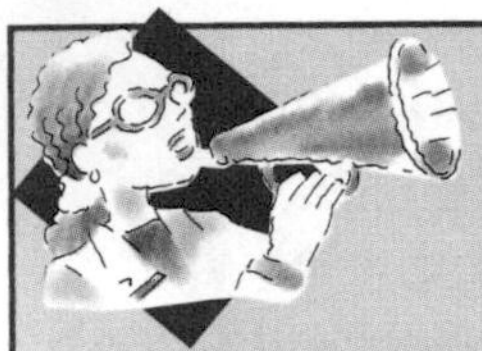

That's a wrap!

Respiratory system review

Structures and functions

Upper airways

- Include the nasopharynx, oropharynx, laryngopharynx, and larynx
- Warm, filter, and humidify inhaled air
- Help to make sound and send air to lower airways

Lower airways

- Trachea—divides into the right and left mainstem bronchi and continues to divide into smaller passages
- Bronchioles—terminate in the alveolar ducts and the alveoli
- Alveoli—gas-exchanging units of the lungs

Thorax

- Includes the clavicles, sternum, scapulae, 12 sets of ribs (which allow the chest to expand and contract during each breath), and 12 thoracic vertebrae

Respiratory muscles

- Diaphragm and external intercostal muscles (primary breathing muscles)—contract on inhalation and relax on exhalation
- Accessory inspiratory muscles (trapezius, sternocleidomastoid, and scalenes)—combine to elevate the scapulae, clavicle, sternum, and upper ribs when primary breathing muscles aren't effective

Health history

- Ask the patient about shortness of breath, and rate his dyspnea on a scale of 0 to 10.
- Determine if the patient has orthopnea, and ask how many pillows he uses to sleep at night.
- Ask if the patient has a cough. If he does, ask him if it's productive or nonproductive. If it's productive, have him describe the sputum.
- Have the patient describe any chest pain, including its location, how it feels, if it radiates, what causes it, and what makes it feel better.
- Ask about the patient's medical history, including smoking, pneumonia, and exposure to irritants.

Assessment

Inspection

- Watch for chest-wall symmetry as the patient breathes. Note any paradoxical, or uneven, chest-wall movement.
- Count the patient's respiratory rate for a full minute (longer if you note abnormalities); normal respiratory rate for an adult is 12 to 20 breaths/minute; up to 40 breaths/minute for infants.
- Observe the patient's respiratory pattern; it should be even, coordinated, and regular with occasional sighs.
- Inspect the skin, tongue, mouth, fingers, and nail beds, which can provide more information about the patient's respiratory status.

Palpation

- Gently use your palms to palpate the chest for crepitus, tenderness, alignment, bulging, or retractions. Palpate the front and back of the chest.
- Use the pads of your fingers to palpate the chest, including over the ribs. Note skin temperature, turgor, and moisture as well as the presence of scars, lumps, lesions, or ulcerations.
- Palpate for tactile fremitus.
- Assess chest-wall symmetry and expansion by placing your hands on the front of the chest with thumbs touching each other, and ask the patient to inhale deeply.

Respiratory system review *(continued)*

Percussion

• Resonant sounds are heard over normal lung tissue.

• Hyperresonance is found over areas of increased air in the lung or pleural space (hyperinflated lung, emphysema).

• Dullness is found over areas of decreased air in the lungs (atelectasis, pneumonia).

• Flatness is found over consolidated areas (atelectasis, pleural effusion).

• Tympany is found over areas where air has collected (large pneumothorax).

Auscultation

• Use the diaphragm of the stethoscope to listen to a full inspiration and a full expiration at each site.

• Ask the patient to breathe through his mouth. (Nose breathing alters the pitch of breath sounds.)

• Wet chest hair to prevent crackles that would be heard if auscultating over dry hair.

Normal breath sounds

• Tracheal—harsh, high-pitched, and discontinuous

• Bronchial—loud, high-pitched, and discontinuous

• Bronchovesicular—medium-pitched and continuous

• Vesicular—soft and low-pitched

Vocal fremitus

• Bronchophony—ask the patient to say "ninety-nine"

• Egophony—ask the patient to say "E"

• Whispered pectoriloquy—ask the patient to whisper "1, 2, 3"

Abnormal findings

Chest-wall abnormalities

• Barrel chest—large front-to-back diameter

• Pigeon chest—sternum protrudes beyond front of abdomen; increased front-to-back diameter of chest

• Funnel chest—depression on all or part of the sternum

• Thoracic kyphoscoliosis—curvature of spine; rotation of vertebrae; distortion of lung tissues

Abnormal respiratory patterns

• Tachypnea—respiratory rate greater than 20 breaths/minute with shallow breathing

• Bradypnea—respiratory rate below 10 breaths/minute

• Apnea—the absence of breathing; may be life-threatening if it lasts long

• Hyperpnea—deep, rapid breathing

• Kussmaul's respirations—rapid, deep, sighing breaths

• Cheyne-Stokes respirations—deep breaths alternating with periods of apnea

• Biot's respirations—rapid, deep breaths that alternate with abrupt apneic periods

Abnormal breath sounds

• Crackles—intermittent, nonmusical, crackling sounds heard during inspiration; classified as fine or coarse

• Wheezes—high-pitched sounds caused by blocked airflow, heard on exhalation

• Rhonchi—low-pitched snoring or rattling sound; heard primarily on exhalation

• Stridor—loud, high-pitched sound heard during inspiration

• Pleural friction rub—low-pitched grating sound heard during inspiration and expiration; accompanied by pain

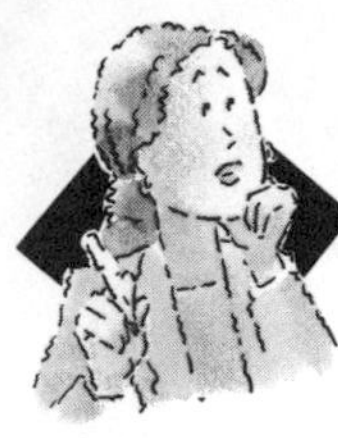

Quick quiz

1. In a patient with COPD, barrel chest indicates:
- A. loss of lung elasticity.
- B. rotation of the spinal column.
- C. increased elasticity of the intercostal muscles.
- D. accessory muscle use.

Answer: A. Barrel chest in patients with COPD is an indication of the loss of elasticity of the lungs and a flattening of the diaphragm.

2. The percussion sound usually heard over most of the lungs is:
- A. dullness.
- B. resonance.
- C. hyperresonance.
- D. tympany.

Answer: B. The lungs, made up of tissue and air, make a resonant percussion sound. Solid tissue is flat or dull; air-filled spaces are hyperresonant or tympanic.

3. When you auscultate the lower lobes of a healthy patient's lungs, you would expect to hear:
- A. tracheal breath sounds.
- B. bronchial breath sounds.
- C. vesicular breath sounds.
- D. bronchovesicular sounds

Answer: C. Vesicular breath sounds are soft, low-pitched, and prolonged during inspiration and can be heard over the lower lobes.

Scoring

☆☆☆ If you answered all three questions correctly, excellent! You've left us breathless with your expertise.

☆☆ If you answered two questions correctly, hoorah! You're our resident respiratory guru.

☆ If you answered fewer than two questions correctly, that's okay! Rereading the chapter is sure to expand your knowledge on the subject.

9

Cardiovascular system

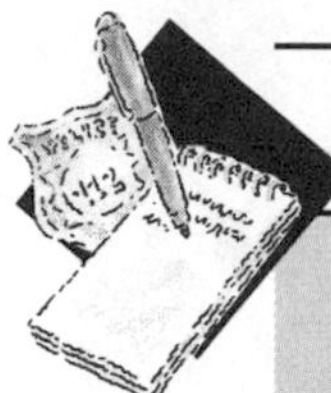

Just the facts

In this chapter, you'll learn:

- structures of the cardiovascular system and their functions
- the proper way to perform an assessment of the cardiovascular system
- normal and abnormal findings.

A look at the cardiovascular system

The cardiovascular system plays an important role in the body. It delivers oxygenated blood to tissues and removes waste products. The heart pumps blood to all organs and tissues of the body. The autonomic nervous system controls how the heart pumps. The vascular network — the arteries and veins — carries blood throughout the body, keeps the heart filled with blood, and maintains blood pressure.

I don't want to brag too much, but pumping blood to all of the organs and tissues in the body is a big job!

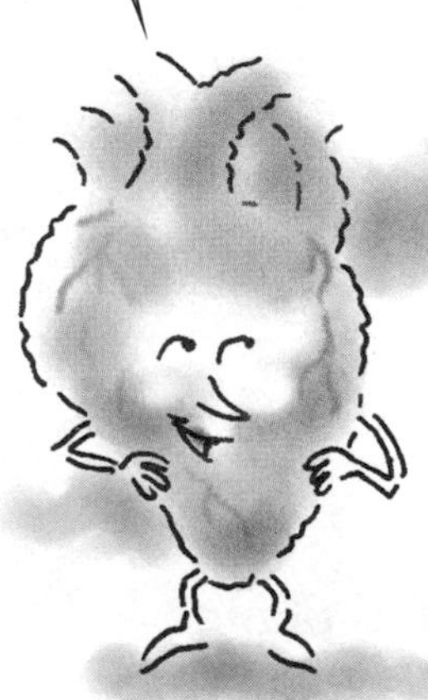

Anatomy and physiology of the cardiovascular system

To make the most of your assessment of the cardiovascular system, you'll need to understand the anatomy and physiology of the heart and the vascular system.

Heart

The heart is a hollow, muscular organ about the size of a closed fist. Located between the lungs in the mediastinum, behind and to the left of the sternum, it's about 5″ (12.5 cm) long and 3½″ (9 cm) in diameter at its widest point. The heart weighs 250 to 300 g.

Anatomy

The heart spans the area from the second to the fifth intercostal space. The right border of the heart aligns with the right border of the sternum. The left border lines up with the left midclavicular line. The exact position of the heart may vary slightly with each patient.

They'rrrrrre great!

Leading into and out of the heart are the great vessels: the inferior vena cava, the superior vena cava, the aorta, the pulmonary artery, and four pulmonary veins.

Remember: the prefix "peri" means "around," and "cardium" means heart. So, "pericardium" literally means "around the heart."

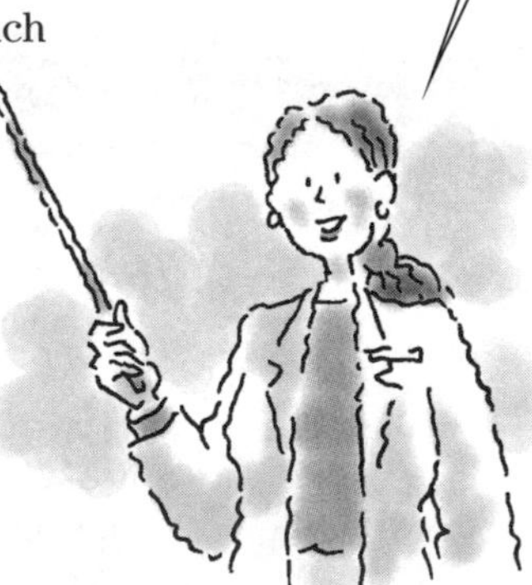

Smooth sliding

The heart is protected by a thin sac called the *pericardium*, which has an inner, or visceral, layer that forms the epicardium and an outer, or parietal, layer. The space between the two layers contains 10 to 30 ml of serous fluid, which prevents friction between the layers as the heart pumps.

Chamber made

The heart has four chambers (two atria and two ventricles) separated by a cardiac septum. The upper atria have thin walls and serve as reservoirs for blood. They also boost the amount of blood moving into the lower ventricles, which fill primarily by gravity. (See *A close look at the heart.*)

Have blood, will travel

Blood moves to and from the heart through specific pathways. Deoxygenated venous blood returns to the right atrium through three vessels: the superior vena cava, inferior vena cava, and coronary sinus.

Blood from the upper body returns to the heart through the superior vena cava. Blood in the lower body returns through the inferior vena cava, and blood from the heart muscle itself returns through the coronary sinus. All of the blood from those vessels empties into the right atrium.

Travel plans

Blood in the right atrium empties into the right ventricle and is then ejected through the pulmonic valve into the pulmonary artery

A close look at the heart

This illustration details the internal structures of the heart.

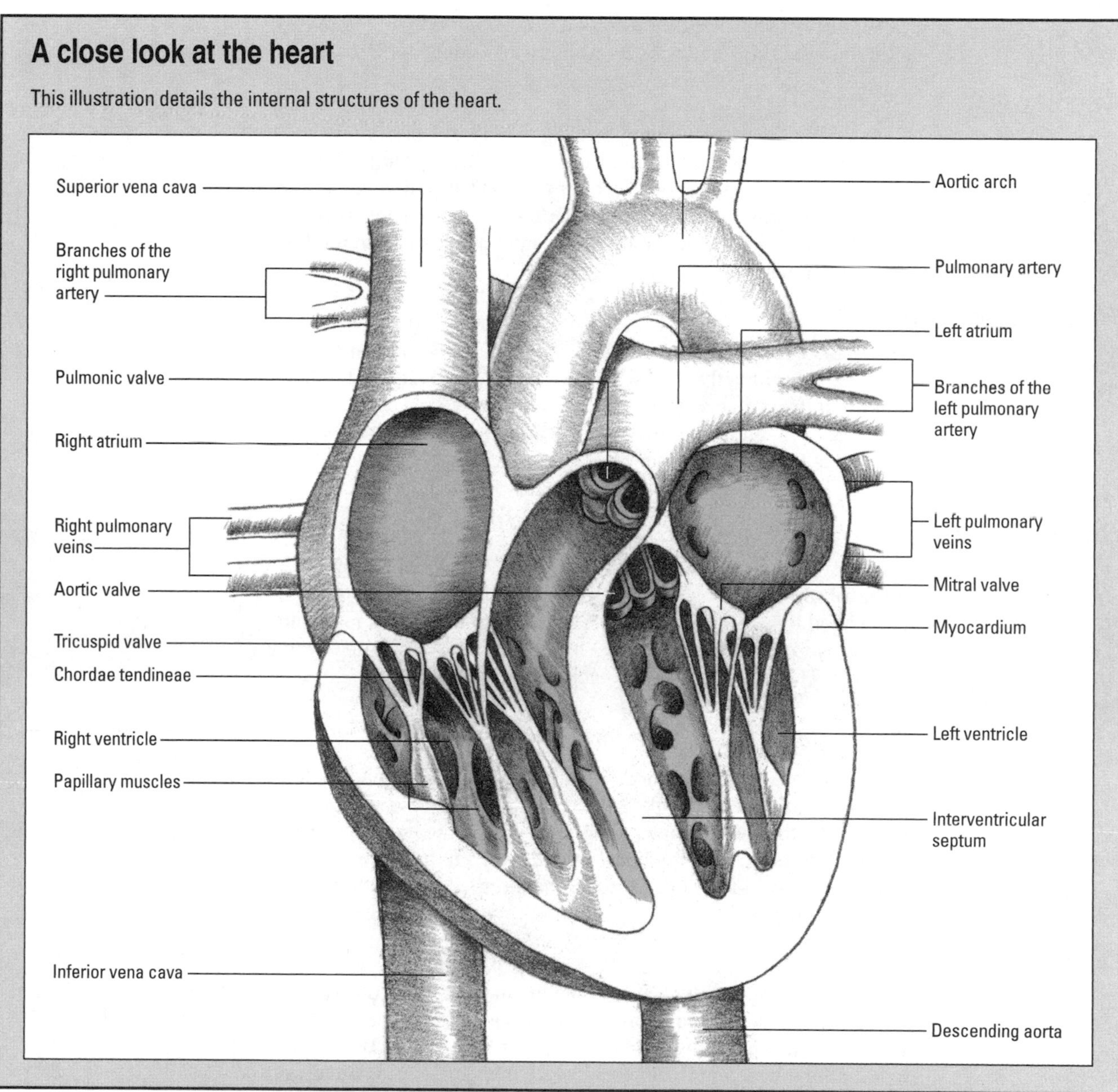

when the ventricle contracts. The blood then travels to the lungs to be oxygenated.

From the lungs, blood travels to the left atrium through the pulmonary veins. The left atrium empties the blood into the left ventricle, which then pumps the blood through the aortic valve into the aorta and throughout the body with each contraction. Because the left ventricle pumps blood against a much higher pressure than the right ventricle, its wall is three times thicker.

Valvular traffic cops

Valves in the heart keep blood flowing in only one direction through the heart. Think of the valves as traffic cops at the entrances to one-way streets, preventing blood from traveling the wrong way despite great pressure to do so. Healthy valves open and close passively as a result of pressure changes within the four heart chambers.

Which valve is where?

Valves between the atria and ventricles are called *atrioventricular valves* and include the tricuspid valve on the right side of the heart and the mitral valve on the left. The pulmonic valve (between the right ventricle and pulmonary artery) and the aortic valve (between the left ventricle and the aorta) are called *semilunar valves.*

On the cusp

Each valve's leaflets, or cusps, are anchored to the heart wall by cords of fibrous tissue. Those cords, called *chordae tendineae*, are controlled by papillary muscles. The cusps of the valves maintain tight closure. The tricuspid valve has three cusps. The mitral valve has two. The semilunar valves each have three cusps.

Physiology

Contractions of the heart occur in a rhythm—the cardiac cycle—and are regulated by impulses that normally begin at the sinoatrial (SA) node, the heart's pacemaker. From there, the impulses are conducted throughout the heart. Impulses from the autonomic nervous system affect the SA node and alter its firing rate to meet the body's needs.

The SA node is the heart's pacemaker. Impulses from this node regulate the heart's rhythm.

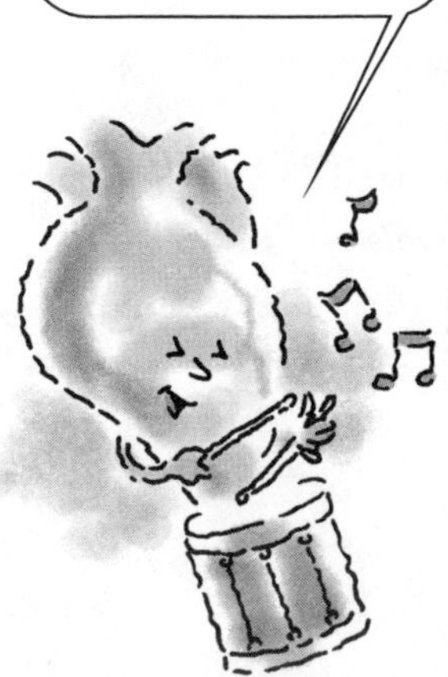

Contract, and then relax

The cardiac cycle consists of systole, the period when the heart contracts and sends blood on its outward journey, and diastole, the period when the heart relaxes and fills with blood. During diastole, the mitral and tricuspid valves are open, and the aortic and pulmonic valves are closed.

Diastole: Parts I and II

Diastole consists of two parts, ventricular filling and atrial contraction. During the first part of diastole, 70% of the blood in the atria drains into the ventricles by gravity, a passive action.

The active period of diastole, atrial contraction (also called the *atrial kick*), accounts for the remaining 30% of blood that passes into the ventricles. Diastole is also when the heart muscle receives its own supply of blood, which is transported by the coronary arteries.

Snap to it

Systole is the period of ventricular contraction. As pressure within the ventricles rises, the mitral and tricuspid valves snap closed. This closure leads to the first heart sound, S_1.

Open flow

When the pressure in the ventricles rises above the pressure in the aorta and pulmonary artery, the aortic and pulmonic valves open. Blood then flows from the ventricles into the pulmonary artery to the lungs and into the aorta to the rest of the body.

Cycle of life

At the end of ventricular contraction, pressure in the ventricles drops below the pressure in the aorta and the pulmonary artery. That pressure difference forces blood to back up toward the ventricles and causes the aortic and pulmonic valves to snap shut, which produces the second heart sound, S_2. As the valves shut, the atria fill with blood in preparation for the next period of diastolic filling, and the cycle begins again. (See *Cardiovascular changes with aging*.)

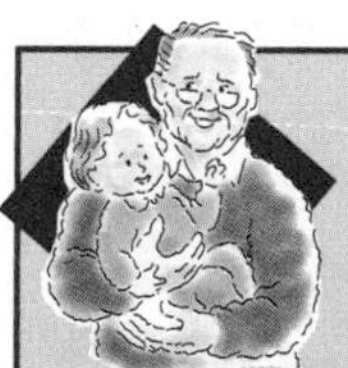

Ages and stages

Cardiovascular changes with aging

Changes in the cardiovascular system occur as a natural part of the aging process. These changes, however, place elderly patients at higher risk for cardiovascular disorders than younger patients. As you assess elderly patients, be aware of these changes that occur with aging:

- slight decrease in heart size
- loss of cardiac contractile strength and efficiency
- decrease in cardiac output of 30% to 35% by age 70
- thickening of heart valve, causing incomplete valve closure (as well as a systolic murmur)
- increase in left ventricular wall thickness of 25% between ages 30 and 80
- fibrous tissue infiltration of sinoatrial node and internodal atrial tracts, causing atrial fibrillation and flutter
- dilation and stretching of veins
- decline in coronary artery blood flow of 35% between the ages 20 and 60
- increased aortic rigidity
- increased amount of time necessary for heart rate to return to normal after exercise
- decreased strength and elasticity of blood vessels, contributing to arterial and venous insufficiency
- decreased ability to respond to physical and emotional stress.

Vascular system

The vascular system delivers oxygen, nutrients, and other substances to the body's cells and removes the waste products of cellular metabolism. The peripheral vascular system consists of a network of arteries, arterioles, capillaries, venules, and veins that's constantly filled with about 5 L of blood. (See *A close look at arteries and veins.*)

Tough travelers

Arteries carry blood away from the heart. Nearly all arteries carry oxygen-rich blood from the heart throughout the rest of the body. The only exception is the pulmonary artery, which carries oxygen-depleted blood from the right ventricle to the lungs.

Arteries are thick-walled because they transport blood under high pressure. Arterial walls contain a tough, elastic layer to help propel blood through the arterial system.

Thin-skinned

The exchange of fluid, nutrients, and metabolic wastes between blood and cells occurs in the capillaries. The exchange can occur because capillaries are thin-walled and highly permeable. About 5% of the circulating blood volume at any given moment is contained within the capillary network. Capillaries are connected to arteries and veins through intermediary vessels called *arterioles* and *venules*, respectively.

Veins are thin and pliable so they can accommodate variations in blood volume.

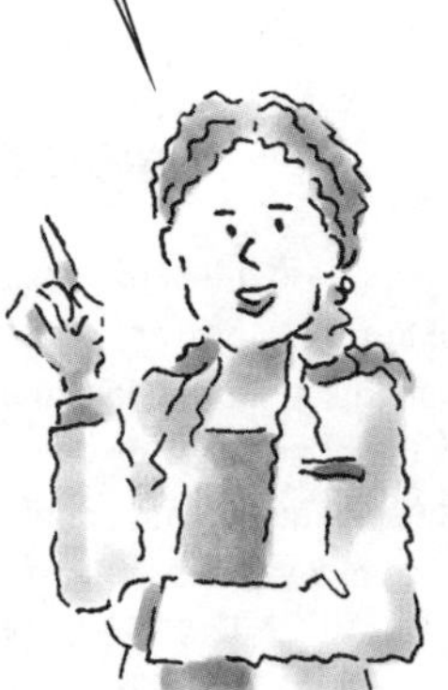

Reservoir veins

Veins carry blood toward the heart. Nearly all veins carry oxygen-depleted blood, the sole exception being the pulmonary vein, which carries oxygenated blood from the lungs to the left atrium. Veins serve as a large reservoir for circulating blood.

The wall of a vein is thinner and more pliable than the wall of an artery. That pliability allows the vein to accommodate variations in blood volume. Veins contain valves at periodic intervals to prevent blood from flowing backward.

Finger on the pulse

Arterial pulses are pressure waves of blood generated by the pumping action of the heart. All vessels in the arterial system have pulsations, but the pulsations can be felt only where an artery lies near the skin. You can palpate for these peripheral pulses: temporal, carotid, brachial, radial, ulnar, femoral, popliteal, posterior tibial, and dorsalis pedis.

The location of pulse points varies between individuals. In older adults, peripheral pulses may be diminished.

A close look at arteries and veins

This illustration shows major arteries and veins of the body.

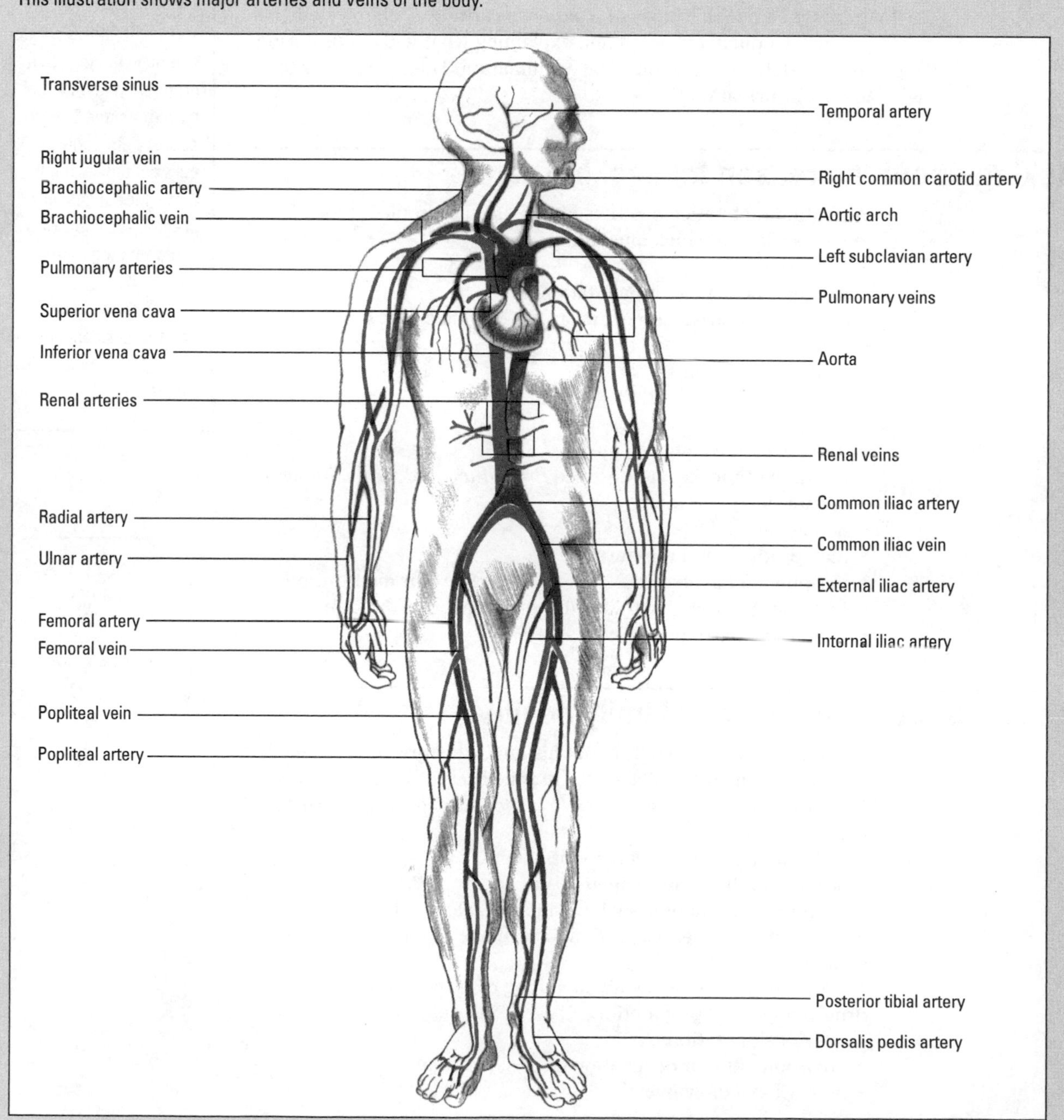

Obtaining a health history

To obtain a health history of a patient's cardiovascular system, begin by introducing yourself and explaining what will occur during the health history and physical examination. Then obtain the following information.

Pregnancy and vein changes

You might find 4+ pitting edema in the legs of a pregnant patient in her third trimester. Severe edema commonly occurs not only in the third trimester but also in pregnant women who stand for long periods of time.

Varicose veins are another common finding during the third trimester.

Asking about the reason for seeking care

You'll find that patients with a cardiovascular problem typically cite specific complaints, including:

- chest pain
- irregular heartbeat or palpitations
- shortness of breath on exertion, when lying down, or at night
- cough
- cyanosis or pallor
- weakness
- fatigue
- unexplained weight change
- swelling of the extremities (see *Pregnancy and vein changes*)
- dizziness
- headache
- high or low blood pressure
- peripheral skin changes, such as decreased hair distribution, skin color changes, or a thin, shiny appearance to the skin
- pain in the extremities, such as leg pain or cramps.

Asking about personal and family health

Ask the patient for details about his family history and past medical history, including diabetes, chronic diseases of the lungs or kidneys, or liver disease. (See *At risk for cardiovascular disease*, page 187.)

Also obtain information about:

- stress and the patient's methods of coping with it
- current health habits, such as smoking, alcohol intake, caffeine intake, exercise, and dietary intake of fat and sodium
- drugs the patient is taking, including over-the-counter drugs and herbal preparations
- previous operations
- environmental or occupational considerations
- activities of daily living.

Does your family have a history of diabetes or lung, kidney, or liver disease?

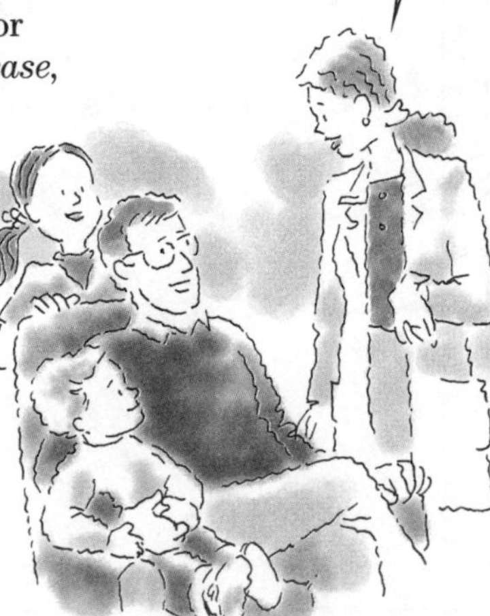

(Text continues on page 187.)

Sites for heart sounds

When auscultating for heart sounds, place the stethoscope over the four sites illustrated below.

Normal heart sounds indicate events in the cardiac cycle, such as the closing of heart valves, and are reflected to specific areas of the chest wall. Auscultation sites are identified by the names of heart valves but aren't located directly over the valves. Rather, these sites are located along the pathway blood takes as it flows through the heart's chambers and valves.

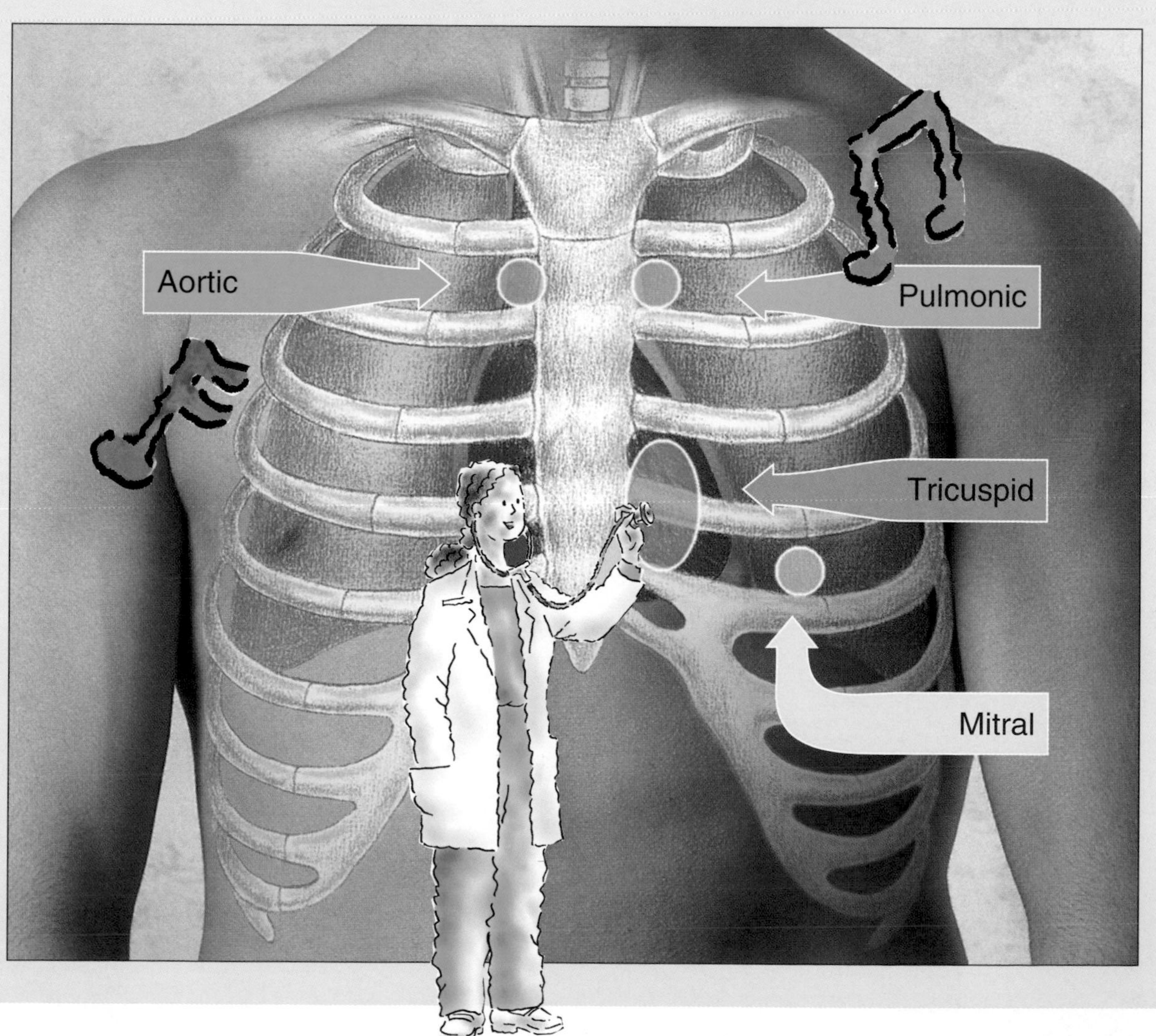

Cycle of heart sounds

When you auscultate a patient's chest and hear that familiar "lub-dub," you're hearing the first and second heart sounds, S_1 and S_2. At times, two other sounds may occur: S_3 and S_4.

Heart sounds are generated by events in the cardiac cycle. When valves close or blood fills the ventricles, vibrations of the heart muscle can be heard through the chest wall.

Varying sound patterns
The phonogram at right shows how heart sounds vary in duration and intensity. For instance, S_2 (which occurs when the semilunar valves snap shut) is a shorter-lasting sound than S_1 because the semilunar valves take less time to close than the atrioventricular valves, which cause S_1.

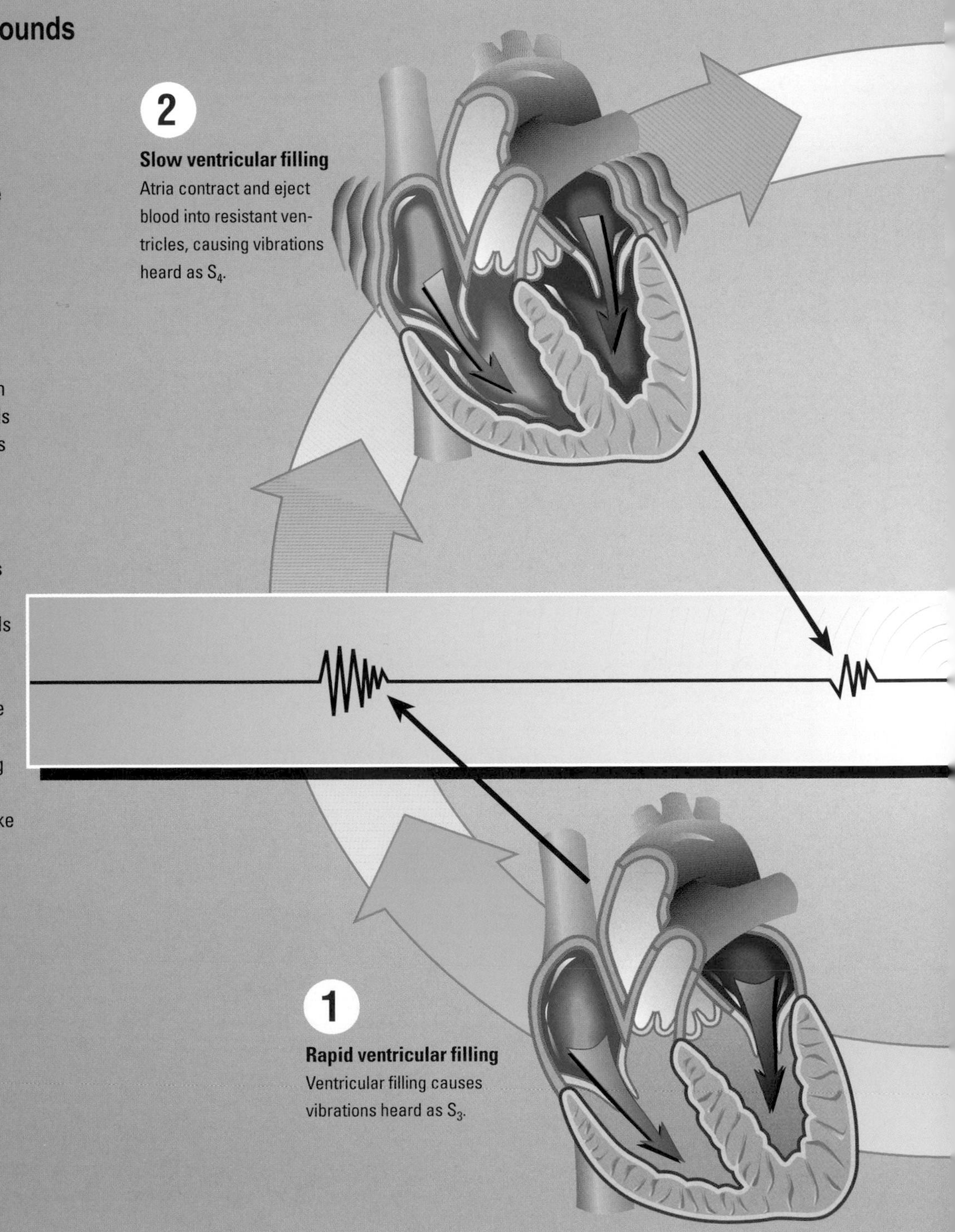

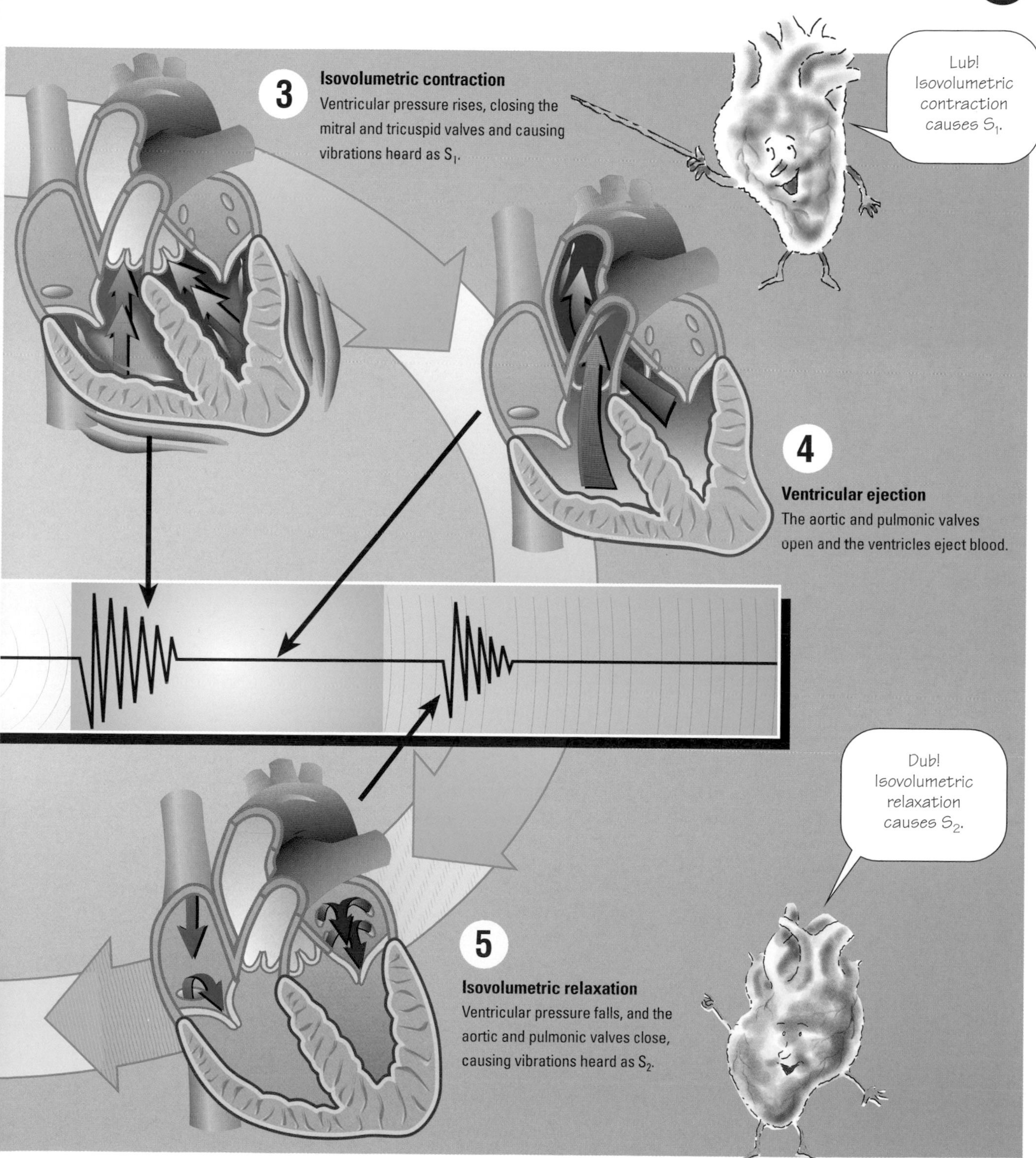

3 Isovolumetric contraction

Ventricular pressure rises, closing the mitral and tricuspid valves and causing vibrations heard as S_1.

4 Ventricular ejection

The aortic and pulmonic valves open and the ventricles eject blood.

5 Isovolumetric relaxation

Ventricular pressure falls, and the aortic and pulmonic valves close, causing vibrations heard as S_2.

Understanding murmurs

Normally, heart valves close tightly and then open completely to let blood flow through. However, various conditions may alter blood flow through the valves, causing murmurs and, in many cases, increasing the workload of the heart.

The first two illustrations show a normal valve open and closed. The other illustrations portray three common reasons for the development of murmurs.

Valve closure is normally an open-and-shut case.

Normal valve open

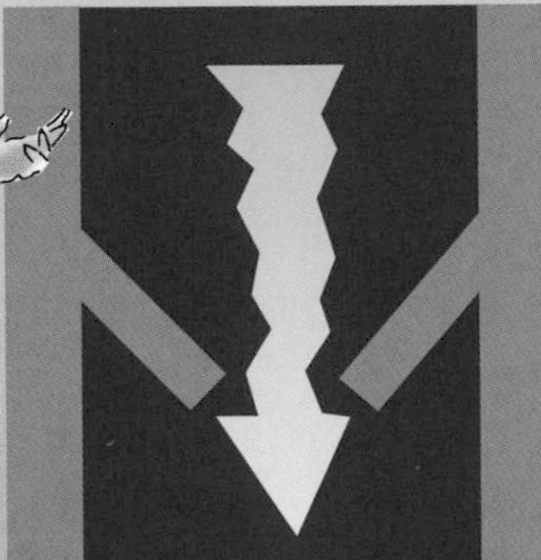

Normal valve closed

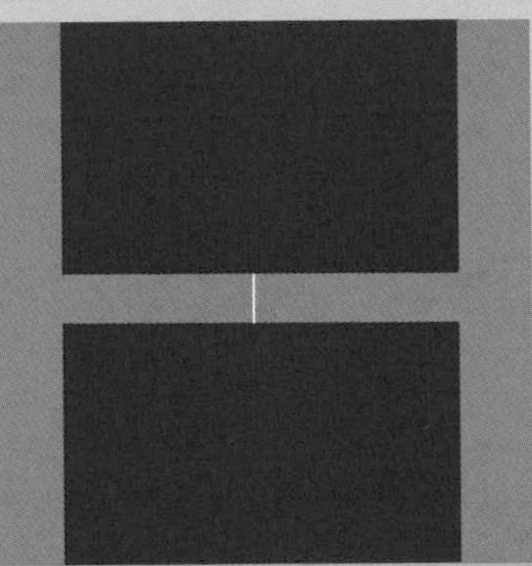

High blood flow

High blood flow through a normal valve may cause a murmur. Examples include an aortic systolic murmur, which can be caused by anemia and a subsequent compensatory increase in cardiac output.

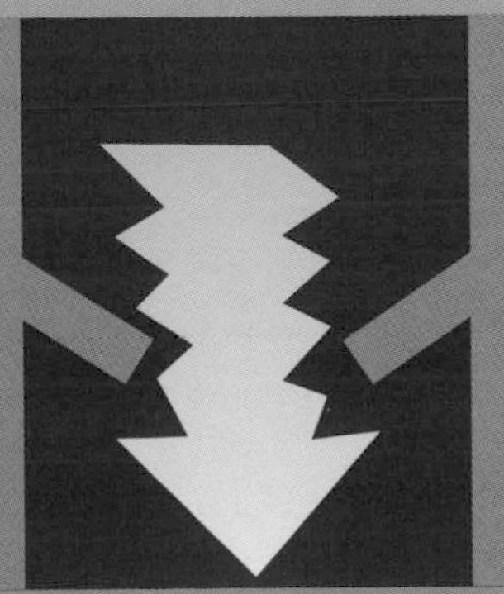

Decreased blood flow

Low blood flow through a stenotic valve can cause a murmur. The valves can't open or close properly because they're thickened, fibrotic, or calcified. Common examples include aortic and mitral stenosis.

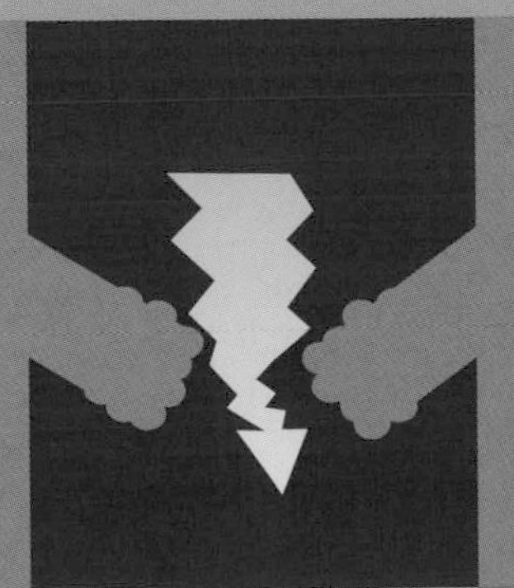

Backflow of blood

A backflow of blood through an insufficient or incompetent valve can cause a murmur. Because the valve can't close properly, blood can leak back or regurgitate into the heart chamber from which it came. Common examples include aortic and mitral insufficiency.

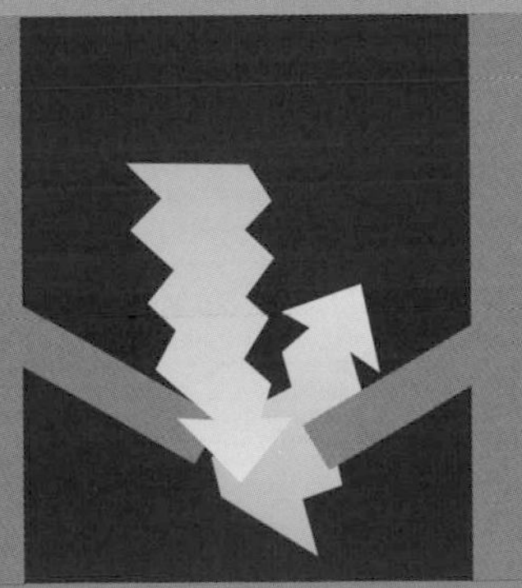

Rating the pain

Many patients with cardiovascular problems complain of chest pain at some point. If your patient has chest pain, ask him to rate the pain on a scale of 0 to 10, in which 0 means no pain and 10 means the worst pain imaginable. Reassess the patient's pain rating frequently during treatment to determine the effectiveness of interventions.

Broadening the scope

In addition to checking for pain, also ask the patient these questions:

- Are you ever short of breath? If so, what activities cause you to be short of breath?
- Do you feel dizzy or fatigued?
- Do your rings or shoes feel tight?
- Do your ankles swell?
- Have you noticed changes in color or sensation in your legs? If so, what are those changes?
- If you have sores or ulcers, how quickly do they heal?
- Do you stand or sit in one place for long periods at work?

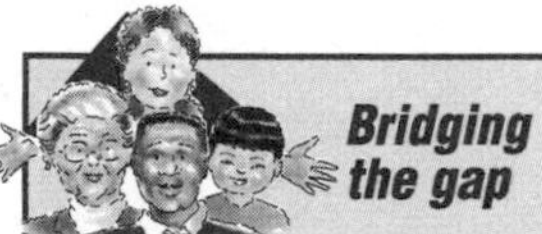

At risk for cardiovascular disease

As you analyze a patient's problems, remember that age, gender, and race are essential considerations in identifying patients at risk for cardiovascular disorders. For example, coronary artery disease most commonly affects white men between ages 40 and 60. Hypertension occurs most often in blacks.

Women are also vulnerable to heart disease, especially postmenopausal women and those with diabetes mellitus.

Assessing the cardiovascular system

Cardiovascular disease affects people of all ages and can take many forms. A consistent, methodical approach to your assessment will help you identify abnormalities. As always, the key to accurate assessment is regular practice, which will help improve technique and efficiency.

Before you begin your physical assessment, you'll need to obtain a stethoscope with a bell and a diaphragm, an appropriate-sized blood pressure cuff, a ruler, and a penlight or other flexible light source. Make sure the room is quiet.

Ask the patient to remove all clothing except his underwear and to put on an examination gown. Have the patient lie on his back, with the head of the examination table at a 30- to 45-degree angle. Stand on the patient's right side if you're right-handed or his left side if you're left-handed so you can auscultate more easily.

Assessing the heart

As with assessment of other body systems, you'll inspect, palpate, percuss, and auscultate in your assessment of the heart.

Inspection

First, take a moment to assess the patient's general appearance. Is he overly thin? Obese? Alert? Anxious? Note his skin color, temperature, turgor, and texture. Are his fingers clubbed? (Clubbing is a sign of chronic hypoxia caused by a lengthy cardiovascular or respiratory disorder.) If the patient is dark-skinned, inspect his mucous membranes for pallor.

Chest check

Next, inspect the chest. Note landmarks you can use to describe your findings as well as structures underlying the chest wall. (See *Identifying cardiovascular landmarks.*)

Look for pulsations, symmetry of movement, retractions, or heaves. A heave is a strong outward thrust of the chest wall and occurs during systole.

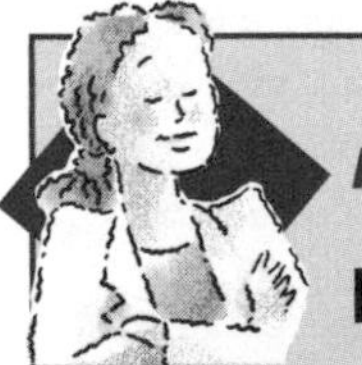

Peak technique

Identifying cardiovascular landmarks

These views show where to find critical landmarks used in cardiovascular assessment.

Anterior thorax

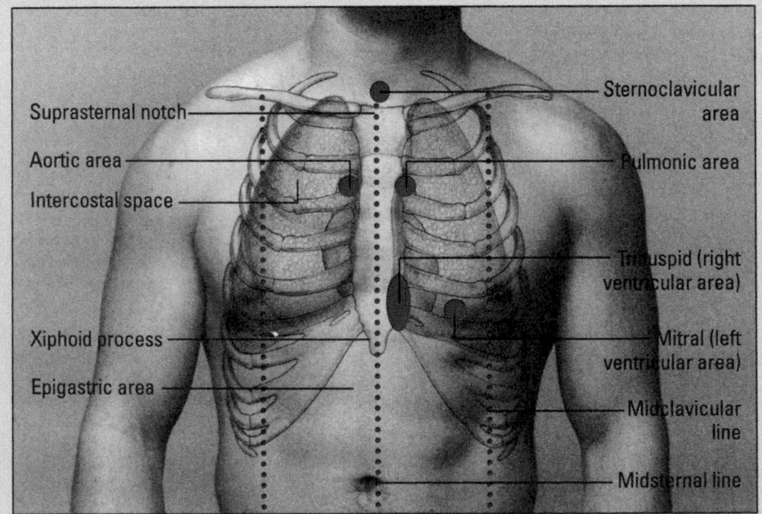

Lateral thorax

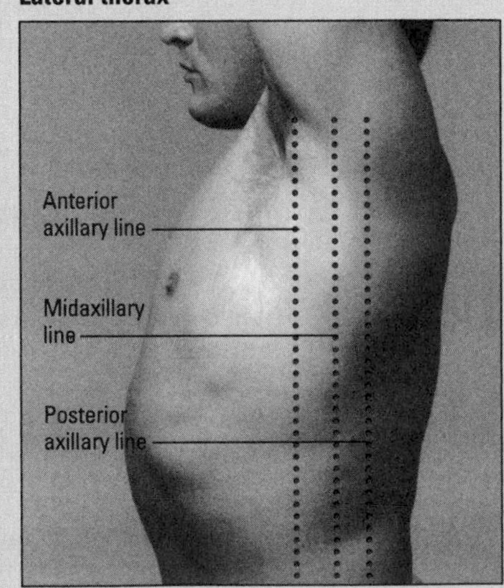

Shed some light on the subject

Position a light source, such as a flashlight or gooseneck lamp, so that it casts a shadow on the patient's chest. Note the location of the apical impulse. This is also usually the point of maximal impulse and should be located in the fifth intercostal space at or just medial to the left midclavicular line.

The apical impulse gives an indication of how well the left ventricle is working because it corresponds to the apex of the heart. The impulse can be seen in about 50% of adults. You'll notice it more easily in children and in patients with thin chest walls. To find the apical impulse in a woman with large breasts, displace the breasts during the examination.

Palpation

Maintain a gentle touch when you palpate so that you won't obscure pulsations or similar findings. Using the ball of your hand, then your fingertips, palpate over the precordium to find the apical impulse. Note heaves or thrills, fine vibrations that feel like the purring of a cat. (See *Assessing the apical impulse.*)

Try to modify

The apical impulse may be difficult to palpate in obese and pregnant patients and in patients with thick chest walls. If it's difficult to palpate with the patient lying on his back, have him lie on his left side or sit upright. It may also be helpful to have the patient exhale completely and hold his breath for a few seconds.

Plentiful places to palpate

Also palpate the sternoclavicular, aortic, pulmonic, tricuspid, and epigastric areas for abnormal pulsations. Normally, you won't feel pulsations in those areas. An aortic arch pulsation in the sternoclavicular area or an abdominal aorta pulsation in the epigastric area may be a normal finding in a thin patient.

Percussing the heart

Although percussion isn't as useful as other methods of assessment, this technique may help you locate cardiac borders. Begin percussing at the anterior axillary line and continue toward the sternum along the fifth intercostal space.

The sound changes from resonance to dullness over the left border of the heart, normally at the midclavicular line. The right border of the heart is usually aligned with the sternum and can't be percussed.

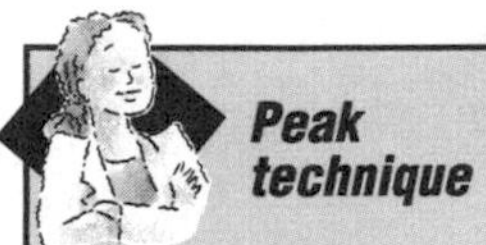

Peak technique

Assessing the apical impulse

The apical impulse is associated with the first heart sound and carotid pulsation. To ensure that you're feeling the apical impulse and not a muscle spasm or some other pulsation, use one hand to palpate the patient's carotid artery and the other to palpate the apical impulse. Then compare the timing and regularity of the impulses. The apical impulse should roughly coincide with the carotid pulsation.

Note the amplitude, size, intensity, location, and duration of the apical impulse. You should feel a gentle pulsation in an area about ½″ to ¾″ (1.5 to 2 cm) in diameter.

If fat or tissue is in the way, take an X-ray

Percussion may be difficult in obese patients because of the fat overlying the chest or in female patients because of breast tissue. In this case, a chest X-ray can provide information about the heart border.

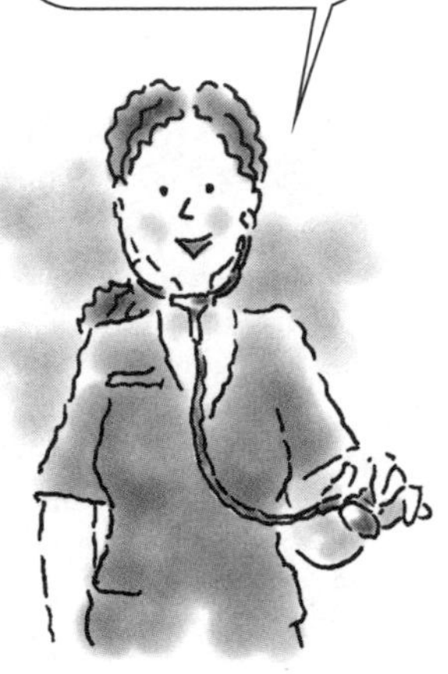

Auscultating for heart sounds

You can learn a great deal about the heart by auscultating for heart sounds. Cardiac auscultation requires a methodical approach and lots of practice. Begin by warming the stethoscope in your hands and then identify the sites where you'll auscultate: over the four cardiac valves and at Erb's point, the third intercostal space at the left sternal border. Use the bell to hear low-pitched sounds and the diaphragm to hear high-pitched sounds. (See *Sites for heart sounds*, page C5.)

Have a plan

Auscultate for heart sounds with the patient in three positions: lying on his back with the head of the bed raised 30 to 45 degrees, sitting up, and lying on his left side. Use a zigzag pattern over the precordium. You can start at the base and work downward or at the apex and work upward. Whichever approach you use, be consistent. (See *Auscultation tips*.)

Use the diaphragm to listen as you go in one direction; use the bell as you come back in the other direction. Be sure to listen over the entire precordium, not just over the valves.

Note the heart rate and rhythm. Always identify S_1 and S_2, and then listen for adventitious sounds, such as third and fourth heart sounds (S_3 and S_4), murmurs, and rubs. (See *Cycle of heart sounds*, pages C6 and C7.)

Listen for the "dub"

Start auscultating at the aortic area where S_2, the second heart sound, is loudest. S_2 is best heard at the base of the heart at the end of ventricular systole. This sound corresponds to closure of the pulmonic and aortic valves and is generally described as sounding like "dub." It's a shorter, higher-pitched, louder sound than S_1. When the pulmonic valve closes later than the aortic valve during inspiration, you'll hear a split S_2.

Listen for the "lub"

From the base of the heart, move to the pulmonic area and then down to the tricuspid area. Then move to the mitral area, where S_1 is the loudest. S_1 is best heard at the apex of the heart. This sound corresponds to closure of the mitral and tricuspid valves and is generally described as sounding like "lub." It's low-pitched and dull. S_1 occurs at the beginning of ventricular systole. It may be split if the mitral valve closes just before the tricuspid.

S_3: Classic sign of heart failure

A third heart sound, S_3, is a normal finding in children and young adults. In addition, S_3 is commonly heard in patients with high cardiac output. Called *ventricular gallop* when it occurs in adults, S_3 may be a cardinal sign of heart failure.

Deep in the heart of Kentucky?

S_3 is best heard at the apex when the patient is lying on his left side. Often compared to the *y* sound in "Ken-tuck-y," S_3 is low-pitched and occurs when the ventricles fill rapidly. It follows S_2 in early ventricular diastole and probably results from vibrations caused by abrupt ventricular distention and resistance to filling. In addition to heart failure, S_3 may also be associated with such conditions as pulmonary edema, atrial septal defect, acute myocardial infarction (MI), and the last trimester of pregnancy.

Gallop poll

S_4 is an adventitious sound called an *atrial gallop* that's heard over the tricuspid or mitral areas with the patient on his left side. You may hear S_4 in patients who are elderly or in those with hypertension, aortic stenosis, or a history of MI. S_4, commonly described as sounding like "Ten-nes-see," occurs just before S_1, after atrial contraction.

The S_4 sound indicates increased resistance to ventricular filling. It results from vibrations caused by forceful atrial ejection of blood into ventricles that are enlarged or hypertrophied and don't move or expand as much as they should.

Auscultating for murmurs

Murmurs occur when structural defects in the heart's chambers or valves cause turbulent blood flow. (See *Understanding murmurs*, page C8.) Turbulence may also be caused by changes in the viscosity of blood or the speed of blood flow. Listen for murmurs over the same precordial areas used in auscultation for heart sounds.

Murmur variations

Murmurs can occur during systole or diastole and are described by several criteria. (See *Tips for describing murmurs*, page 192.) Their pitch can be high, medium, or low. They can vary in intensity, growing louder or softer. (See *Grading murmurs*, page 192.) They can vary by location, sound pattern (blowing, harsh, or musi-

Auscultation tips

Follow these tips when you auscultate a patient's heart:

- Concentrate as you listen for each sound.
- Avoid auscultating through clothing or wound dressings because they can block sound.
- Avoid picking up extraneous sounds by keeping the stethoscope tubing off the patient's body and other surfaces.
- Until you become proficient at auscultation and can examine a patient quickly, explain to him that even though you may listen to his chest for a long period, it doesn't mean anything is wrong.
- Ask the patient to breathe normally and to hold his breath periodically to enhance sounds that may be difficult to hear.

Grading murmurs

Use the system outlined here to describe the intensity of a murmur. When recording your findings, use Roman numerals as part of a fraction, always with VI as the denominator. For example, a grade III murmur would be recorded as "grade III/VI."

- Grade I is a barely audible murmur.
- Grade II is audible but quiet and soft.
- Grade III is moderately loud, without a thrust or thrill.
- Grade IV is loud, with a thrill.
- Grade V is very loud, with a thrust or a thrill.
- Grade VI is loud enough to be heard before the stethoscope comes into contact with the chest.

Tips for describing murmurs

Describing murmurs can be tricky. After you've auscultated a murmur, list the terms you would use to describe it. Then check the patient's chart to see how others have described it or ask an experienced colleague to listen and describe the murmur. Compare the descriptions and then auscultate for the murmur again, if necessary, to confirm the description.

cal), radiation (to the neck or axillae), and period during which they occur in the cardiac cycle (pansystolic or midsystolic).

Sit up, please

The best way to hear murmurs is with the patient sitting up and leaning forward. You can also have him lie on his left side. (See *Positioning the patient for auscultation.*)

Auscultating for pericardial friction rub

To listen for a pericardial friction rub, have the patient sit upright, lean forward, and exhale. Listen with the diaphragm of the stethoscope over the third intercostal space on the left side of the chest. A pericardial friction rub has a scratchy, rubbing quality. If you suspect a rub but have trouble hearing one, ask the patient to hold his breath.

Leg veins should be evaluated while the patient is standing.

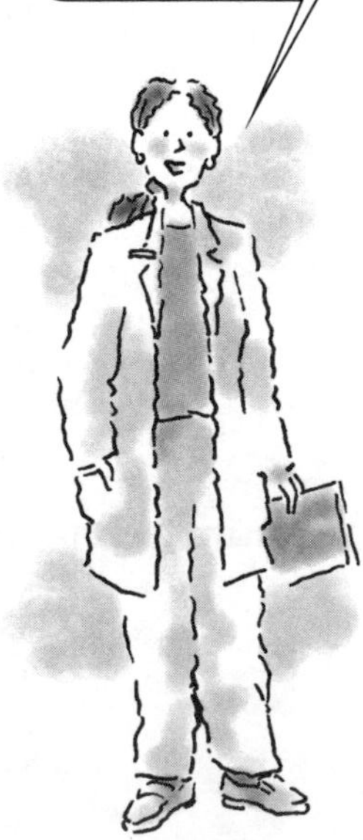

Assessing the vascular system

Assessment of the vascular system is an important part of a full cardiovascular assessment. Examination of the patient's arms and legs can reveal arterial or venous disorders. Examine the patient's arms when you take his vital signs. Check the legs later during the physical examination, when the patient is lying on his back. Remember to evaluate leg veins when the patient is standing.

Inspection

Start your assessment of the vascular system the same way you start an assessment of the cardiac system — by making general observations. Are the arms equal in size? Are the legs symmetrical?

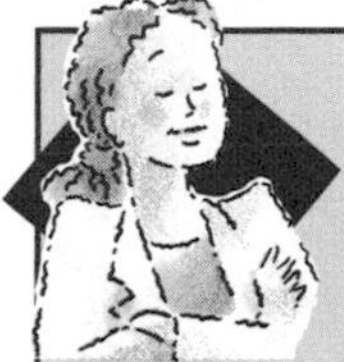

Peak technique

Positioning the patient for auscultation

If heart sounds are faint or undetectable, try listening to them with the patient seated and leaning forward or lying on his left side, which brings the heart closer to the surface of the chest. These illustrations show how to position the patient for high- and low-pitched sounds.

Forward-leaning

The forward-leaning position is best suited for hearing high-pitched sounds related to semilunar valve problems, such as aortic and pulmonic valve murmurs. To auscultate for these sounds, place the diaphragm of the stethoscope over the aortic and pulmonic areas in the right and left second intercostal spaces, as shown below.

Left lateral recumbent

The left lateral recumbent position is best suited for hearing low-pitched sounds, such as mitral valve murmurs and extra heart sounds. To hear these sounds, place the bell of the stethoscope over the apical area, as shown below.

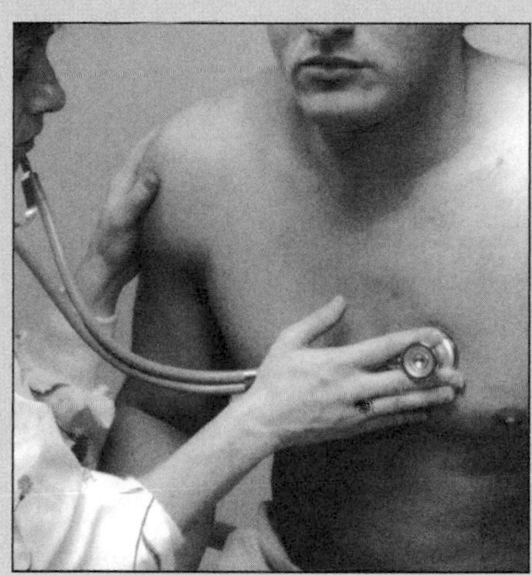

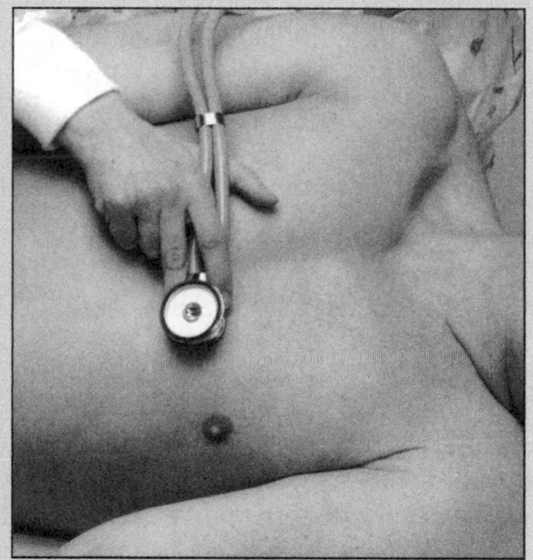

Inspect the skin color. Note how body hair is distributed. Note lesions, scars, clubbing, and edema of the extremities. If the patient is confined to bed, check the sacrum for swelling. Examine the fingernails and toenails for abnormalities.

Start at the top

Start your inspection by observing vessels in the neck. The carotid artery should have a brisk, localized pulsation. The internal jugular vein has a softer, undulating pulsation. The carotid pulsation doesn't decrease when the patient is upright, when he inhales, or when you palpate the carotid. The internal jugular pulsation, on the other hand, changes in response to position, breathing, and palpation.

Check carotid artery pulsations. Are they weak or bounding? Inspect the jugular veins. Inspection of these vessels can provide information about blood volume and pressure in the right side of the heart.

Take this lying down

To check the jugular venous pulse, have the patient lie on his back. Elevate the head of the bed 30 to 45 degrees and turn the patient's head slightly away from you. Normally, the highest pulsation occurs no more than 1½" (4 cm) above the sternal notch. If pulsations appear higher, it indicates elevation in central venous pressure and jugular vein distention.

Palpation

The first step in palpation is to assess skin temperature, texture, and turgor. Then check capillary refill by assessing the nail beds on the fingers and toes. Refill time should be no more than 3 seconds, or long enough to say "capillary refill."

Swell scale

Palpate the patient's arms and legs for temperature and edema. Edema is graded on a four-point scale. If your finger leaves a slight imprint, the edema is recorded as +1. If your finger leaves a deep imprint that only slowly returns to normal, the edema is recorded as +4.

Artery check!

Palpate for arterial pulses by gently pressing with the pads of your index and middle fingers. Start at the top of the patient's body at the temporal artery and work your way down. Check the carotid, brachial, radial, femoral, popliteal, posterior tibial, and dorsalis pedis pulses.

Palpate for the pulse on each side, comparing pulse volume and symmetry. *Don't palpate both carotid arteries at the same time or press too firmly. If you do, the patient may faint or become bradycardic.* If you haven't put on gloves for the examination, do so when you palpate the femoral arteries.

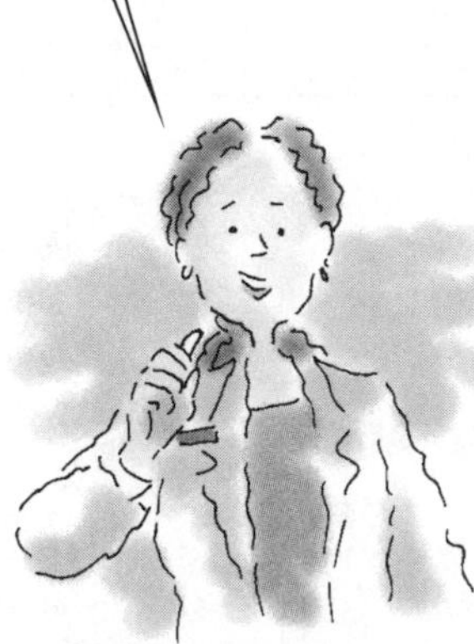

Making the grade

All pulses should be regular in rhythm and equal in strength. Pulses are also graded on a four-point scale: 4+ is bounding, 3+ is increased, 2+ is normal, 1+ is weak, and 0 is absent. (See *Assessing arterial pulses.*)

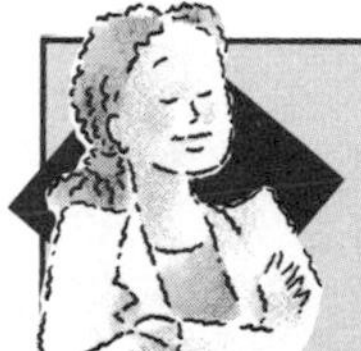

Peak technique

Assessing arterial pulses

To assess arterial pulses, apply pressure with your index and middle fingers. These illustrations show where to position your fingers when palpating for various pulses.

Carotid pulse

Lightly place your fingers just lateral to the trachea and below the jaw angle. Never palpate both carotid arteries at the same time.

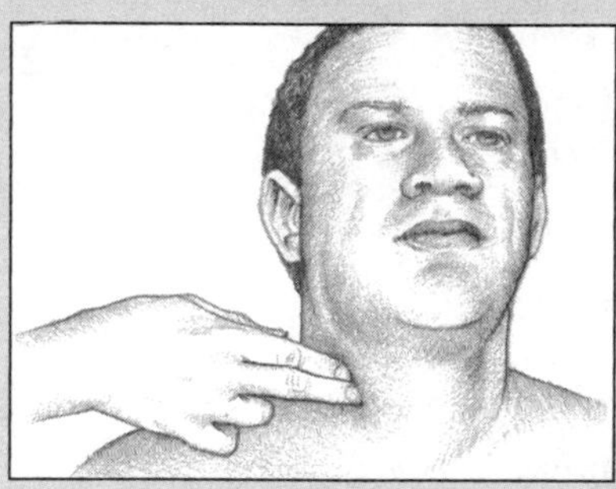

Brachial pulse

Position your fingers medial to the biceps tendon.

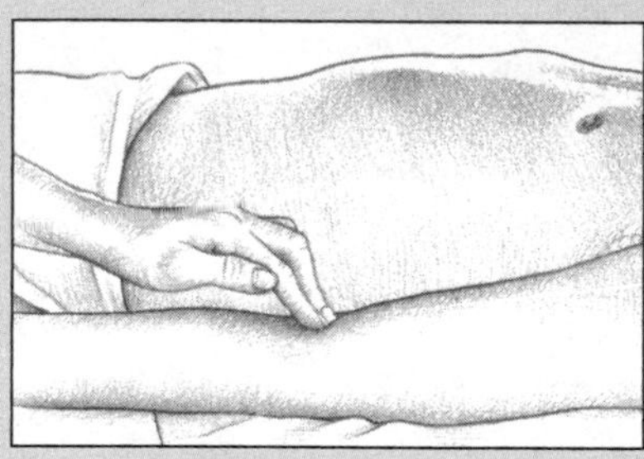

Radial pulse

Apply gentle pressure to the medial and ventral side of the wrist, just below the base of the thumb.

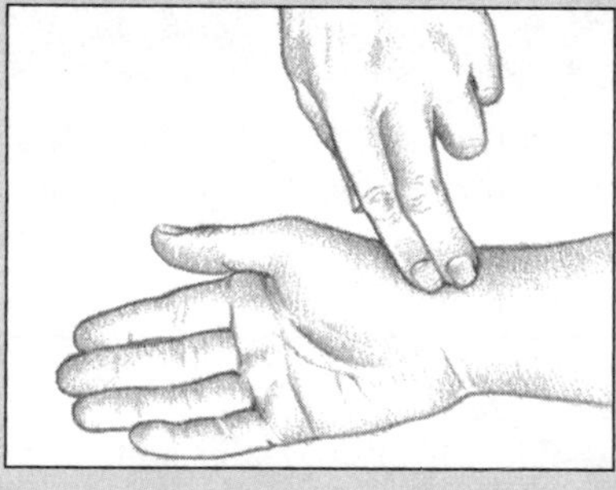

Femoral pulse

Press relatively hard at a point inferior to the inguinal ligament. For an obese patient, palpate in the crease of the groin, halfway between the pubic bone and the hip bone.

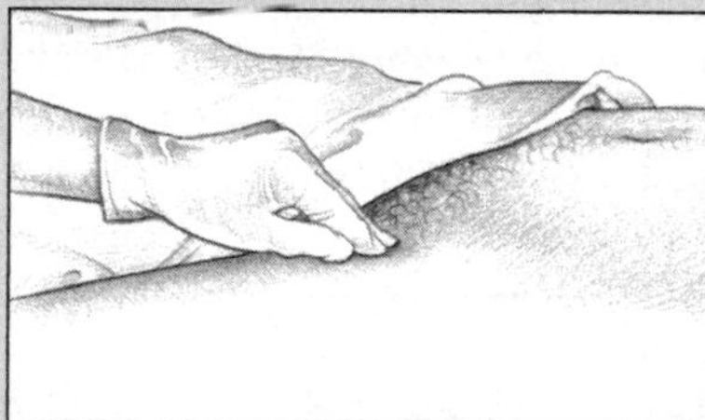

Popliteal pulse

Press firmly in the popliteal fossa at the back of the knee.

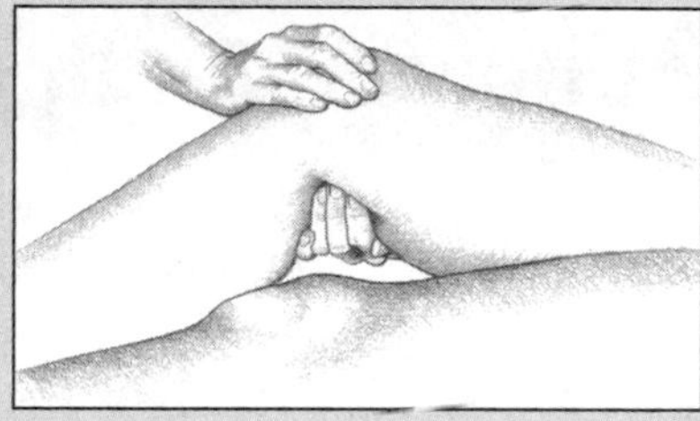

Posterior tibial pulse

Apply pressure behind and slightly below the malleolus of the ankle.

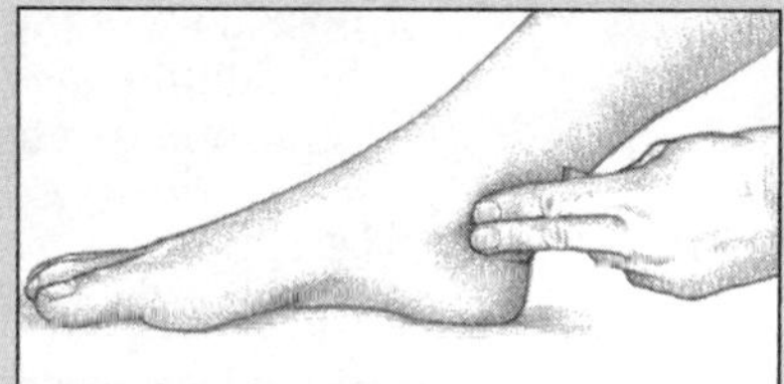

Dorsalis pedis pulse

Place your fingers on the medial dorsum of the foot while the patient points his toes down. The pulse is difficult to palpate here and may seem to be absent in healthy patients.

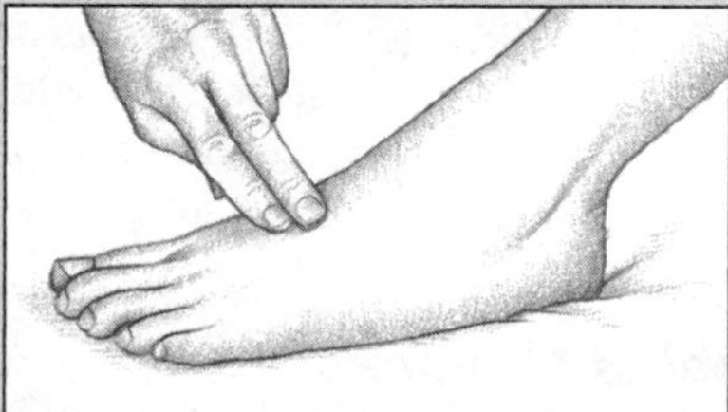

Auscultation

After you palpate, use the bell of the stethoscope to begin auscultation; then follow the palpation sequence and listen over each artery. You shouldn't hear sounds over the carotid arteries. A hum, or bruit, sounds like buzzing or blowing and could indicate arteriosclerotic plaque formation.

Assess the upper abdomen for abnormal pulsations, which could indicate the presence of an abdominal aortic aneurysm. Finally, auscultate for the femoral and popliteal pulses, checking for a bruit or other abnormal sounds.

Abnormal findings

This section outlines some of the most common cardiovascular abnormalities and their causes. (See *Cardiovascular abnormalities*.)

Chest pain

Chest pain can arise suddenly or gradually, and its cause may be difficult to ascertain initially. The pain can radiate to the arms, neck, jaw, or back. It can be steady or intermittent, mild or acute. In addition, the pain can range in character from a sharp, shooting sensation to a feeling of heaviness, fullness, or even indigestion.

Common culprits

Chest pain may be caused by various disorders. Common cardiovascular causes include angina, myocardial infarction, and cardiomyopathy. Chest pain may be provoked or aggravated by stress, anxiety, exertion, deep breathing, or eating certain foods. (See *Chest pain*, pages 199 and 200.)

Palpitations

Palpitations — defined as a conscious awareness of one's heartbeat — are usually felt over the precordium or in the throat or neck. The patient may describe them as pounding, jumping, turning, fluttering or flopping, or as missed or skipped beats. Palpitations may be regular or irregular, fast or slow, paroxysmal or sustained.

Behind the beat

Although usually insignificant, palpitations may result from a cardiac or metabolic disorder or from the effects of certain drugs.

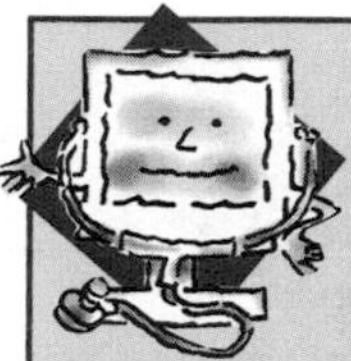

Interpretation station

Cardiovascular abnormalities

This chart shows some common groups of findings for signs and symptoms of the cardiovascular system, along with their probable causes.

Sign or symptom and findings	Probable cause
Fatigue	
• Fatigue following mild activity • Pallor • Tachycardia • Dyspnea	Anemia
• Persistent fatigue unrelated to exertion • Headache • Anorexia • Constipation • Sexual dysfunction • Loss of concentration • Irritability	Depression
• Progressive fatigue • Cardiac murmur • Exertional dyspnea • Cough • Hemoptysis	Valvular heart disease
Palpitations	
• Paroxysmal palpitations • Diaphoresis • Facial flushing • Trembling • Impending sense of doom • Hyperventilation • Dizziness	Acute anxiety attack
***Palpitations** (continued)*	
• Paroxysmal or sustained palpitations • Dizziness • Weakness • Fatigue • Irregular, rapid, or slow pulse rate • Decreased blood pressure • Confusion • Diaphoresis	Cardiac arrhythmias
• Sustained palpitations • Fatigue • Irritability • Hunger • Cold sweats • Tremors • Anxiety	Hypoglycemia
Peripheral edema	
• Headache • Bilateral leg edema with pitting ankle edema • Weight gain despite anorexia • Nausea • Chest tightness • Hypotension • Pallor • Palpitations • Inspiratory crackles	Heart failure

(continued)

Cardiovascular abnormalities *(continued)*

Sign or symptom and findings	Probable cause
Peripheral edema *(continued)*	
• Bilateral arm edema accompanied by facial and neck edema • Edematous areas marked by dilated veins • Headache • Vertigo • Visual disturbances	Superior vena cava syndrome
• Moderate to severe, unilateral or bilateral leg edema • Darkened skin • Stasis ulcers around the ankle	Venous insufficiency

Nonpathologic palpitations may occur with a newly implanted prosthetic valve because the valve's clicking sound heightens the patient's awareness of his heartbeat. Transient palpitations may accompany emotional stress (such as fright, anger, or anxiety) or physical stress (such as exercise or fever). Stimulants such as tobacco and caffeine may also cause palpitations.

Fatigue

Fatigue is a feeling of excessive tiredness, lack of energy, or exhaustion accompanied by a strong desire to rest or sleep. Fatigue is a normal and important response to physical overexertion, prolonged emotional stress, and sleep deprivation. However, it can also be a nonspecific symptom of cardiovascular disease, especially heart failure and valvular heart disease.

Skin and hair abnormalities

Cyanosis, pallor, or cool skin may indicate poor cardiac output and tissue perfusion. Conditions causing fever or increased cardiac output may make the skin warmer than is normal. Absence of body hair on the arms or legs may indicate diminished arterial blood flow to those areas. (See *Findings in arterial and venous insufficiency*, page 201.)

That's just swell

Swelling, or edema, may indicate heart failure or venous insufficiency. It may also result from varicosities or thrombophlebitis.

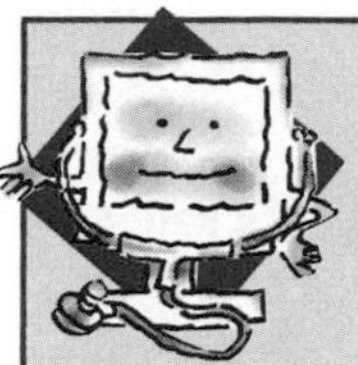

Interpretation station

Chest pain

Use this chart to help you more accurately assess chest pain.

What it feels like	Where it's located	What makes it worse	What causes it	What makes it better
Aching, squeezing, pressure, heaviness, burning pain; usually subsides within 10 minutes	Substernal; may radiate to jaw, neck, arms, and back	Eating, physical effort, smoking, cold weather, stress, anger, hunger, lying down	Angina pectoris	Rest, nitroglycerin, oxygen (*Note:* Unstable angina appears even at rest.)
Tightness or pressure; burning, aching pain, possibly accompanied by shortness of breath, diaphoresis, weakness, anxiety, or nausea; sudden onset; lasts 30 minutes to 2 hours	Typically across chest but may radiate to jaw, neck, arms, or back	Exertion, anxiety	Acute myocardial infarction	Opioid analgesics such as morphine sulfate, nitroglycerin, oxygen, reperfusion of blocked coronary artery
Sharp and continuous; may be accompanied by friction rub; sudden onset	Substernal; may radiate to neck or left arm	Deep breathing, supine position	Pericarditis	Sitting up, leaning forward, anti-inflammatory drugs
Excruciating, tearing pain; may be accompanied by blood pressure difference between right and left arm; sudden onset	Retrosternal, upper abdominal, or epigastric; may radiate to back, neck, or shoulders	Not applicable	Dissecting aortic aneurysm	Analgesics, surgery
Sudden, stabbing pain; may be accompanied by cyanosis, dyspnea, or cough with hemoptysis	Over lung area	Inspiration	Pulmonary embolus	Analgesics
Sudden and severe pain, sometimes accompanied by dyspnea, increased pulse rate, decreased breath sounds (especially on one side), or deviated trachea	Lateral thorax	Normal respiration	Pneumothorax	Analgesics, chest tube insertion
Dull, pressurelike, squeezing pain	Substernal, epigastric areas	Food, cold liquids, exercise	Esophageal spasm	Nitroglycerin, calcium channel blockers
Sharp, severe pain	Lower chest or upper abdomen	Eating a heavy meal, bending, lying down	Hiatal hernia	Antacids, walking, semi-Fowler's position

(continued)

Chest pain *(continued)*

What it feels like	Where it's located	What makes it worse	What causes it	What makes it better
Burning feeling after eating sometimes accompanied by hematemesis or tarry stools; sudden onset that generally subsides within 15 to 20 minutes	Epigastric	Lack of food or highly acidic foods	Peptic ulcer	Food, antacids
Gripping, sharp pain; possibly nausea and vomiting	Right epigastric or abdominal areas; possible radiation to shoulders	Eating fatty foods, lying down	Cholecystitis	Rest and analgesics, surgery
Continuous or intermittent sharp pain; possibly tender to touch; gradual or sudden onset	Anywhere in chest	Movement, palpation	Chest-wall syndrome	Time, analgesics, heat applications
Dull or stabbing pain usually accompanied by hyperventilation or breathlessness; sudden onset; lasting less than 1 minute or as long as several days	Anywhere in chest	Increased respiratory rate, stress or anxiety	Acute anxiety	Slowing of respiratory rate, stress relief

Chronic right-sided heart failure may cause ascites and generalized edema. Right-sided heart failure may cause swelling in the lower legs. If the patient has compression of a vein in a specific area, he may have localized swelling along the path of the compressed vessel.

Abnormal pulsations

A displaced apical impulse may indicate an enlarged left ventricle, which may be caused by heart failure or hypertension. A forceful apical impulse, or one lasting longer than a third of the cardiac cycle, may point to increased cardiac output. If you find a pulsation in the patient's aortic, pulmonic, or tricuspid area, his heart chamber may be enlarged or he may have valvular disease.

Pulses here, there, everywhere

Increased cardiac output or an aortic aneurysm may also produce pulsations in the aortic area. A patient with an epigastric pulsation may have early heart failure or an aortic aneurysm. A pulsation in the sternoclavicular area suggests an aortic aneurysm. A patient

Findings in arterial and venous insufficiency

Assessment findings differ in patients with arterial insufficiency and those with chronic venous insufficiency. These illustrations show those differences.

Arterial insufficiency

In a patient with arterial insufficiency, pulses may be decreased or absent. The skin will be cool, pale, and shiny, and the patient may have pain in the legs and feet. Ulcerations typically occur in the area around the toes, and the foot usually turns deep red when dependent. Nails may be thick and ridged.

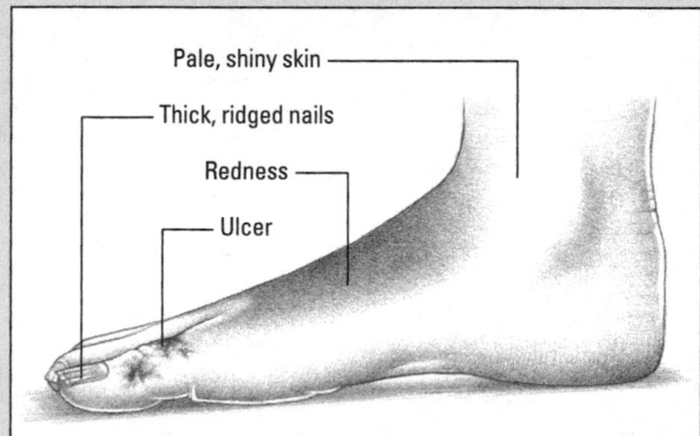

Chronic venous insufficiency

In a patient with chronic venous insufficiency, check for ulcerations around the ankle. Pulses are present but may be difficult to find because of edema. The foot may become cyanotic when dependent.

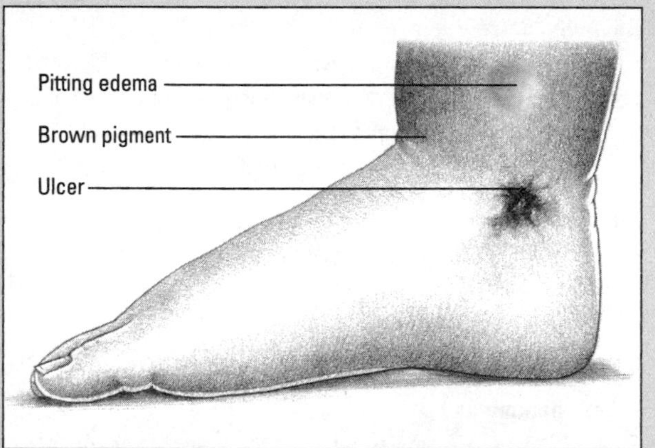

with anemia, anxiety, increased cardiac output, or a thin chest wall may have slight pulsations to the right and left of the sternum.

Weak ones, strong ones

A weak arterial pulse may indicate decreased cardiac output or increased peripheral vascular resistance, both of which point to arterial atherosclerotic disease. Many elderly patients have weak pedal pulses.

Strong or bounding pulsations usually occur in a patient with a condition that causes increased cardiac output, such as hypertension, hypoxia, anemia, exercise, or anxiety. (See *Pulse waveforms*, page 202.)

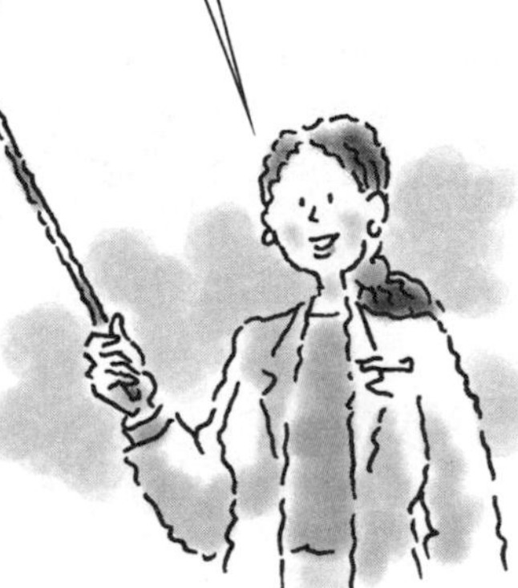

Thrills and heaves

A thrill, which is a palpable vibration, usually suggests a valvular dysfunction. A heave, lifting of the chest wall felt during palpation, along the left sternal border may mean

Pulse waveforms

To identify abnormal arterial pulses, check these waveforms and see which one matches the patient's peripheral pulse.

Weak pulse
A weak pulse has a decreased amplitude with a slower upstroke and downstroke. Possible causes of a weak pulse include increased peripheral vascular resistance, as occurs in cold weather or with severe heart failure, and decreased stroke volume, as occurs with hypovolemia or aortic stenosis.

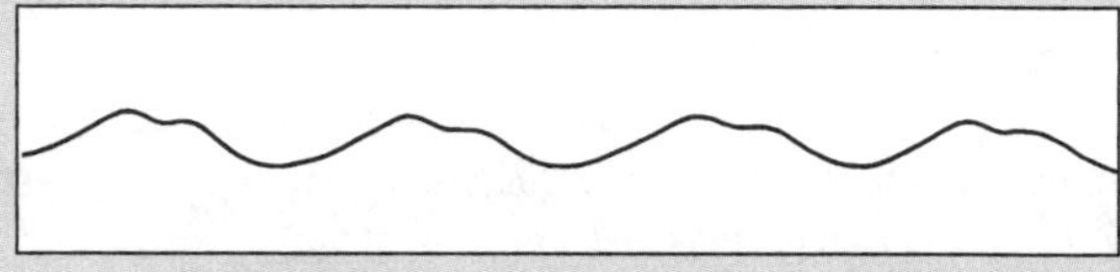

Bounding pulse
A bounding pulse has a sharp upstroke and downstroke with a pointed peak. The amplitude is elevated. Possible causes of a bounding pulse include increased stroke volume, as with aortic insufficiency, or stiffness of arterial walls, as with aging.

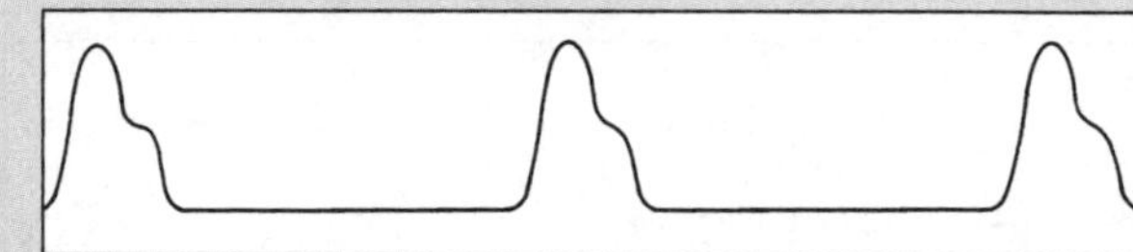

Pulsus alternans
Pulsus alternans has a regular, alternating pattern of a weak and a strong pulse. This pulse is associated with left-sided heart failure.

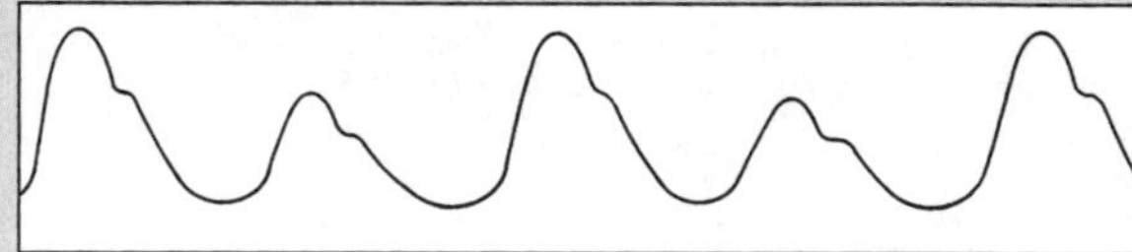

Pulsus bigeminus
Pulsus bigeminus is similar to pulsus alternans but occurs at irregular intervals. This pulse is caused by premature atrial or ventricular beats.

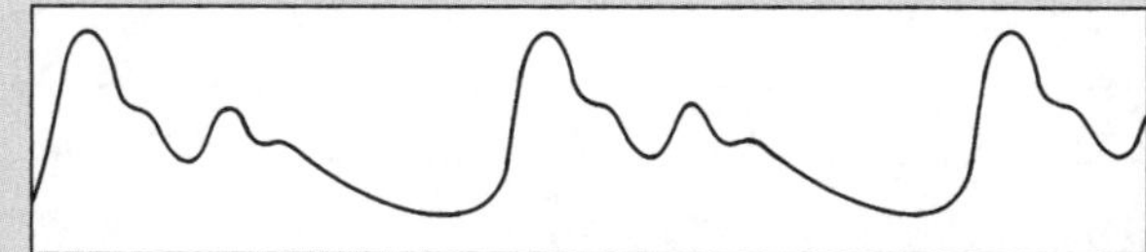

Pulsus paradoxus
Pulsus paradoxus has increases and decreases in amplitude associated with the respiratory cycle. Marked decreases occur when the patient inhales. Pulsus paradoxus is associated with pericardial tamponade, advanced heart failure, and constrictive pericarditis.

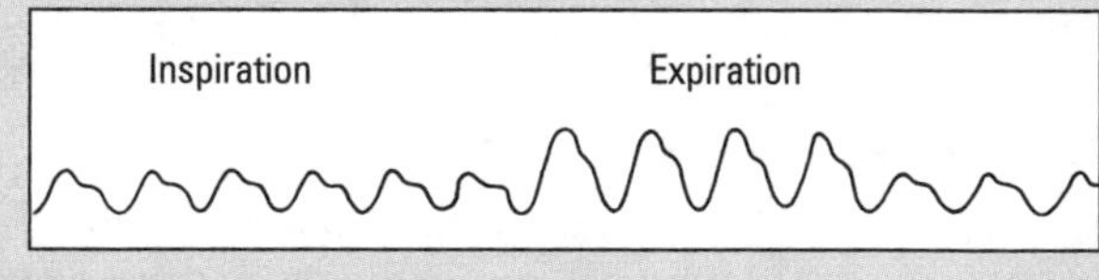

Pulsus biferiens
Pulsus biferiens shows an initial upstroke, a subsequent downstroke, and then another upstroke during systole. Pulsus biferiens is caused by aortic stenosis and aortic insufficiency.

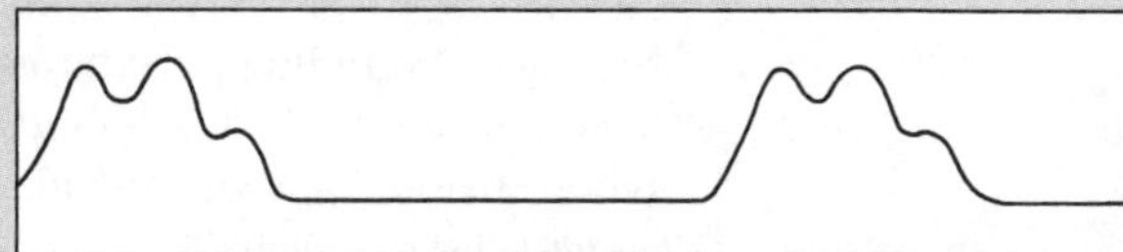

right ventricular hypertrophy; over the left ventricular area, a ventricular aneurysm.

Abnormal sounds

Abnormal auscultation findings include abnormal heart sounds (see *Abnormal heart sounds*, page 204), heart murmurs, and bruits.

Murmurs

Murmurs can occur as a result of a number of conditions and have widely varied characteristics. Here's a rundown on some of the more common murmur types.

Low-pitched murmur

Aortic stenosis, a condition in which the aortic valve has calcified and restricts blood flow, causes a midsystolic, low-pitched, harsh murmur that radiates from the valve to the carotid artery.

Going back and forth

This murmur shifts from crescendo to decrescendo and back. *Crescendo* is a term used to describe the configuration of a murmur that increases in intensity. Likewise, a *decrescendo* murmur decreases in intensity. The crescendo-decrescendo murmur of aortic stenosis results from the turbulent, highly pressured flow of blood across stiffened leaflets and through a narrowed opening.

Medium-pitched murmur

During auscultation, listen for a murmur near the pulmonic valve. This murmur might indicate pulmonic stenosis, a condition in which the pulmonic valve has calcified and interferes with the flow of blood out of the right ventricle.

That sounds so harsh

This murmur is medium-pitched, systolic, and harsh and shifts from crescendo to decrescendo and back. It's caused by turbulent blood flow across a stiffened, narrowed valve.

High-pitched murmurs

In a patient with aortic insufficiency, the blood flows backward through the aortic valve and causes a high-pitched, blowing, decrescendo, diastolic murmur. This murmur radiates from the aortic valve area to the left sternal border.

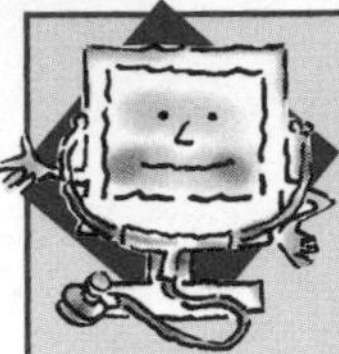

Interpretation station

Abnormal heart sounds

Whenever auscultation reveals an abnormal heart sound, try to identify the sound and its timing in the cardiac cycle. Knowing those characteristics can help you identify the possible cause for the sound. Use this chart to put all that information together.

Abnormal heart sound	Timing	Possible causes
Accentuated S_1	Beginning of systole	Mitral stenosis or fever
Diminished S_1	Beginning of systole	Mitral insufficiency, heart block, or severe mitral insufficiency with a calcified, immobile valve
Split S_1	Beginning of systole	Right bundle-branch block (BBB) or premature ventricular contractions
Accentuated S_2	End of systole	Pulmonary or systemic hypertension
Diminished or inaudible S_2	End of systole	Aortic or pulmonic stenosis
Persistent S_2 split	End of systole	Delayed closure of the pulmonic valve, usually from overfilling of the right ventricle, causing prolonged systolic ejection time
Reversed or paradoxical S_2 split that appears during exhalation and disappears during inspiration	End of systole	Delayed ventricular stimulation, left BBB, or prolonged left ventricular ejection time
S_3 (ventricular gallop)	Early diastole	Overdistention of the ventricles during the rapid-filling segment of diastole or mitral insufficiency of ventricular failure (normal in children and young adults)
S_4 (atrial or presystolic gallop)	Late diastole	Pulmonic stenosis, hypertension, coronary artery disease, aortic stenosis, or forceful atrial contraction due to resistance to ventricular filling late in diastole (resulting from left ventricular hypertrophy)
Pericardial friction rub (grating or leathery sound at the left sternal border; usually muffled, high-pitched, and transient)	Throughout systole and diastole	Pericardial inflammation

Wrong way!

In a patient with pulmonic insufficiency, the blood flows backward through the pulmonic valve, causing a blowing, diastolic, decrescendo murmur at Erb's point (at the left sternal border of the third intercostal space). If the patient has a higher-than-normal pulmonary pressure, the murmur is high-pitched. If not, it will be low-pitched.

A murmur is never just a murmur. Variations in sound provide clues about the patient's underlying heart condition.

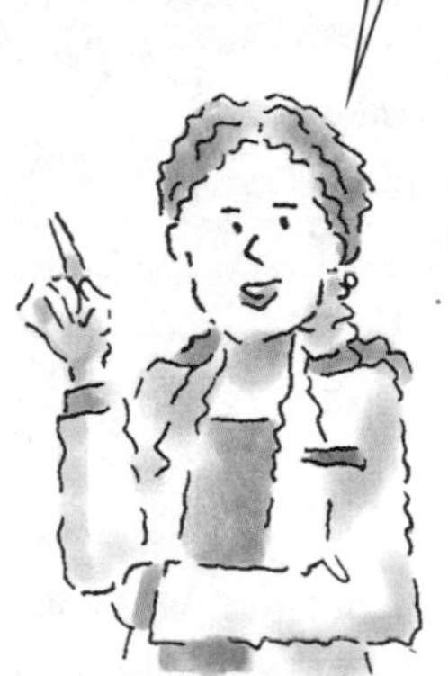

Rumbling murmur

Mitral stenosis is a condition in which the mitral valve has calcified and is blocking blood flow out of the left atrium. Listen for a low-pitched, rumbling, crescendo-decrescendo murmur in the mitral valve area. This murmur results from turbulent blood flow across the stiffened, narrowed valve.

Blowing murmur

In a patient with mitral insufficiency, blood regurgitates into the left atrium. The regurgitation produces a high-pitched, blowing murmur throughout systole (pansystolic or holosystolic). This murmur may radiate from the mitral area to the left axillary line. You can hear it best at the apex.

Low, rumbling murmur

Tricuspid stenosis is a condition in which the tricuspid valve has calcified and is blocking blood flow through the valve from the right atrium. Listen for a low, rumbling, crescendo-decrescendo murmur in the tricuspid area. This murmur results from turbulent blood flow across the stiffened, narrowed valvular leaflets.

High-pitched, blowing murmur

In a patient with tricuspid insufficiency, blood regurgitates into the right atrium. This backflow of blood through the valve causes a high-pitched, blowing murmur throughout systole in the tricuspid area. This murmur becomes louder when the patient inhales.

Bruits

A murmurlike sound of vascular (rather than cardiac) origin is called a *bruit.* If you hear a bruit during arterial auscultation, the patient may have occlusive arterial disease or an arteriovenous fistula. Various high cardiac output conditions—such as anemia, hyperthyroidism, and pheochromocytoma—may also cause bruits.

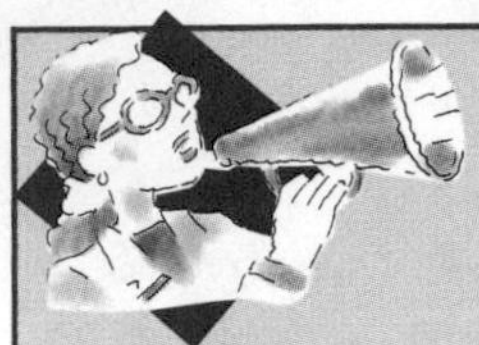

That's a wrap!

Cardiovascular system review

Structures

Heart

- A hollow, muscular organ that pumps blood to all organs and tissues of the body
- Protected by a thin sac called the *pericardium*
- Consists of four chambers: two atria and two ventricles
- Contains valves to keep blood flowing in only one direction
- Contracts to send blood out (systole), then relaxes and fills with blood (diastole)

Vascular system

- Arteries: thick-walled vessels that carry oxygenated blood away from the heart
- Veins: thin-walled vessels that carry deoxygenated blood toward the heart
- Pulses: pressure waves of blood generated by the pumping action of the heart

Blood circulation

- Deoxygenated venous blood flows from the superior vena cava, inferior vena cava, and coronary sinus into the right atrium.
- Blood flows from the right atrium through the tricuspid valve and into the right ventricle.
- Blood is then ejected through the pulmonic valve into the pulmonary artery, where it travels to the lungs for oxygenation.
- Oxygenated blood then flows through the pulmonary veins and returns to the left atrium.
- Blood passes through the mitral valve and into the left ventricle.
- Blood is pumped through the aortic valve and into the aorta for delivery to the rest of the body.

Obtaining a health history

- Ask about current problems, including chest pain, palpitations, shortness of breath, peripheral skin changes, and changes in extremities.
- Have the patient rate his chest pain on a scale of 0 to 10, with 0 being no pain and 10 being the worst pain imaginable.
- Ask about a family history of cardiovascular disease, diabetes, and chronic diseases of the lungs or kidneys.

Assessing the heart

- Inspect the patient's general appearance, noting skin color, temperature, turgor, and texture.
- Inspect the chest, noting the location of the apical impulse.
- Palpate over the precordium to find the apical impulse.
- Palpate the sternoclavicular, aortic, pulmonic, tricuspid, and epigastric areas for abnormal pulsations.
- Percuss the chest wall to locate cardiac borders.
- Auscultate for heart sounds with the patient lying on his back with the head of the bed raised 30 to 45 degrees, with him sitting up, and with him lying on his left side.
- Auscultate for murmurs by asking the patient to sit up and lean forward or having him lie on his left side.
- Auscultate for a pericardial friction rub by asking the patient to sit upright, lean forward, and exhale.

Cardiovascular system review *(continued)*

Heart sounds

- S_1: best heard at the apex of the heart; corresponds to closure of the mitral and tricuspid valves
- S_2: best heard at the base of the heart; corresponds to closure of the pulmonic and aortic valves
- S_3: commonly heard in patients with high cardiac output or heart failure (called *ventricular gallop*); a normal finding in children and young adults
- S_4: adventitious sound called *atrial gallop;* heard in patients who are elderly or in those with hypertension, aortic stenosis, or a history of myocardial infarction

Assessing the vascular system

- Inspect the patient's general appearance, skin, and fingernails and toenails.
- Check the carotid artery pulsations and the jugular venous pulse.
- Palpate the patient's skin over the upper and lower extremities for temperature, texture, and turgor.
- Check capillary refill time (should be less than 3 seconds).
- Palpate arterial pulses on each side of the body, moving from head-to-toe (temporal, carotid, brachial, radial, femoral, popliteal, posterior tibial, and dorsalis pedis arteries, in that order).
- Auscultate over each artery in this same order, listening for hums or bruits.

Abnormal findings

- Chest pain: sensation that varies in severity and presentation depending on the cause
- Palpitations: a conscious awareness of one's heartbeat
- Fatigue: a feeling of excessive tiredness, lack of energy, or exhaustion accompanied by a strong desire to rest or sleep
- Thrill: palpable vibration indicating valvular dysfunction
- Heave: lifting of the chest wall felt during palpation; indicates ventricular hypertrophy (when felt on the sternal border) or ventricular aneurysm (when felt over the left ventricle)
- Murmur: sound made by turbulent blood flow; may increase in intensity (crescendo) or decrease in intensity (decrescendo)
- Bruit: a murmurlike sound heard over blood vessels

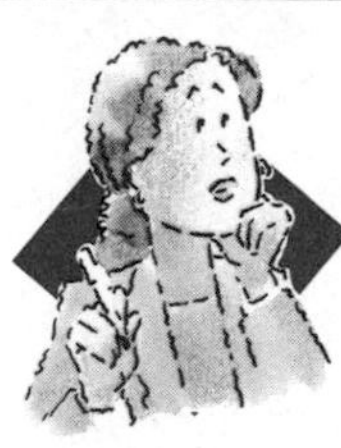

Quick quiz

1. When listening to heart sounds, you can hear S_1 best at the:
A. base of the heart.
B. apex of the heart.
C. second intercostal space to the right of the sternum.
D. fifth intercostal space to the right of the sternum.

Answer: B. S_1 is best heard at the apex of the heart.

2. You're auscultating for heart sounds in a 3-year-old girl and hear an S_3. You assess this sound to be a:

A. normal finding.
B. probable sign of heart failure.
C. possible sign of atrial septal defect.
D. possible sign of patent ductus arteriosus.

Answer: A. S_3 is a normal finding in a child. This sound can indicate heart failure in an adult.

3. Capillary refill time is normally:

A. 1 to 3 seconds.
B. 4 to 6 seconds.
C. 7 to 10 seconds.
D. 11 to 15 seconds.

Answer: A. Capillary refill time that's longer than 3 seconds is considered delayed and indicates decreased perfusion.

4. As you auscultate heart sounds in a 53-year-old patient you hear an S_4. This sound may indicate:

A. heart failure.
B. a normal finding in the last trimester of pregnancy.
C. ventricular gallop
D. hypertension.

Answer: D. An S_4 may be heard in patients who are elderly or in those with hypertension, aortic stenosis, or a history of MI.

5. You suspect that your patient has a pericardial friction rub but you have trouble hearing it. What should you do?

A. Ask the patient to hold his breath.
B. Ask the patient to exhale forcefully.
C. Ask the patient to lie on his left side.
D. Ask the patient to lie flat on his back.

Answer: A. If you suspect a pericardial rub but have trouble hearing one, ask the patient to hold his breath.

Scoring

☆☆☆ If you answered all five questions correctly, take a bow! You're a star of the heart.

☆☆ If you answered four questions correctly, sensational! You're pumped with information.

☆ If you answered fewer than four questions correctly, keep at it! You're just getting into the rhythm.

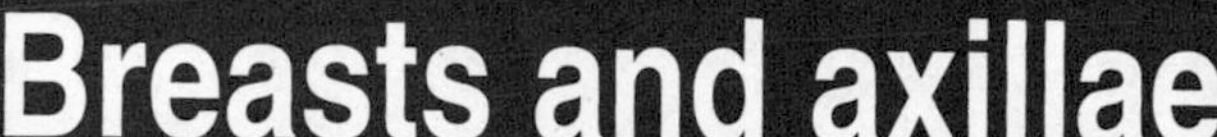

Breasts and axillae

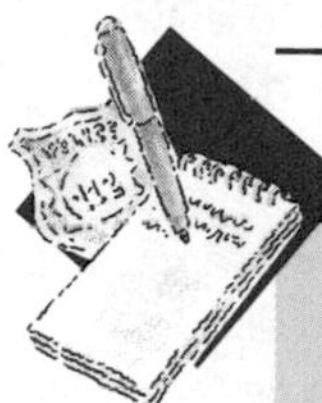

Just the facts

In this chapter, you'll learn:

- structures that make up the breasts
- breast changes that occur with age, pregnancy, and other conditions
- the proper way to obtain a patient history about breasts
- techniques for performing a physical assessment of the breasts and axillae
- causes of breast and axillae abnormalities and how to recognize them.

A look at the breasts and axillae

With breast cancer becoming increasingly prominent in the news, more women are aware of the disease's risk factors, treatments, and diagnostic measures. By staying informed and performing breast self-examinations regularly, women can take control of their health and seek medical care when they notice a change in their breasts.

Breast self-examinations empower the patient to take control of her own health.

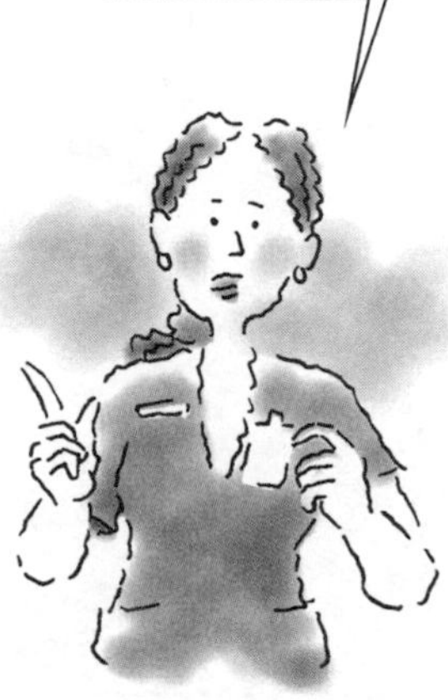

A delicate matter

No matter how informed a woman is, she can still feel anxious during breast examinations, even if she hasn't noticed a problem. That's because the social and psychological significance of female breasts goes far beyond their biological function. The breast is more than just a delicate structure; it's a delicate subject. Keep this in mind during your assessment. It will let you proceed carefully and professionally, helping your patient feel more at ease.

Anatomy of the breasts

The breasts, also called *mammary glands* in women, lie on the anterior chest wall. (See *The female breast.*) They're located vertically between the second or third and the sixth or seventh ribs over the pectoralis major muscle and the serratus anterior muscle, and horizontally between the sternal border and the midaxillary line.

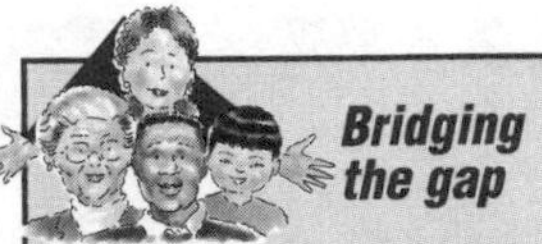

Differences in areola pigmentation

The pigment of the nipple and areola vary among different races, getting darker as skin tone darkens. Whites have light-colored nipples and areolae, usually pink or light beige. People with darker complexions, such as Blacks and Asians, have medium brown to almost black nipples and areolae.

Breast structures

Each breast has a centrally located nipple of pigmented erectile tissue ringed by an areola that's darker than the adjacent tissue. (See *Differences in areola pigmentation.*) Sebaceous glands, also called *Montgomery's tubercles*, are scattered on the areola surface, along with hair follicles.

Support structures

Beneath the skin are glandular, fibrous, and fatty tissues that vary in proportion with age, weight, gender, and other factors such as pregnancy. A small triangle of tissue, called the *tail of Spence*, projects into the axilla. Attached to the chest wall musculature are

The female breast

This illustration shows a lateral cross section of the female breast.

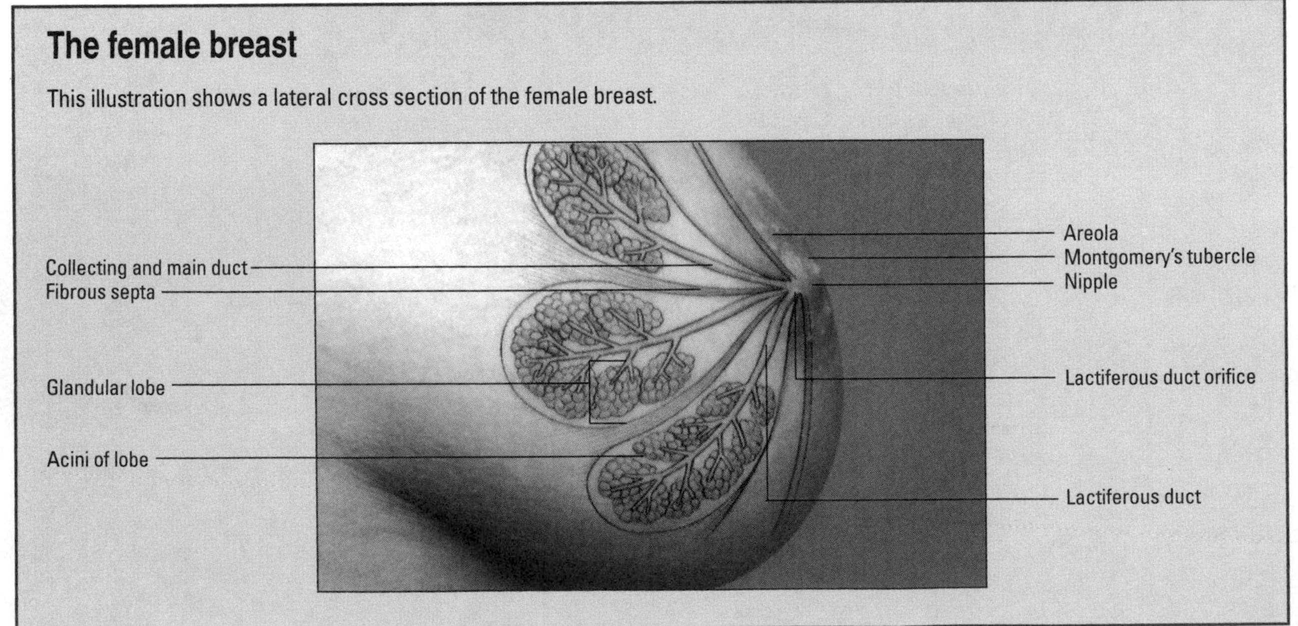

fibrous bands, called *Cooper's ligaments*, that support each breast.

The breasts have several lymph node chains that drain various areas, including the chest wall and arms.

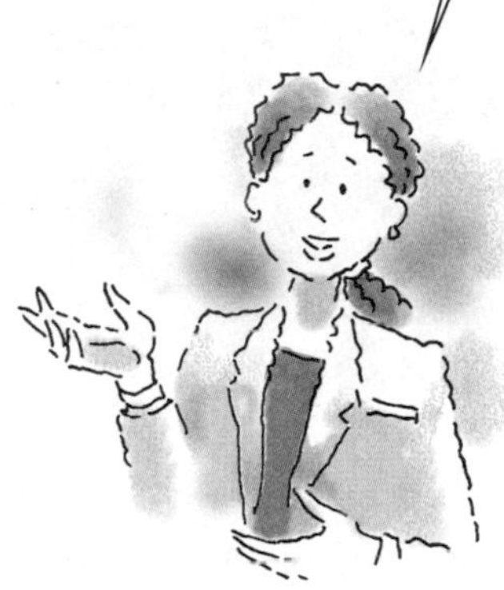

Lobes and ducts

In women, each breast is surrounded by 12 to 25 glandular lobes containing alveoli that produce milk. The lactiferous ducts from each lobe transport milk to the nipple. In men, the breast has a nipple, an areola, and mostly flat tissue bordering the chest wall.

Lymph nodes

The breasts also hold several lymph node chains, each serving different areas. The pectoral lymph nodes drain lymph fluid from most of the breast and anterior chest. The brachial nodes drain most of the arm. The subscapular nodes drain the posterior chest wall and part of the arm. The midaxillary nodes, located near the ribs and the serratus anterior muscle high in the axilla, are the central draining nodes for the pectoral, brachial, and subscapular nodes.

For the ladies

In women, the internal mammary nodes drain the mammary lobes. The superficial lymphatic vessels drain the skin.

Cancer route

In both men and women, the lymphatic system is the most common route of spread of cells that cause breast cancer. (See *Lymph node chains*, page 212.)

How the breasts change with age

A woman's breasts make many transformations throughout the life cycle. Their appearance starts changing at puberty and continues changing during the reproductive years, pregnancy, and menopause. (See *Breast changes throughout life*, page 213.)

Changes during puberty

Breast development is an early sign of puberty in girls. It usually occurs between ages 8 and 13. Menarche, the start of the menstrual cycle, typically occurs about 2 years later. Development of breast tissue in girls younger than age 8 is abnormal, and the patient should be referred to a doctor.

Lymph node chains

This illustration shows the different lymph node chains in the breast, axilla, and upper arm.

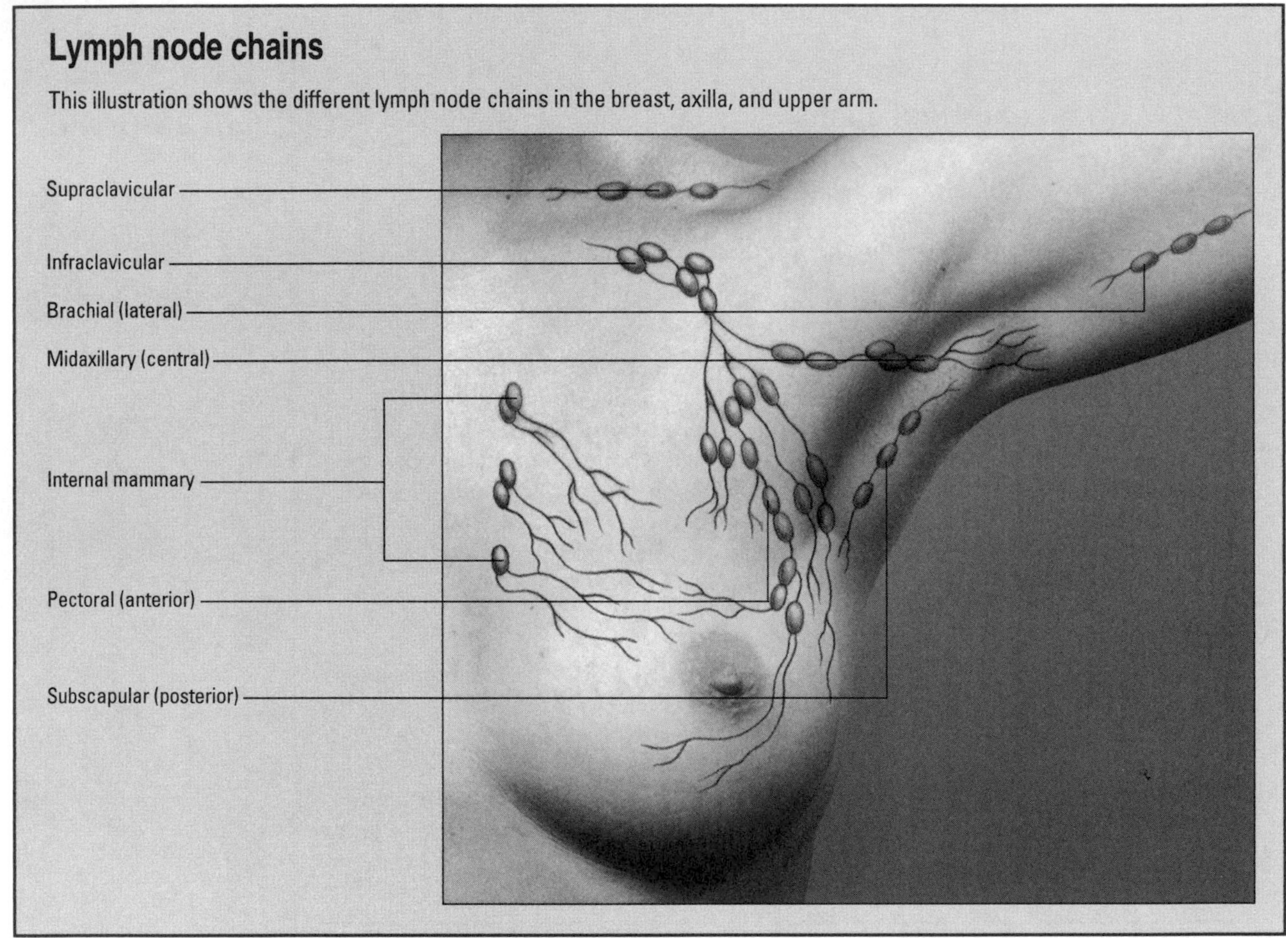

In the beginning…

Breast development usually starts with the breast and nipple protruding as a single mound of flesh. The shape of the adult female breast is formed gradually. During puberty, breast development is commonly unilateral or asymmetrical.

Changes during the reproductive years

During the reproductive years, a woman's breasts may become full or tender in response to hormonal fluctuations during the menstrual cycle.

Altered state

During pregnancy, breast changes occur in response to hormones from the corpus luteum and the placenta. The areola becomes

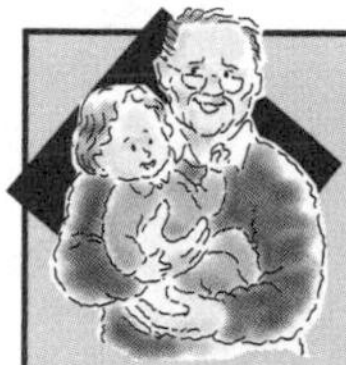

Ages and stages

Breast changes throughout life

These illustrations show how a woman's breasts typically change from before puberty through menopause.

Before age 8

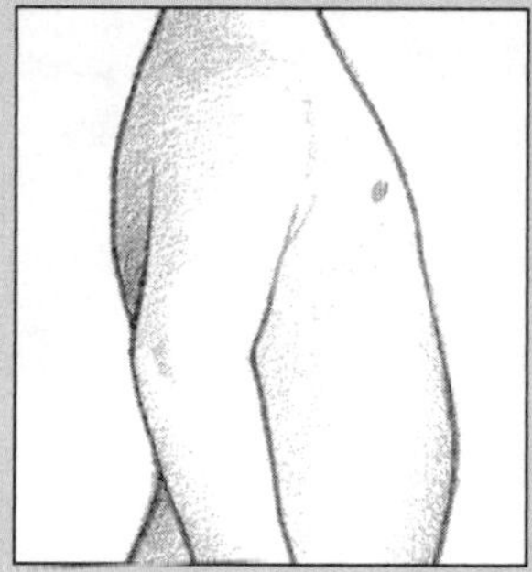

Between ages 10 and 14

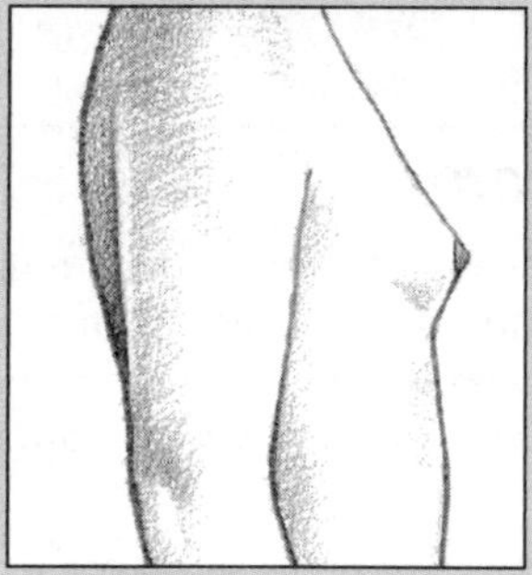

During adulthood (having never given birth)

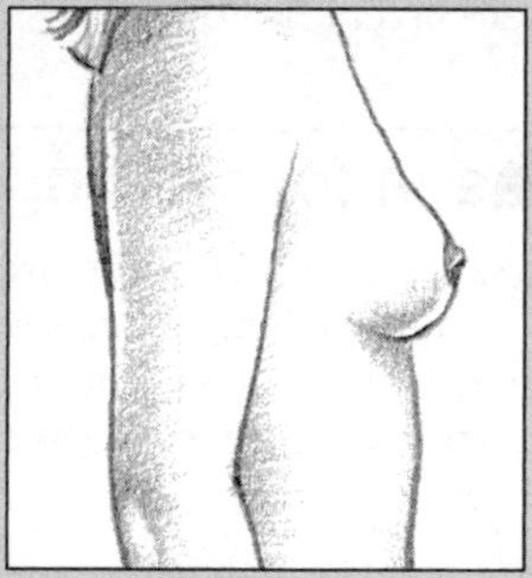

During pregnancy

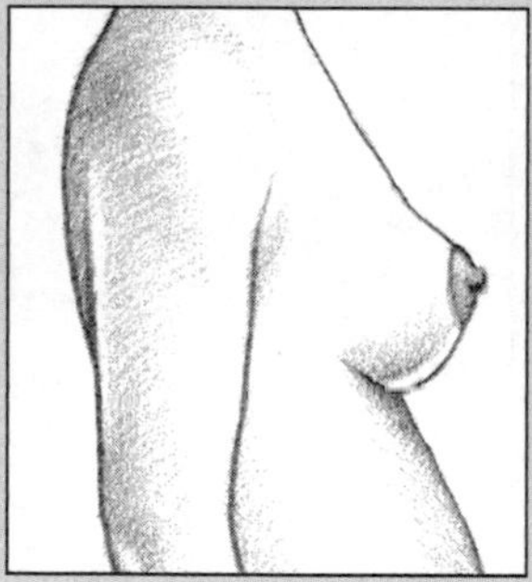

After pregnancy

After menopause

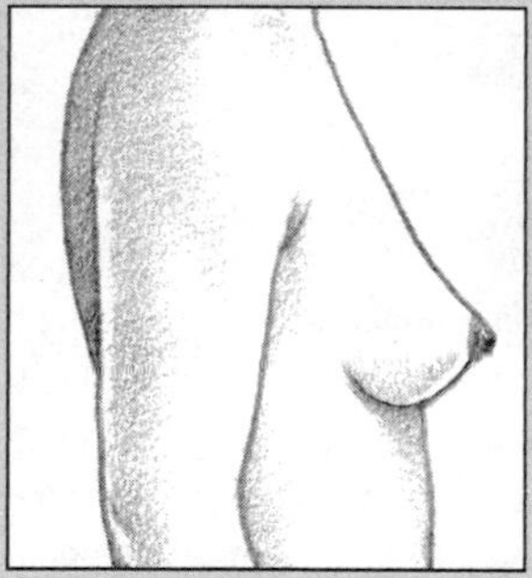

After menopause, decreased estrogen levels cause glandular tissue in the breast to atrophy.

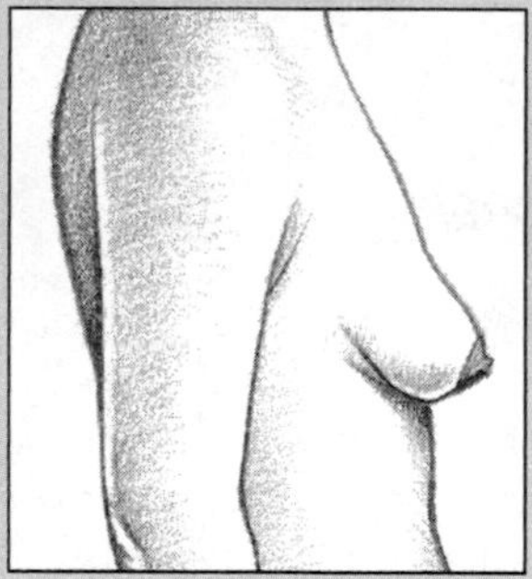

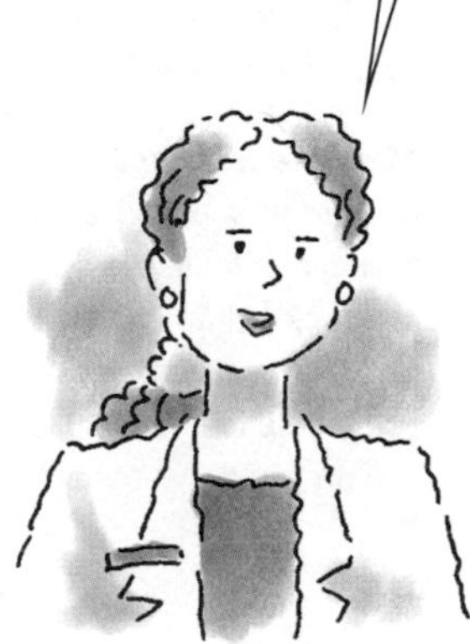

deeply pigmented and increases in diameter. The nipple becomes darker, more prominent, and erect. The breasts enlarge because of the proliferation and hypertrophy of the alveolar cells and lactiferous ducts. As veins engorge, a venous pattern may become visible. In addition, striae may appear as a result of stretching, and Montgomery's tubercles may become prominent.

Changes after menopause

After menopause, estrogen levels decrease, causing glandular tissue to atrophy and be replaced with fatty deposits. The breasts become flabbier and smaller than they were before menopause. As the ligaments relax, the breasts hang loosely from the chest. The nipples flatten, losing some of their erectile quality. The ducts around the nipples may feel like firm strings.

Obtaining a health history

You'll typically begin your health history by asking the patient about her reason for seeking care. You'll then want to ask the patient questions about her personal and family medical history as well as her current health.

Asking about the reason for seeking care

Common complaints about the breasts include breast pain, nipple discharge and rash, lumps, masses, and other changes. Complaints such as these — whether they come from women or men — warrant further investigation. (See *Male concerns* and *Evaluating breast lumps*.)

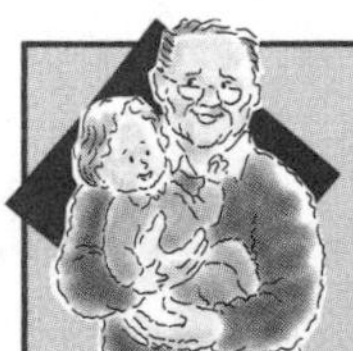

Ages and stages

Male concerns

Keep in mind that men also need breast examinations and that the incidence of breast cancer in males is rising. Men with breast disorders may feel uneasy or embarrassed about being examined because they see their condition as being unmanly. Remember that a man needs a gentle, professional hand as much as a woman does.

Male breast cancer and gynecomastia

Be sure to examine a man's breasts thoroughly during a complete physical assessment. Don't overlook palpation of the nipple and areola in male patients; assess for the same changes you would in a woman. Breast cancer in men usually occurs in the areolar area.

Gynecomastia is abnormal enlargement of the male breast. It may be caused by cirrhosis, leukemia, thyrotoxicosis, the administration of a hormone, illicit drug use (especially marijuana and heroin), alcohol consumption, or a hormonal imbalance.

Breasts in boys and older men

Adolescent boys may have temporary stimulation of breast tissue caused by the hormone estrogen, which is produced in males *and* females. Breast enlargement in boys usually stops when they begin producing adequate amounts of the male sex hormone testosterone. Older men may experience gynecomastia as a result of age-related hormonal alterations or an adverse effect of certain medications.

Evaluating breast lumps

If you find a breast lump during your assessment, evaluate it using this flowchart. Masses may be further investigated with a biopsy.

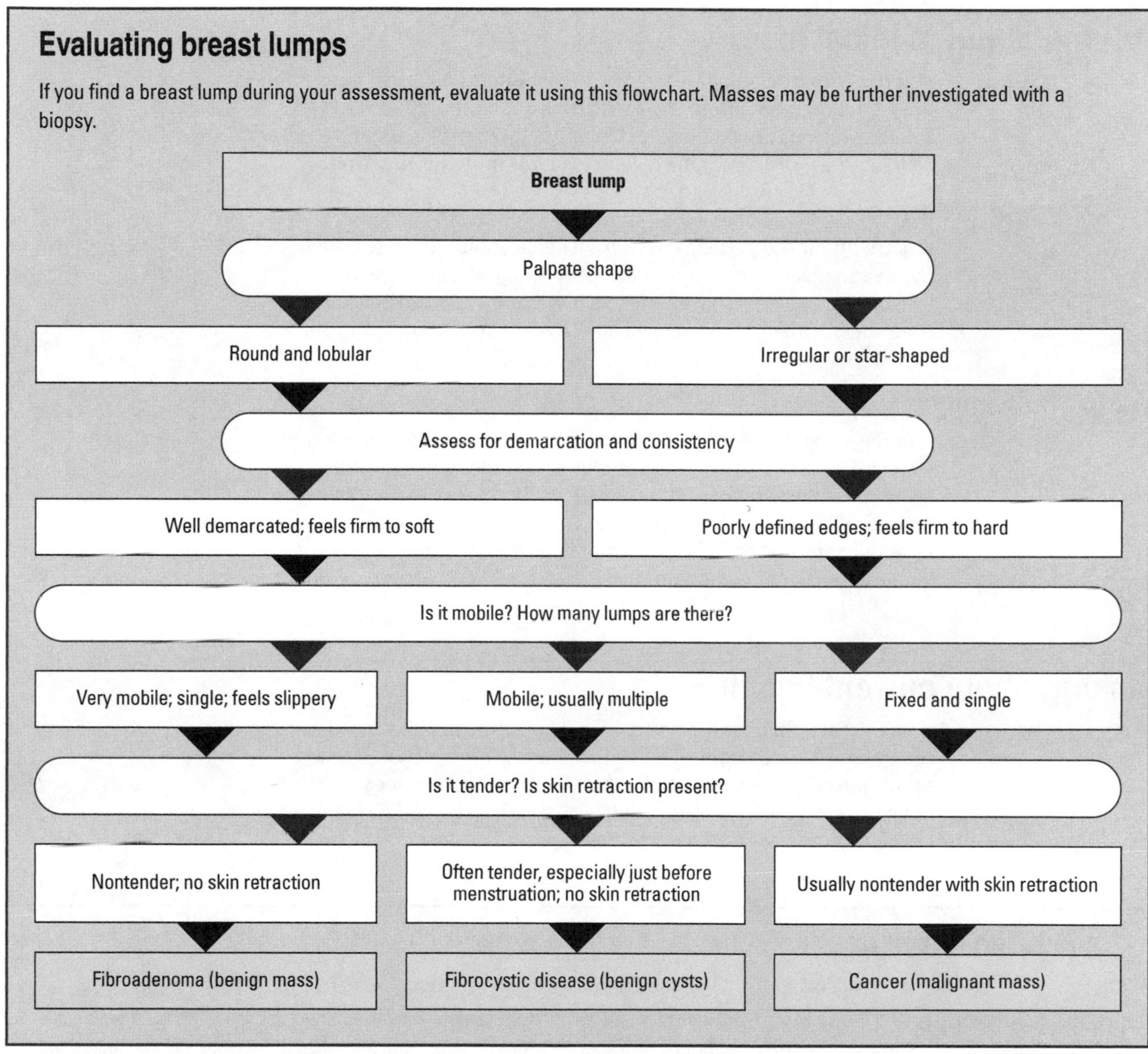

Dig deeper

To investigate these complaints, ask about the symptom's onset, duration, and severity. What day of the menstrual cycle do the signs or symptoms appear, if applicable? What relieves or worsens them?

Asking about medical history

Ask the patient if she has ever had breast lumps, a biopsy, or breast surgery, including enlargement or reduction. Also ask if she has a history of breast disease. If she has had breast cancer, fibroadenoma, or fibrocystic disease, ask for more information.

Periods and pregnancies

Inquire about the patient's menstrual cycle and record the date of her last menses. If the patient has been pregnant, ask how many pregnancies and live births she has had. How old was she each time she became pregnant? Did she have complications? Did she breast-feed?

All in the family

Ask the patient if any family members have had breast disorders, especially breast cancer. Also ask about the incidence of other types of cancer. Having a close relative with breast cancer greatly increases the patient's risk of having the disease. Teach the patient how to examine her breasts and the importance of regular breast examinations and mammograms. (See *Scheduling breast examinations.*)

Asking about current health

Some breast changes are a normal part of aging, so be sure to ask the patient how old she is. If she has noticed breast changes, ask her to describe them in detail. When did they occur? Does she have pain, tenderness, discharge, or rash? Has she had changes in her underarm area?

Scheduling breast examinations

The American Cancer Society and the American College of Radiology recommend the schedule shown here for regular breast examinations. Depending on their needs, some patients may follow schedules that have been modified by their doctors. Women with a family history of or a genetic predisposition for breast cancer—as well as women who have a personal history of cancer—may need earlier or more frequent screening tests and examinations.

Age	Breast self-examination (optional)	Mammography	Clinical breast examination
20 to 39	Monthly, 7 to 10 days after menses begins	Not recommended	Every 3 years
40 and older	Monthly, 7 to 10 days after menses begins	Yearly	Yearly

Down on the pharm

Ask the patient what drugs she takes regularly, such as birth control pills, contraceptive patches, or a vaginal ring with estrogen. Birth control pills can cause breast swelling and tenderness. Ask about her diet, especially caffeine intake. Caffeine has been linked to fibrocystic disease of the breasts. Ask the patient if she's under a lot of stress, smokes, or drinks alcohol. Discuss the possible link between those factors and breast cancer.

Hear ye! Hear ye! Let it be known that birth control pills can make the breasts swollen and tender!

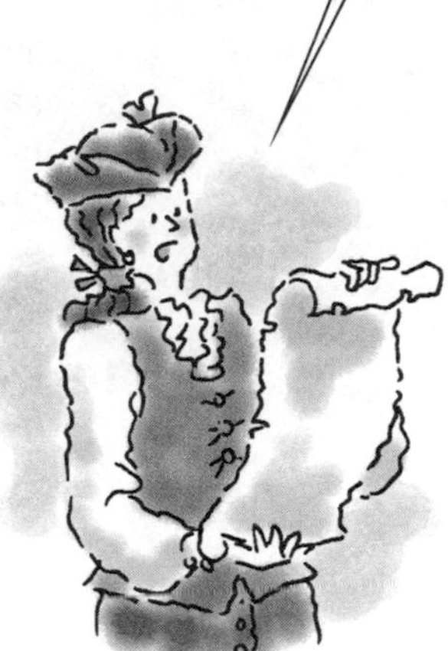

Assessing the breasts and axillae

Having a breast examination can be stressful for a woman. To reduce your patient's anxiety, provide privacy, make her as comfortable as possible, and explain what the examination involves.

Examining the breasts

Before examining the breasts, make sure the room is well lighted. Have the patient disrobe from the waist up and sit with her arms at her sides. Keep both breasts uncovered so you can observe them simultaneously to detect differences.

Inspection

Breast skin should be smooth, undimpled, and the same color as the rest of the skin. Check for edema, which can accompany lymphatic obstruction and may signal cancer. Note breast size and symmetry. Asymmetry may occur normally in some adult women, with the left breast usually larger than the right. Inspect the nipples, noting their size and shape. If a nipple is inverted, dimpled, or creased, ask the patient when she first noticed the abnormality.

Assume the position

Next, inspect the patient's breasts while she holds her arms over her head, and then again while she has her hands on her hips. Having the patient assume these positions will help you detect skin or nipple dimpling that might not have been obvious before.

Alternate pose

If the patient has large or pendulous breasts, have her stand with her hands on the back of a chair and lean forward. This position helps reveal subtle breast or nipple asymmetry.

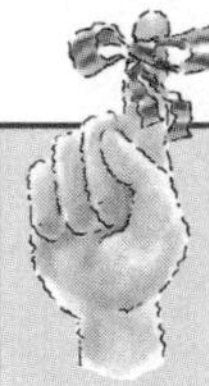

Memory jogger

To remember what to look for as you assess the nipple, think of the word **DISC.**

Discharge

Inversion

Skin changes

Compare with the other side

Palpation

Before palpating the breasts, ask the patient to lie in a supine position, and place a small pillow under her shoulder on the side you're examining. This causes the breast on that side to protrude. (See *Palpating the breast.*)

Hands behind your head! You're under examination.

Have the patient put her hand behind her head on the side you're examining. This spreads the breast more evenly across the chest and makes finding nodules easier. If her breasts are small, she can leave her arm at her side.

A circuitous route

To perform palpation, place your fingers flat on the breast and compress the tissues gently against the chest wall, palpating in concentric circles outward from the nipple. Palpate the entire breast, including the periphery, tail of Spence, and areola. For a patient with pendulous breasts, palpate down or across the breast with the patient sitting upright.

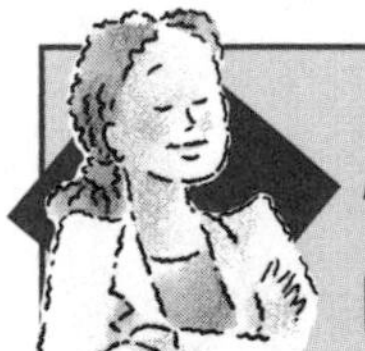

Peak technique

Palpating the breast

Use your three middle fingers to palpate the breast systematically. Rotating your fingers gently against the chest wall, move in concentric circles. Make sure you include the tail of Spence in your examination.

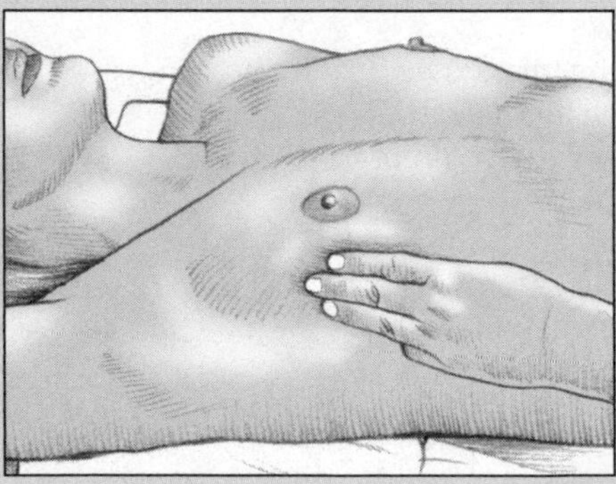

Examining the areola and nipple

After palpating the breast, put on a glove and then palpate the areola and nipple. Gently squeeze the nipple between your thumb and index finger to check for discharge.

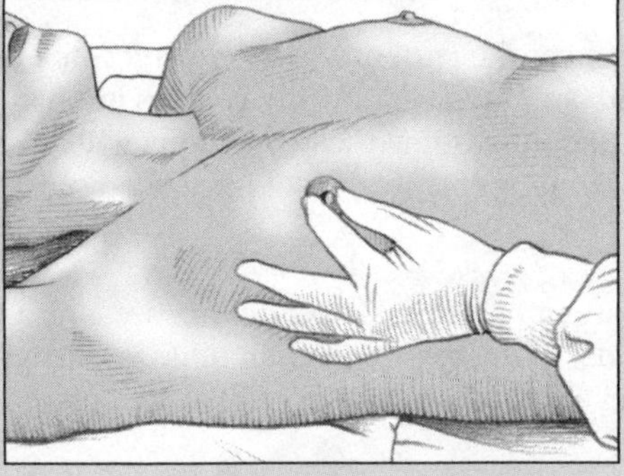

Check the consistency

As you palpate, note the consistency of the breast tissue. Normal consistency varies widely, depending in part on the proportions of fat and glandular tissue. Check for nodules and unusual tenderness. Tenderness may be related to cysts and cancer. However, nodularity, fullness, and mild tenderness are also premenstrual symptoms. Be sure to ask your patient where she is in her menstrual cycle.

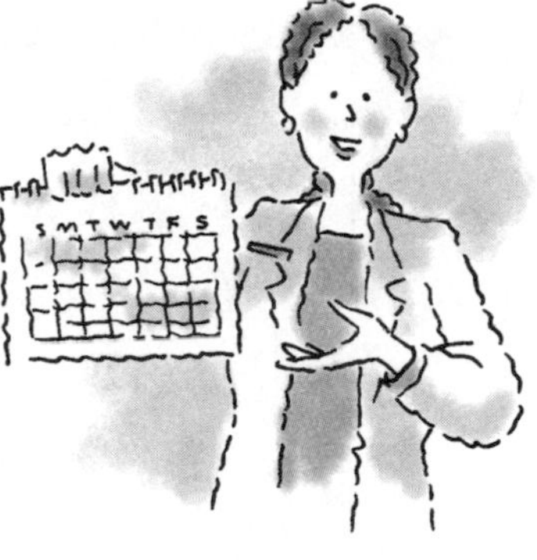

Compare and contrast

A lump or mass that feels different from the rest of the breast tissue may indicate a pathologic change and warrants further investigation by a doctor. If you find what you think is an abnormality, check the other breast, too. Keep in mind that the inframammary ridge at the lower edge of the breast is normally firm and may be mistaken for a tumor.

Sizing up the situation

If you palpate a mass, record these characteristics:

- size in centimeters
- shape — round, discoid, regular, or irregular
- consistency — soft, firm, or hard
- mobility
- degree of tenderness
- location, using the quadrant or clock method (see *Identifying locations of breast lesions*, page 220).

When to get a smear

Finally, palpate the nipple, noting its elasticity. It should be rough, elastic, and round. The nipple also typically protrudes from the breast. Compress the nipple and areola to detect discharge. If discharge is present and the patient isn't pregnant or lactating, assess the color, consistency, and quantity of the discharge. If possible, obtain a cytologic smear.

To obtain a smear, put on gloves, place a glass slide over the nipple, and smear the discharge on the slide. Spray the slide with a fixative, label it with the patient's name and the date, and send it to the laboratory, according to your facility's policy.

Examining the axillae

To examine the axillae, use the techniques of inspection and palpation. With the patient sitting or standing, inspect the skin of the axillae for rashes, infections, or unusual pigmentation.

Identifying locations of breast lesions

Mentally divide the breast into four quadrants and a fifth segment, the tail of Spence. Describe your findings according to the appropriate quadrant or segment. You can also think of the breast as a clock, with the nipple in the center. Then specify locations according to the time (2 o'clock, for example). Either way, specify the location of a lesion or other findings by the distance in centimeters from the nipple.

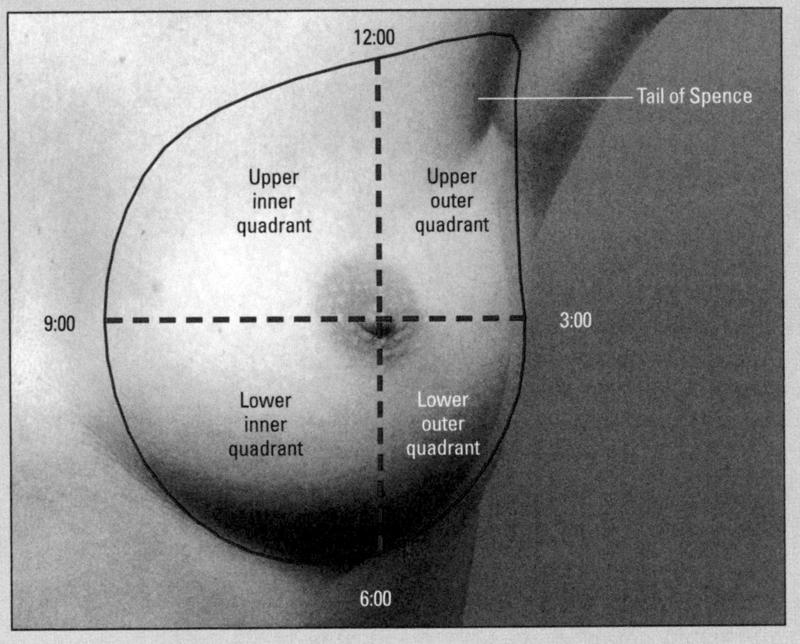

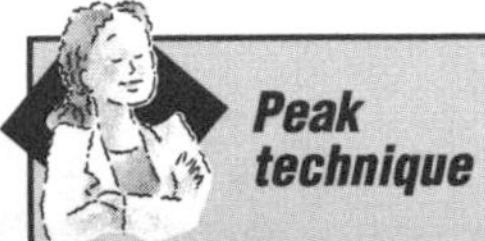

Palpating the axilla

To palpate the axilla, have the patient sit or lie down. Wear gloves if an ulceration or discharge is present. Ask her to relax her arm, and support it with your nondominant hand.

Keeping the fingers of your dominant hand together, reach high into the apex of the axilla, as shown below. Position your fingers so they're directly behind the pectoral muscles, pointing toward the midclavicle. Sweep your fingers downward against the ribs and serratus anterior muscle to palpate the midaxillary or central lymph nodes.

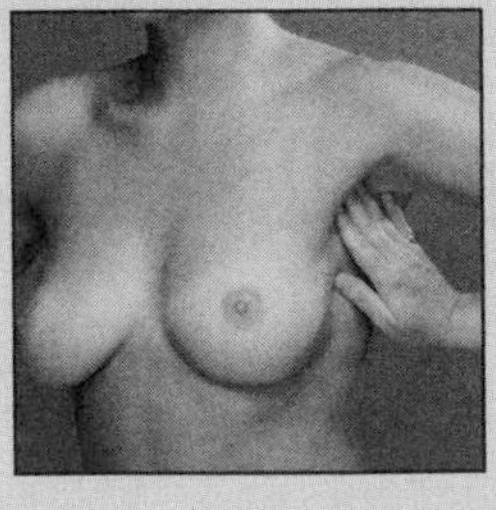

Prepare to palpate

Before palpating, ask the patient to relax her arm on the side you're examining. Support her elbow with one of your hands. Cup the fingers of your other hand, and reach high into the apex of the axilla. Place your fingers directly behind the pectoral muscles, pointing toward the midclavicle. (See *Palpating the axilla.*)

Assessing the axillary nodes

First, try to palpate the central nodes by pressing your fingers downward and in toward the chest wall. You can usually palpate one or more of the nodes, which should be soft, small, and nontender. If you feel a hard, large, or tender lesion, try to palpate the other groups of lymph nodes for comparison.

It's the pits

To palpate the pectoral and anterior nodes, grasp the anterior axillary fold between your thumb and fingers and palpate inside the borders of the pectoral muscles. Palpate the lateral nodes by pressing your fingers along the upper inner arm. Try to compress these nodes against the humerus. To palpate the subscapular or posterior nodes, stand behind the patient and press your fingers to feel the inside of the muscle of the posterior axillary fold.

Assessing the clavicular nodes

If the axillary nodes appear abnormal, assess the nodes in the clavicular area. To do this, have the patient relax her neck muscles by flexing her head slightly forward. Stand in front of her and hook your fingers over the clavicle beside the sternocleidomastoid muscle. Rotate your fingers deeply into this area to feel the supraclavicular nodes.

Abnormal findings

The menstrual cycle, certain prescription drugs, pregnancy, and other conditions can cause breast changes; therefore, you might have trouble differentiating abnormal changes from those that are normal. To help you, this section describes several common abnormal findings. (See also *Breast abnormalities*, pages 222 and 223.)

Breast nodule

A breast nodule, or lump, may be found in any part of the breast, including the axilla. Breast nodules may range in clinical significance from the benign lumps of fibrocystic breast disease to the malignant masses of breast cancer.

Dimpling

Breast dimpling — the puckering or retraction of skin on the breast — results from abnormal attachment of the skin to underlying tissue. It suggests an inflammatory or malignant mass beneath the skin surface and usually represents a late sign of breast cancer. (See *Dimpling and peau d'orange.*)

Dimpling and peau d'orange

These illustrations show two common abnormalities in breast tissue: dimpling and peau d'orange.

Dimpling

Dimpling usually suggests an inflammatory or malignant mass beneath the skin's surface. The illustration shows breast dimpling and nipple inversion caused by a malignant mass above the areola.

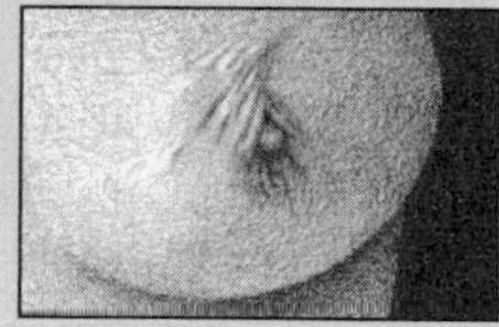

Peau d'orange

Peau d'orange is usually a late sign of breast cancer, but it can also occur with breast or axillary lymph node infection. The skin's orange-peel appearance comes from lymphatic edema around deepened hair follicles.

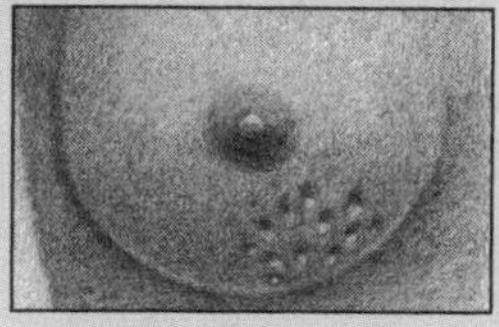

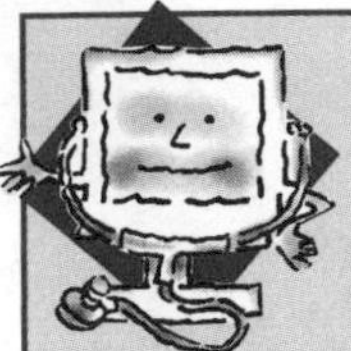

Interpretation station

Breast abnormalities

This chart shows you some common groups of findings for the chief signs and symptoms of the breasts and axillae, along with their probable causes.

Sign or symptom and findings	Probable cause
Breast dimpling	
• Firm, irregular, nontender lump • Nipple retraction, deviation, inversion, or flattening • Enlarged axillary lymph nodes	Breast abscess
• History of trauma to fatty tissue of the breast (patient may not remember such trauma) • Tenderness and erythema • Bruising • Hard, indurated, poorly delineated lump that's fibrotic and fixed to underlying tissue or overlying skin • Nipple retraction	Fat necrosis
• Heat • Erythema • Swelling • Pain and tenderness • Flulike signs and symptoms, such as fever, malaise, fatigue, and aching	Mastitis
Breast nodule	
• Single nodule that feels firm, elastic, and round or lobular, with well-defined margins • Extremely mobile, "slippery" feel • No pain or tenderness • Size varies from pinpoint to very large • Grows rapidly • Usually located around the nipple or the lateral side of the upper outer quadrant	Adeno-fibroma
***Breast nodule** (continued)*	
• Hard, poorly delineated nodule • Fixed to the skin or underlying tissue • Breast dimpling • Nipple deviation or retraction • Located in the upper outer quadrant (50% of cases) • Nontender • Serous or bloody discharge • Edema or peau d'orange of the skin overlying the mass • Axillary lymphadenopathy	Breast cancer
• Smooth, round, slightly elastic nodules • Increased size and tenderness just before menstruation • Mobile • Clear, watery (serous), or sticky nipple discharge • Bloating • Irritability • Abdominal cramping	Fibrocystic breast disease
Breast pain	
• Tender, palpable abscesses on the periphery of the areola • Fever • Inflamed sebaceous Montgomery's glands	Areolar gland abscess

Breast abnormalities *(continued)*

Sign or symptom and findings	Probable cause
Breast pain *(continued)*	
• Unilateral breast pain or tenderness • Serous or bloody nipple discharge, usually only from one duct • Small, soft, poorly delineated mass in the ducts beneath the areola	Intraductal papilloma
• Small, well-delineated nodule • Localized erythema • Induration	Sebaceous cyst (infection)
Nipple retraction	
• Unilateral nipple retraction • Hard, fixed, nontender breast nodule • Nipple itching, burning, or erosion • Watery or bloody nipple discharge • Altered breast contour • Dimpling or peau d'orange • Tenderness, redness, and warmth	Breast cancer
• Unilateral nipple retraction, deviation, cracking, or flattening • Firm and indurated or tender, discrete breast nodule • Warmth, erythema, tenderness, and edema • Possible fatigue, fever, and chills	Mastitis

Peau d'orange

Usually another late sign of breast cancer, peau d'orange (orange peel skin) is the edematous thickening and pitting of breast skin. This sign can also occur with breast or axillary lymph node infection of Graves' disease. Its striking orange peel appearance stems from lymphatic edema around deepened hair follicles.

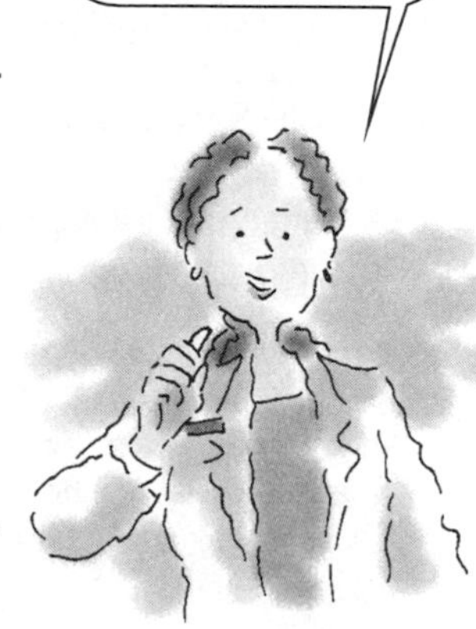

"Orange" you glad you know how to spot breast abnormalities such as peau d'orange?

Nipple retraction

Nipple retraction, the inward displacement of the nipple below the level of surrounding breast tissue, may indicate an inflammatory breast lesion or cancer. It results from scar tissue formation within a lesion or large mammary duct. As the scar tissue shortens, it pulls adjacent tissue inward, causing nipple deviation, flattening, and finally retraction.

Nipple discharge

Nipple discharge can occur spontaneously or can be elicited by nipple stimulation. It's characterized as intermittent or constant, unilateral or bilateral, and by color, consistency, and composition. It can be a normal finding; however, nipple discharge can also signal serious underlying disease, particularly when accompanied by other breast changes. Significant causes include endocrine disorders, cancer, certain drugs, and blocked lactiferous ducts.

Breast pain

Breast pain commonly results from benign breast disease, such as mastitis or fibrocystic breast disease. It may occur during rest or movement and may be aggravated by manipulation or palpation. Breast tenderness refers to pain elicited by physical contact.

Visible veins

Prominent veins in the breast may indicate cancer in some patients; however, they're considered normal in pregnant women because of engorgement.

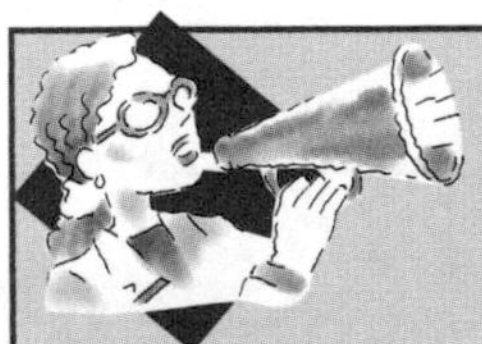

That's a wrap!

Breasts and axillae review

Structures

- Nipple: pigmented erectile tissue located in the center of each breast
- Areola: ringed area that surrounds the nipple; darker in color than adjacent tissue
- Cooper's ligaments: fibrous bands that support each breast
- Glandular lobes: contain the alveoli that produce milk
- Lactiferous ducts: transport milk from each lobe to the nipple

Health history

- Ask the patient about a history of breast lumps, breast surgery, breast cancer, fibrocystic breast disease, or other breast disorders.
- Ask about the patient's menstrual and pregnancy history.
- Ask about a family history of breast disorders, especially breast cancer.

Assessment

- Inspect the breast, noting breast size and symmetry and skin condition.
- Palpate each breast in concentric circles outward from the nipple, including the periphery, tail of Spence, and areola.
- Palpate the nipple and compress to check for discharge.
- Inspect and palpate the axilla.
- Palpate lymph node chains.

Documenting a breast mass

Note these characteristics:

- Diameter
- Shape
- Consistency

Breasts and axillae review *(continued)*

- Mobility
- Degree of tenderness
- Location

Abnormal findings

- Breast nodule—breast lump that may be benign or malignant
- Breast dimpling—the puckering or retraction of skin on the breast
- Peau d'orange (orange peel skin)—the edematous thickening and pitting of breast skin
- Nipple retraction—inward displacement of the nipple below the level of surrounding breast tissue
- Nipple discharge—may be a normal finding or can signal serious disease
- Pain—may occur during rest or movement; may be aggravated by manipulation or palpation
- Visible veins—may indicate cancer but also occur normally in pregnant women

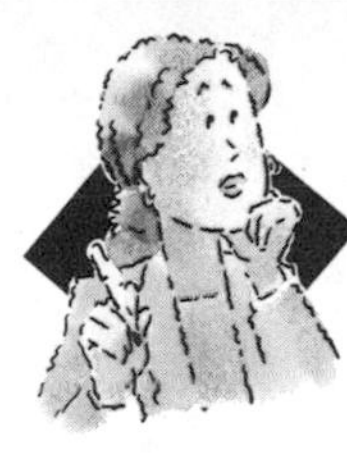

Quick quiz

1. Most malignant breast cancers occur in the region of the breast known as the:

A. lower inner quadrant.
B. lower outer quadrant.
C. upper inner quadrant.
D. upper outer quadrant.

Answer: D. Although a malignancy can occur in any part of the breast, it usually occurs in the upper outer quadrant and appears as a hard, immobile, irregular lump.

2. Normal changes in the breasts of a premenstrual woman include:

A. a single hard, fixed mass.
B. nipple inversion and skin dimpling.
C. tenderness and soft, mobile cysts.
D. redness and scaling over a portion of the breast.

Answer: C. A week before menses, both breasts are usually tender with soft, benign, mobile, fluid-filled cysts.

3. After obtaining a smear of nipple discharge on a glass slide, you would:

A. freeze the slide before sending it to the laboratory.
B. let the smear air-dry before sending it to the laboratory.
C. spray the slide with a cytologic fixative before sending it to the laboratory.
D. spread the smear with a cotton swab, apply a cover slip to the slide, and send it to the laboratory.

Answer: C. To obtain a culture of nipple discharge, place a glass slide over the nipple and smear the discharge on the slide. Then spray the slide with a cytologic fixative before sending it to the laboratory.

4. The tail of Spence is located:
- A. above the nipple at the midclavicular line.
- B. in the upper outer quadrant, toward the axilla.
- C. in the upper inner quadrant, near the sternum.
- D. in the lower outer quadrant, close to the ribs.

Answer: B. The tail of Spence is a small triangle of tissue located in the upper outer quadrant of the breast, toward the axilla.

Scoring

☆☆☆ If you answered all four questions correctly, way to go! You're an impeccable inspector and a precision palpator.

☆☆ If you answered three questions correctly, good job! When it comes to palpation, you're more than passable.

☆ If you answered fewer than three questions correctly, that's okay! With more preparation, you'll be poised on the edge of palpation perfection.

Gastrointestinal system

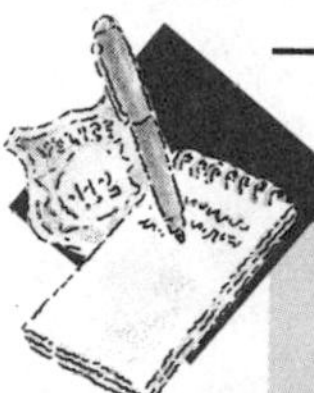

Just the facts

In this chapter, you'll learn:

- organs and structures that make up the GI system
- methods to obtain a patient history of the GI system
- techniques for performing a physical assessment of the GI system
- causes and characteristics of abnormalities in the GI system.

A look at the GI system

The GI system's major functions include ingestion and digestion of food and elimination of waste products. When these processes are interrupted, the patient can experience problems ranging from loss of appetite to acid-base imbalances.

Anatomy and physiology of the GI system

The GI system consists of two major divisions: the GI tract and the accessory organs. (See *Parts of the GI system*, page 228.)

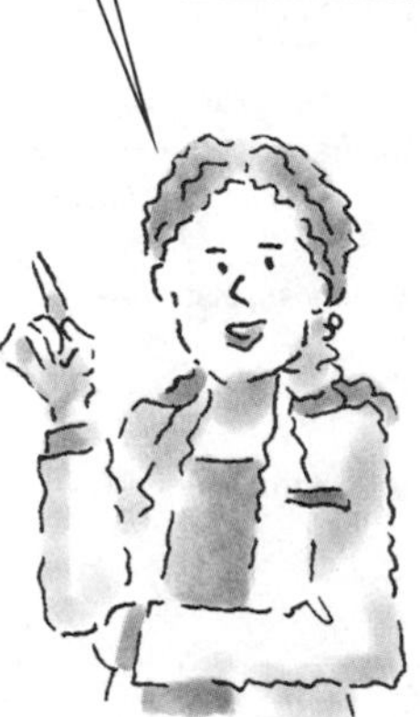

GI tract

The GI tract is a hollow tube that begins at the mouth and ends at the anus. About 25′ (7.5 m) long, the GI tract consists of smooth muscle alternating with blood vessels and nerve tissue. Specialized circular and longitudinal fibers contract, causing peristalsis, which aids in propelling food through the GI tract. The GI tract in-

Parts of the GI system

This illustration shows the GI system's major anatomic structures. Knowing these structures will help you conduct an accurate physical assessment.

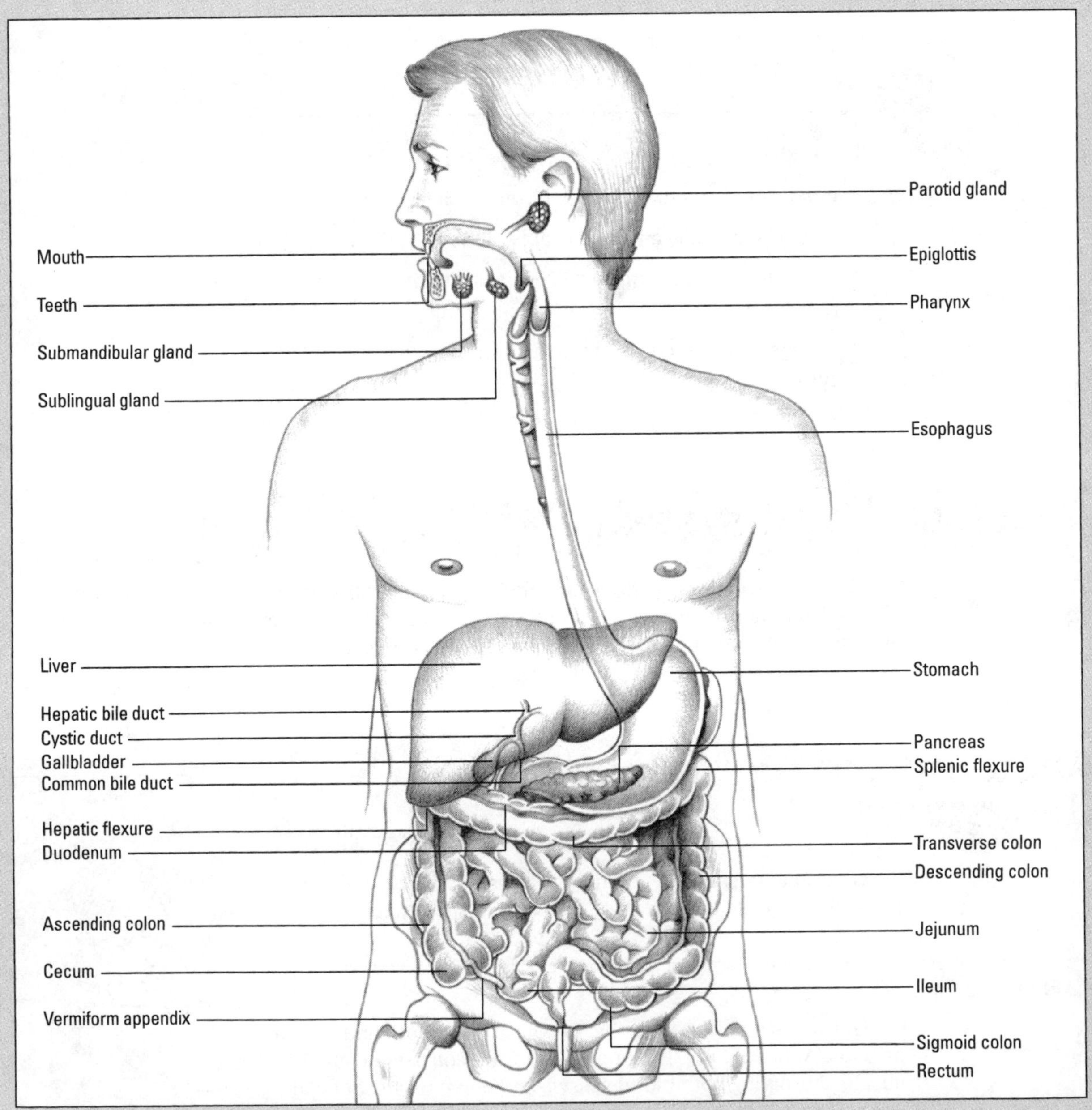

cludes the pharynx, esophagus, stomach, small intestine, and large intestine.

Start at the mouth

Digestive processes begin in the mouth with chewing, salivating, and swallowing. The tongue provides the sense of taste. Saliva is produced by three pairs of glands: the parotid, submandibular, and sublingual.

Proceed to the pharynx

The pharynx, or throat, allows the passage of food from the mouth to the esophagus. The pharynx assists in the swallowing process and secretes mucus that aids in digestion. The epiglottis—a thin, leaf-shaped structure made of fibrocartilage—is directly behind the root of the tongue. When food is swallowed, the epiglottis closes over the larynx and the soft palate lifts to block the nasal cavity. These actions keep food and fluid from being aspirated into the airway.

Down the esophagus

The esophagus is a muscular, hollow tube about 10″ (25.5 cm) long that moves food from the pharynx to the stomach. When food is swallowed, the upper esophageal sphincter relaxes, and the food moves into the esophagus. Peristalsis then propels the food toward the stomach. The gastroesophageal sphincter at the lower end of the esophagus normally remains closed to prevent the reflux of gastric contents. The sphincter opens during swallowing, belching, and vomiting.

Stay awhile in the stomach

The stomach, a reservoir for food, is a dilated, saclike structure that lies obliquely in the left upper quadrant below the esophagus and diaphragm, to the right of the spleen, and partly under the liver. The stomach contains two important sphincters: the cardiac sphincter, which protects the entrance to the stomach, and the pyloric sphincter, which guards the exit.

The stomach has three major functions. It:

- stores food
- mixes food with gastric juices (hydrochloric acid)
- passes chyme—a watery mixture of partly digested food and digestive juices—into the small intestine for further digestion and absorption.

An average meal can remain in the stomach for 3 to 4 hours. Rugae, accordion-like folds in the stomach lining, allow the stomach to expand when large amounts of food and fluid are ingested.

Once this food reaches my stomach, it will remain there for 3 or 4 hours before moving on to the small intestine.

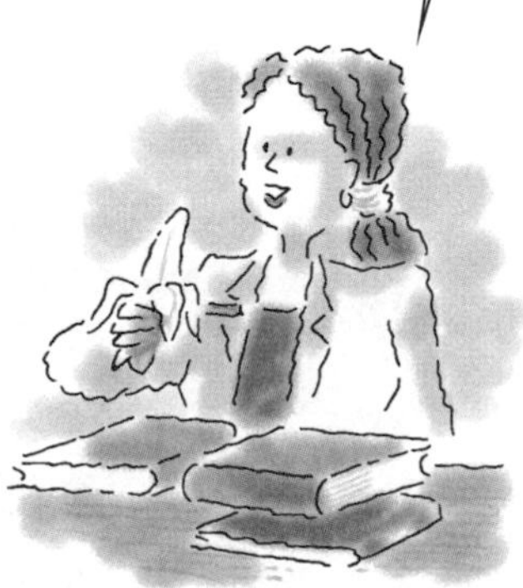

Slip through the small intestine

The small intestine is about 20′ (6 m) long and is named for its diameter, not its length. It has three sections: the duodenum, the jejunum, and the ileum. As chyme passes into the small intestine, the end products of digestion are absorbed through its thin mucous membrane lining into the bloodstream.

Carbohydrates, fats, and proteins are broken down in the small intestine. Enzymes from the pancreas, bile from the liver, and hormones from glands of the small intestine all aid digestion. These secretions mix with the chyme as it moves through the intestines by peristalsis.

And finally head through the large intestine

The large intestine, or colon, is about 5′ (1.5 m) long. It includes the cecum; the ascending, transverse, descending, and sigmoid colons; the rectum; and the anus — in that order — and is responsible for:

- absorbing excess water and electrolytes
- storing food residue
- eliminating waste products in the form of feces.

The appendix, a fingerlike projection, is attached to the cecum. Bacteria in the colon produce gas, or flatus.

Accessory organs

Accessory GI organs include the liver, pancreas, gallbladder, and bile ducts. The abdominal aorta and the gastric and splenic veins also aid the GI system.

You'd think with all my functions I'd lose a little weight, but I'm the heaviest organ in the body!

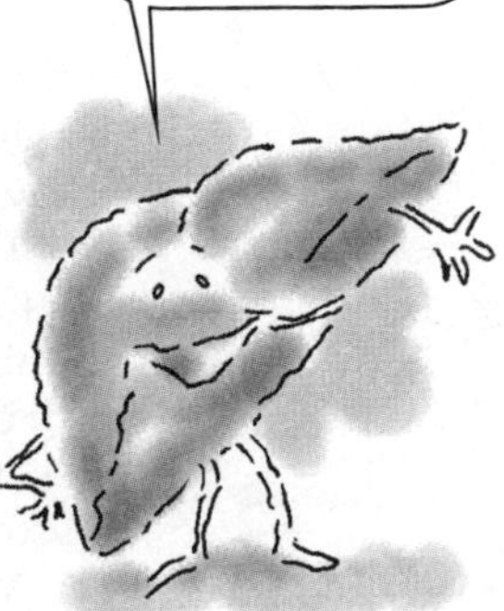

Look at the liver

The liver is located in the right upper quadrant under the diaphragm. It has two major lobes, divided by the falciform ligament. The liver is the heaviest organ in the body, weighing about 3 lb (1.5 kg) in an adult.

The liver's functions include:

- metabolizing carbohydrates, fats, and proteins
- detoxifying blood
- converting ammonia to urea for excretion
- synthesizing plasma proteins, nonessential amino acids, vitamin A, and essential nutrients, such as iron and vitamins D, K, and B_{12}.

The liver also secretes bile, a greenish fluid that helps digest fats and absorb fatty acids, cholesterol, and other lipids. Bile also gives stool its color.

Gape at the gallbladder

The gallbladder is a small, pear-shaped organ about 4″ (10 cm) long that lies halfway under the right lobe of the liver. Its main function is to store bile from the liver until the bile is emptied into the duodenum. This process occurs when the small intestine initiates chemical impulses that cause the gallbladder to contract.

Probe the pancreas

The pancreas, which measures 6″ to 8″ (15 to 20.5 cm) in length, lies horizontally in the abdomen, behind the stomach. It consists of a head, tail, and body. The body of the pancreas is located in the right upper quadrant, and the tail is in the left upper quadrant, attached to the duodenum. The tail of the pancreas touches the spleen.

The pancreas releases insulin and glycogen into the bloodstream and produces pancreatic enzymes that are released into the duodenum for digestion.

Behold the bile ducts

The bile ducts provide passageways for bile to travel from the liver to the intestines. Two hepatic ducts drain the liver and the cystic duct drains the gallbladder. These ducts converge into the common bile duct, which then empties into the duodenum.

Visualize the vascular structures

The abdominal aorta supplies blood to the GI tract. It enters the abdomen, separates into the common iliac arteries, and then branches into many arteries extending the length of the GI tract.

The gastric and splenic veins drain absorbed nutrients into the portal vein of the liver. After entering the liver, the venous blood circulates and then exits the liver through the hepatic vein, emptying into the inferior vena cava.

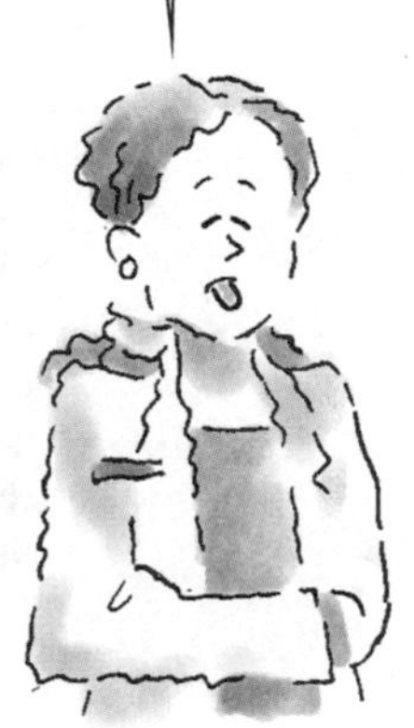

Obtaining a health history

If your patient has a GI problem, he'll usually complain about pain, heartburn, nausea, vomiting, or altered bowel habits. To investigate these and other signs and symptoms, ask him about the location, quality, onset, duration, frequency, and severity of each.

Knowing what precipitates and relieves the patient's symptoms will help you perform a more accurate physical assessment and better plan your care.

Asking about past health

To determine if your patient's problem is new or recurring, ask about past GI illnesses, such as an ulcer; liver, pancreas, or gallbladder disease; inflammatory bowel disease; rectal or GI bleeding; hiatal hernia; irritable bowel syndrome; diverticulitis; gastroesophageal reflux disease; or cancer. Also ask if he has had abdominal surgery or trauma.

Asking about current health

Ask the patient if he's taking any medications. Several drugs — especially aspirin, nonsteroidal anti-inflammatory drugs, antibiotics, and opioid analgesics — can cause nausea, vomiting, diarrhea, constipation, and other GI signs and symptoms.

Be sure to ask about laxative use; habitual use may cause constipation. Also ask the patient if he's allergic to medications or foods. Such allergies commonly cause GI symptoms.

Gnawing problems

In addition, ask the patient about changes in appetite, difficulty chewing or swallowing, and changes in bowel habits. Does he have excessive belching or passing of gas? Has he noticed a change in the color, amount, and appearance of his stool? Has he ever seen blood in his stool?

Travel plans

If the patient's reason for seeking care is diarrhea, find out if he recently traveled abroad. Diarrhea, hepatitis, and parasitic infections can result from ingesting contaminated food or water.

Asking about family health

Because some GI disorders are hereditary, ask the patient whether anyone in his family has had a GI disorder. (See *Culture and the GI history*.)

Disorders with a familial link include:

- ulcerative colitis
- colorectal cancer
- peptic ulcers
- gastric cancer
- diabetes
- alcoholism
- Crohn's disease.

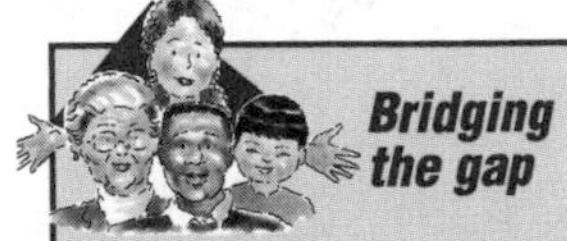

Culture and the GI history

When taking a health history, consider your patient's ethnic background. For example, patients from Japan, Iceland, Chile, and Austria are at higher risk of death from gastric cancer than patients from other countries. Also, Crohn's disease is more common in patients who are Jewish.

Asking about psychosocial health

Inquire about your patient's occupation, home life, financial situation, stress level, and recent life changes. Be sure to ask about alcohol, caffeine, and tobacco use as well as food consumption, exercise habits, and oral hygiene. Also ask about sleep patterns: How many hours of sleep does he feel he needs? How many does he get?

Assessing the GI system

A physical assessment of the GI system should include a thorough examination of the mouth, abdomen, and rectum. To perform an abdominal assessment, use this sequence: inspection, auscultation, percussion, and palpation. Palpating or percussing the abdomen before you auscultate can change the character of the patient's bowel sounds and lead to an inaccurate assessment.

Before beginning your examination, explain the techniques you'll be using and warn the patient that some procedures might be uncomfortable. Perform the examination in a private, quiet, warm, and well-lighted room.

Examining the mouth

Use inspection and palpation to assess the mouth. Be sure to put on gloves before examining the patient.

Open wide

First, inspect the patient's mouth and jaw for asymmetry and swelling. Check his bite, noting malocclusion from an overbite or underbite. Inspect the inner and outer lips, teeth, gums, and oral mucosa with a penlight. Note bleeding; ulcerations; carious, loose, missing, or broken teeth; and color changes, including rashes. Palpate the gums, inner lips, and cheeks for tenderness, lumps, and lesions.

Assess the tongue, checking for coating, tremors, swelling, and ulcerations. Note unusual breath odors. Finally, examine the pharynx by pressing a tongue blade firmly down on the middle of the tongue and asking the patient to say "Ahh." Look for uvular deviation, tonsillar abnormalities, lesions, plaques, and exudate.

Examining the abdomen

Use inspection, auscultation, percussion, and palpation to examine the abdomen. To ensure an accurate assessment, take these actions before the examination:

- Ask the patient to empty his bladder.
- Drape the genitalia and, if the patient is female, her breasts.
- Place a small pillow under the patient's knees to help relax the abdominal muscles.
- Ask the patient to keep his arms at his sides.
- Keep the room warm. Chilling can cause abdominal muscles to become tense.
- Warm your hands and the stethoscope.
- Speak softly, and encourage the patient to perform breathing exercises or use imagery during uncomfortable procedures.
- Ask the patient to point to any areas of pain.
- Assess painful areas last to help prevent the patient from becoming tense.

Hold the ice! A cold room can make the abdominal muscles tense, which may affect your examination.

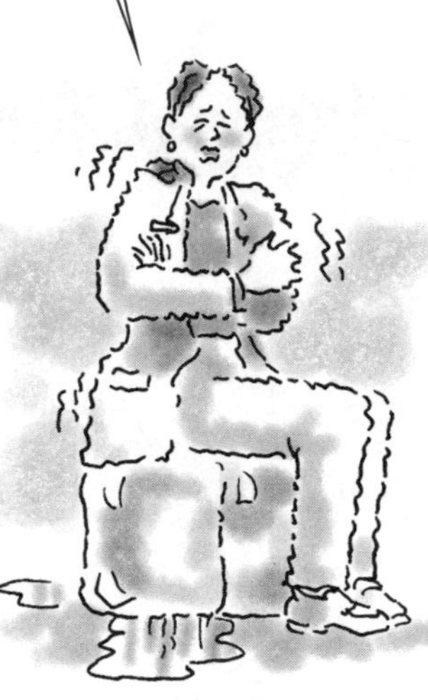

Inspection

Begin by mentally dividing the abdomen into four quadrants and then imagining the organs in each quadrant. (See *Abdominal quadrants.*)

It's all in the terms

You can more accurately pinpoint your physical findings by knowing these three terms:

- epigastric — above the umbilicus and between the costal margins
- umbilical — around the navel
- suprapubic — above the symphysis pubis.

Battle of the bulge

Observe the abdomen for symmetry, checking for bumps, bulges, or masses. A bulge may indicate bladder distention or hernia.

Also note the patient's abdominal shape and contour. The abdomen should be flat to rounded in people of average weight. A protruding abdomen may be caused by obesity, pregnancy, ascites, or abdominal distention. A slender person may have a slightly concave abdomen.

Innie or outie?

Assess the umbilicus, which should be inverted and located midline in the abdomen. Conditions such as pregnancy, ascites, or an underlying mass can cause the umbilicus to protrude. Have the pa-

Abdominal quadrants

To perform a systematic GI assessment, try to visualize the abdominal structures by dividing the abdomen into four quadrants, as shown here.

Right upper quadrant
- Right lobe of liver
- Gallbladder
- Pylorus
- Duodenum
- Head of the pancreas
- Hepatic flexure of the colon
- Portions of the ascending and transverse colon

Right lower quadrant
- Cecum and appendix
- Portion of the ascending colon

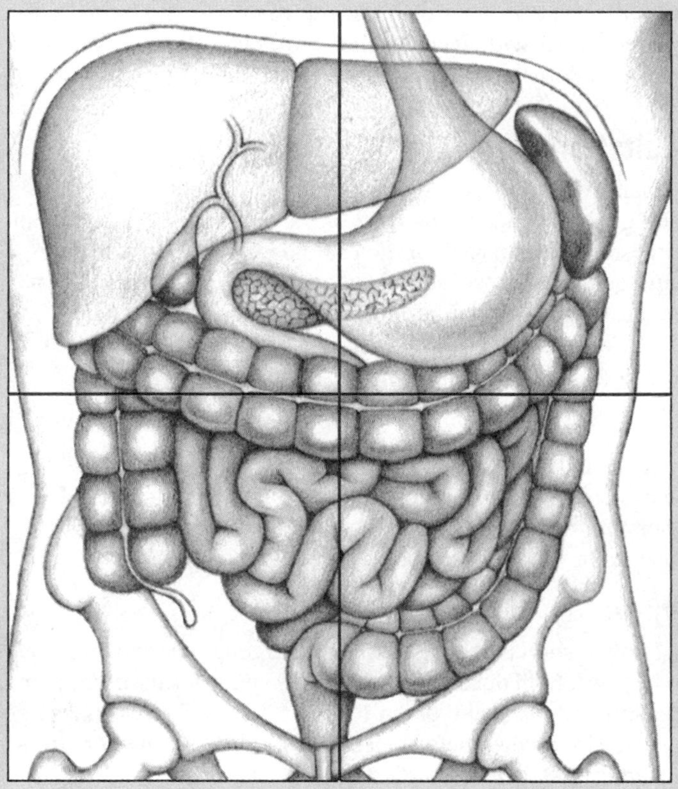

Left upper quadrant
- Left lobe of the liver
- Stomach
- Body of the pancreas
- Splenic flexure of the colon
- Portions of the transverse and descending colon

Left lower quadrant
- Sigmoid colon
- Portion of the descending colon

tient raise his head and shoulders. If his umbilicus protrudes, he may have an umbilical hernia.

Stretched to the limit

The skin of the abdomen should be smooth and uniform in color. Striae, or stretch marks, can be caused by pregnancy, excessive weight gain, or ascites. New striae are pink or blue; old striae are silvery white (in patients with darker skin, striae may be dark brown). Note dilated veins. Record the length of any surgical scars on the abdomen.

Riding the peristaltic wave

Note abdominal movements and pulsations. Usually, waves of peristalsis can't be seen; if they're visible, they look like slight, wavelike motions. Visible rippling waves may indicate bowel obstruction and should be reported immediately. In thin patients, pulsation of the aorta is visible in the epigastric area. Marked pulsations may occur with hypertension, aortic insufficiency, aortic aneurysm, and other conditions causing widening pulse pressure.

Visible, rippling waves of peristalsis may signal a bowel obstruction. Be sure to report such a finding immediately.

Auscultation

Lightly place the stethoscope diaphragm in the right lower quadrant, slightly below and to the right of the umbilicus. Auscultate in a clockwise fashion in each of the four quadrants. Note the character and quality of bowel sounds in each quadrant. In some cases, you may need to auscultate for 5 minutes before you hear sounds. Be sure to allow enough time to listen in each quadrant before you decide that bowel sounds are absent.

Silence the suction

Before auscultating the abdomen of a patient with a nasogastric tube or another abdominal tube connected to suction, briefly clamp the tube or turn off the suction. Suction noises can obscure or mimic actual bowel sounds.

Pardon my borborygmus

Normal bowel sounds are high-pitched, gurgling noises caused by air mixing with fluid during peristalsis. The noises vary in frequency, pitch, and intensity and occur irregularly from 5 to 34 times per minute. They're loudest before mealtimes. Borborygmus, or stomach growling, is the loud, gurgling, splashing bowel sound heard over the large intestine as gas passes through it.

Too much activity or not enough?

Bowel sounds are classified as normal, hypoactive, or hyperactive. Hyperactive bowel sounds — loud, high-pitched, tinkling sounds that occur frequently — may be caused by diarrhea, constipation, or laxative use.

Hypoactive bowel sounds are heard infrequently. They're associated with ileus, bowel obstruction, or peritonitis and indicate diminished peristalsis. Paralytic ileus, torsion of the bowel, or the use of opioid analgesics and other medications can decrease peristalsis.

Voice of the vessels

Auscultate for vascular sounds with the bell of the stethoscope. (See *Vascular sounds.*) Using firm pressure, listen over the aorta and renal, iliac, and femoral arteries for bruits, venous hums, and friction rubs.

Percussion

Direct or indirect percussion is used to detect the size and location of abdominal organs and to detect air or fluid in the abdomen, stomach, or bowel.

In direct percussion, strike your hand or finger directly against the patient's abdomen. With indirect percussion, use the middle finger of your dominant hand or a percussion hammer to strike a finger resting on the patient's abdomen. Begin percussion in the right lower quadrant and proceed clockwise, covering all four quadrants.

Don't percuss the abdomen of a patient with an abdominal aortic aneurysm or a transplanted abdominal organ. Doing so can precipitate a rupture or organ rejection.

Hollow or dull?

You normally hear two sounds during percussion of the abdomen: tympany and dullness. When you percuss over hollow organs, such as an empty stomach or bowel, you hear a clear, hollow sound like a drum beating. This sound, tympany, predominates because air is normally present in the stomach and bowel. The degree of tympany depends on the amount of air and gastric dilation.

When you percuss over solid organs, such as the liver, kidney, or feces-filled intestines, the sound changes to dullness. Note where percussed sounds change from tympany to dullness. (See *Sites of tympany and dullness*, page 238.)

How large is the liver?

Percussion of the liver can help you estimate its size. (See *Percussing and measuring the liver*, page 238.) Hepatomegaly is commonly associated with hepatitis and other liver diseases. Liver borders may be obscured and difficult to assess.

Splenic dullard

The spleen is located at about the level of the 10th rib, in the left midaxillary line. Percussion may produce a small area of dullness, generally 7″ (17.8 cm) or less in adults. However, the spleen usually can't be percussed because tympany from the colon masks the dullness of the spleen. It's also difficult to distinguish between the dullness of the posterior flank and the dullness of the spleen.

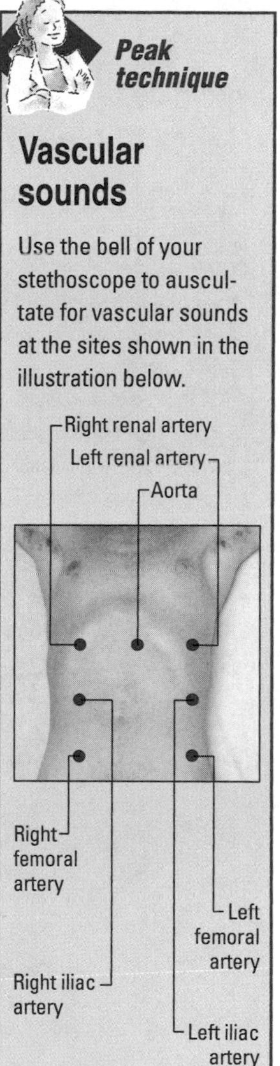

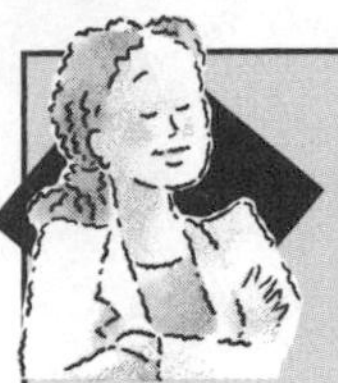

Peak technique

Percussing and measuring the liver

To percuss and measure the liver, follow these steps:

- Identify the upper border of liver dullness. Start in the right midclavicular line in an area of lung resonance, and percuss downward toward the liver. Use a pen to mark the spot where the sound changes to dullness.
- Start in the right midclavicular line at a level below the umbilicus, and lightly percuss upward toward the liver. Mark the spot where the sound changes from tympany to dullness.
- Use a ruler to measure the vertical span between the two marked spots, as shown aove. In an adult, a normal liver span ranges from 2½″ to 4¾″ (6.5 to 12 cm).

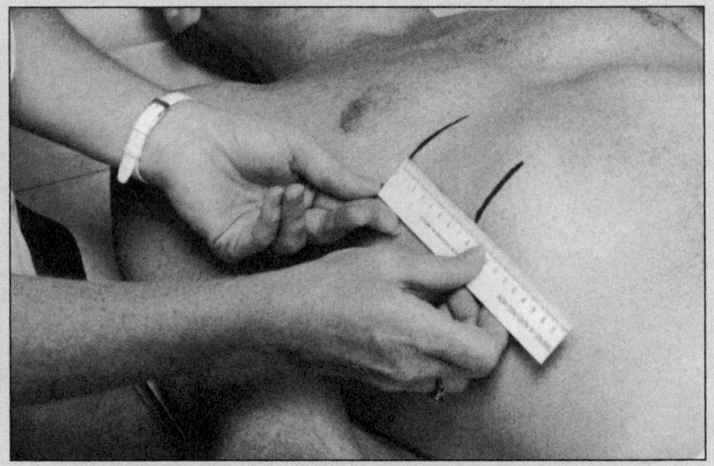

Growing problem

Conditions that cause splenomegaly include mononucleosis, trauma, and illnesses that destroy red blood cells, such as sickle cell anemia and some cancers. (See *Spleen or kidney enlargement?*) To assess a patient for splenic enlargement, ask him to breathe deeply. Then percuss along the 9th to 11th intercostal spaces on the left, listening for a change from tympany to dullness. Measure the area of dullness. This is called a *positive splenic percussion sign.*

Palpation

Abdominal palpation includes light and deep touch to help determine the size, shape, position, and tenderness of major abdominal organs and to detect masses and fluid accumulation. Palpate all four quadrants, leaving painful and tender areas for last.

Light touch

Light palpation helps identify muscle resistance and tenderness as well as the location of some superficial organs. To palpate, put the fingers of one hand close together, depress the skin about ½″ (1.5 cm) with your fingertips, and make gentle, rotating movements. Avoid short, quick jabs.

Sites of tympany and dullness

Expect to auscultate tympany and dullness in the areas shown here.

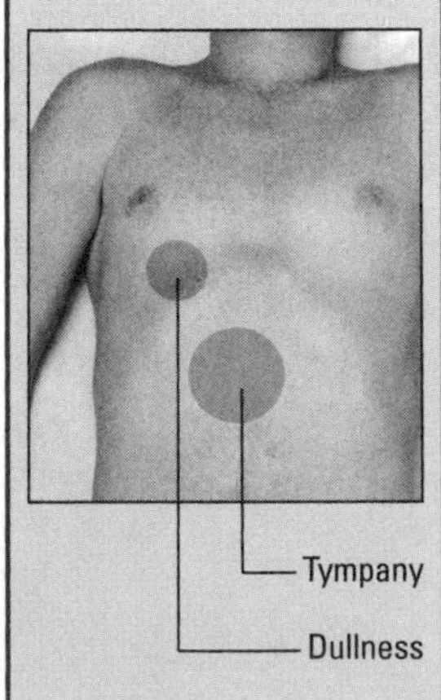

What you're feeling for

The abdomen should be soft and nontender. As you palpate the four quadrants, note organs, masses, and areas of tenderness or increased resistance. Determine whether resistance is due to the patient's being cold, tense, or ticklish, or if it's due to involuntary guarding or rigidity from muscle spasms or peritoneal inflammation.

Tickled pink?

Help the ticklish patient relax by putting his hand over yours as you palpate. If he complains of abdominal tenderness even before you touch him, palpate by placing your stethoscope lightly on his abdomen.

Pressing the issue

To perform deep palpation, push the abdomen down 2″ to 3″ (5 to 7.5 cm). In an obese patient, put one hand on top of the other and push. Palpate the entire abdomen in a clockwise direction, checking for tenderness, pulsations, organ enlargement, and masses.

Please do not touch

If the patient's abdomen is rigid, don't palpate it. He could have peritoneal inflammation, and palpation could cause pain or could rupture an inflamed organ.

Feeling out the situation

Palpate the patient's liver to check for enlargement and tenderness. (See *Palpating the liver*, page 240.) Unless the spleen is enlarged, it isn't palpable. If you do feel the spleen, stop palpating immediately because compression can cause rupture. (See *Palpating the spleen*, page 241.)

Spleen or kidney enlargement?

To differentiate between spleen and kidney enlargement, ask your patient to take a deep breath. Then percuss along the 9th and 11th intercostal spaces. You should hear tympany produced by colonic or gastric air. If you hear dullness instead, the patient's spleen may be enlarged. If you hear resonance, his left kidney may be enlarged.

Special assessment procedures

To check for rebound tenderness or ascites, follow these guidelines.

On the rebound

Perform the test for rebound tenderness when you suspect peritoneal inflammation. Check for rebound at the end of your examination.

Choosing a site away from the painful area, position your hand at a 90-degree angle to the abdomen. Push down slowly and deeply into the abdomen; then withdraw your hand quickly. Rapid

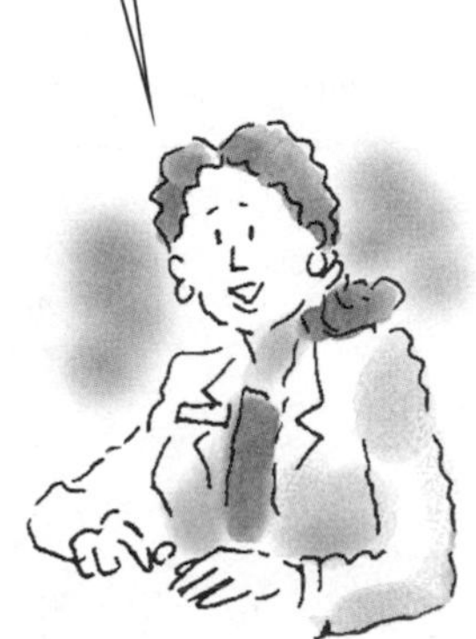

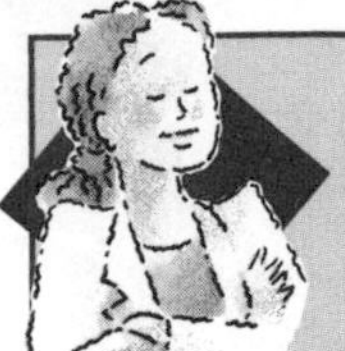

Peak technique

Palpating the liver

These illustrations show the correct hand positions for two ways of palpating the liver.

Method 1: Standard palpation

- Place the patient in the supine position. Standing at his right side, place your left hand under his back at the approximate location of the liver.
- Place your right hand slightly below the mark you made earlier at the liver's upper border. Point the fingers of your right hand toward the patient's head just under the right costal margin.
- As the patient inhales deeply, gently press in and up on the abdomen until the liver brushes under your right hand. The edge should be smooth, firm, and somewhat round. Note any tenderness.

Method 2: Hooking the liver

- Hooking is an alternate way of palpating the liver. To hook the liver, stand next to the patient's right shoulder, facing his feet. Place your hands side by side, and hook your fingertips over the right costal margin, below the lower mark of dullness.
- Ask the patient to take a deep breath as you push your fingertips in and up. If the liver is palpable, you may feel its edge as it slides down in the abdomen as he breathes in.

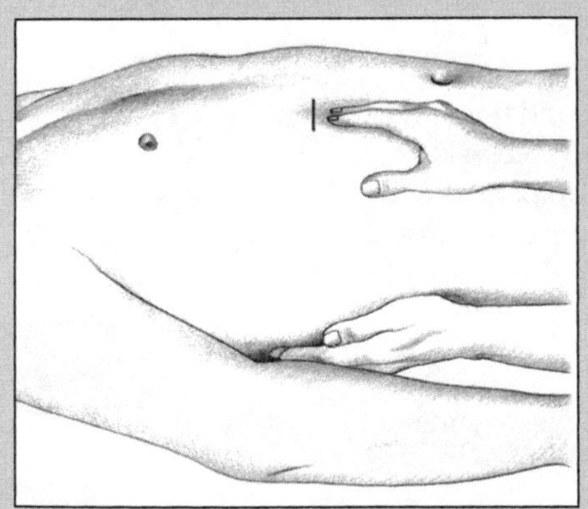

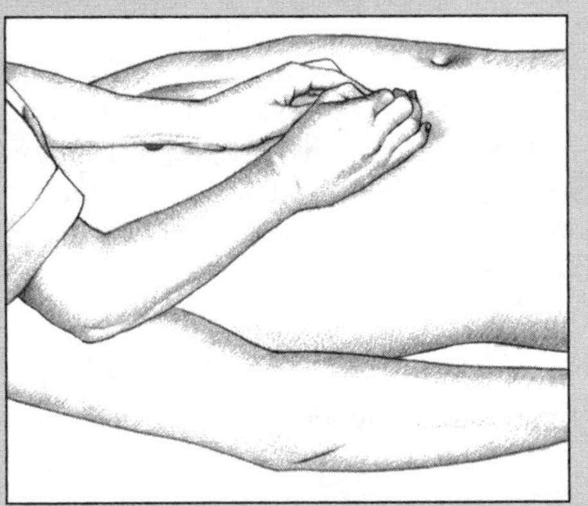

withdrawal causes the underlying structures to rebound suddenly and results in a sharp, stabbing pain on the inflamed side. Don't repeat this maneuver because you may rupture an inflamed appendix. (See *Eliciting rebound tenderness in children.*)

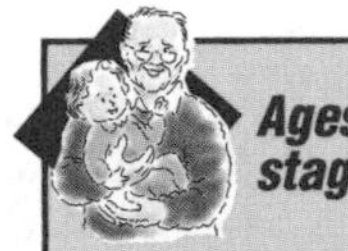

Ages and stages

Eliciting rebound tenderness in children

Eliciting rebound tenderness in young children who can't verbalize how they feel may be difficult. Be alert for such clues as an anguished facial expression, grimace, or intensified crying.

When attempting to assess this symptom, use techniques that elicit minimal tenderness. For example, have the child hop or jump to allow tissue to rebound gently while you watch closely for signs of pain. With this technique, the child won't associate the exacerbation of his pain with your actions, and you may gain the child's cooperation.

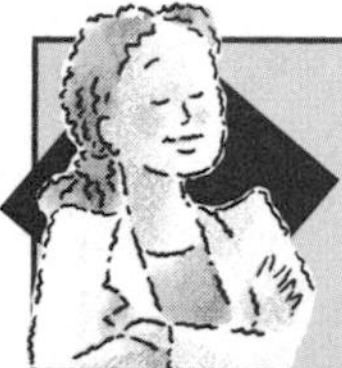

Peak technique

Palpating the spleen

Although a normal spleen isn't palpable, an enlarged spleen is. To palpate the spleen, stand on the patient's right side. Use your left hand to support his posterior left lower rib cage. Ask him to take a deep breath. Then, with your right hand on his abdomen, press up and in toward the spleen.

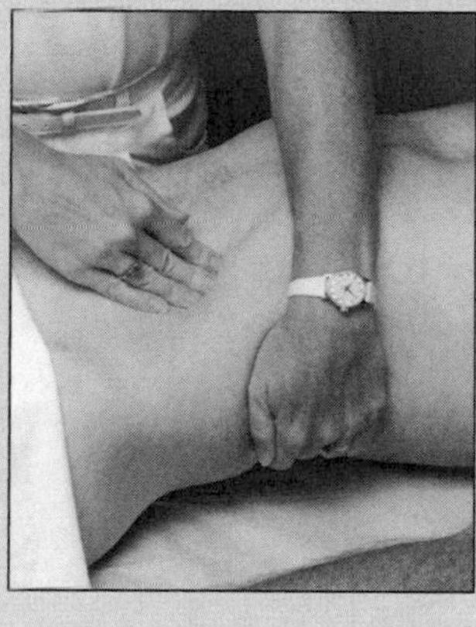

Water logged

Ascites, a large accumulation of fluid in the peritoneal cavity, can be caused by advanced liver disease, heart failure, pancreatitis, or cancer.

If ascites is present, use a tape measure to measure the fullest part of the abdomen. Mark this point on the patient's abdomen with indelible ink so you'll be sure to measure it consistently. This measurement is important, especially if fluid removal or paracentesis is performed. (See *Checking for ascites*, page 242.)

Examining the rectum and anus

If your patient is age 40 or older, perform a rectal examination as part of your GI assessment. Be sure to explain the procedure to the patient.

Inspect the outside

First, inspect the perianal area. Put on gloves and spread the buttocks to expose the anus and surrounding tissue, checking for fissures, lesions, scars, inflammation, discharge, rectal prolapse, and external hemorrhoids. Ask the patient to strain as if he's having a bowel movement; this may reveal internal hemorrhoids, polyps, or fissures.

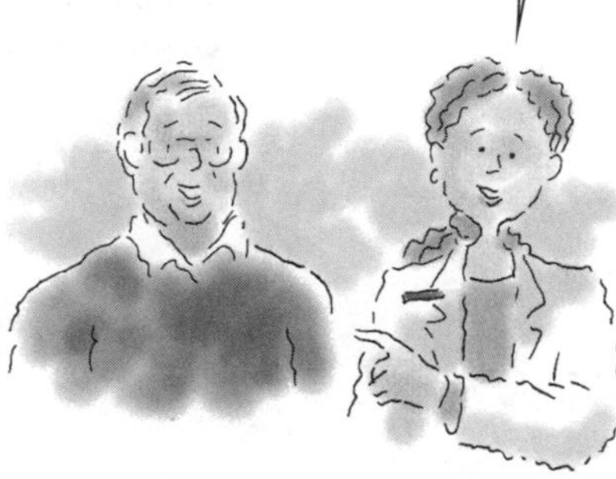

The skin in the perianal area is normally somewhat darker than that of the surrounding area.

Palpate the inside

Next palpate the rectum. Apply a water-soluble lubricant to your gloved index finger. Tell the patient to relax and warn him that he'll feel some pressure. Ask the patient to bear down. As the sphincter opens, gently insert your finger into the rectum, toward the umbilicus. To palpate as much of the rectal wall as possible, rotate your finger clockwise and then counterclockwise. The rectal walls should feel soft and smooth, without masses, fecal impaction, or tenderness.

Inspect and test

Remove your finger from the rectum, and inspect the glove for stool, blood, and mucus. Test fecal matter adhering to the glove for occult blood using a guaiac test.

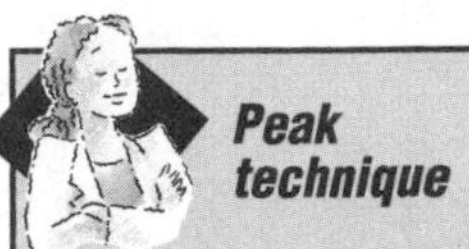

Peak technique

Checking for ascites

To check for ascites, have an assistant place the ulnar edge of her hand firmly on the patient's abdomen at its midline. Then, as you stand facing the patient's head, place the palm of your right hand against the patient's left flank, as shown below. Give the right abdomen a firm tap with your left hand. If ascites is present, you may see and feel a "fluid wave" ripple across the abdomen.

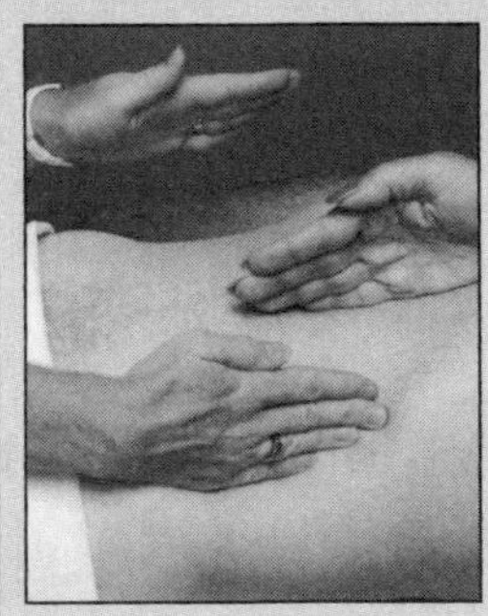

Abnormal findings

GI disorders can affect a patient's ingestion, digestion, and elimination. This section describes common abnormalities you might uncover during a GI assessment. (See *GI abnormalities*.)

Nausea and vomiting

Usually occurring together, nausea and vomiting can be caused by existing illnesses, such as myocardial infarction, gastric and peritoneal irritation, appendicitis, bowel obstruction, cholecystitis, acute pancreatitis, and neurologic disturbances, or by some medications.

Dysphagia

Dysphagia, or difficulty swallowing, may be accompanied by weight loss. It can be caused by an obstruction, achalasia of the lower esophagogastric junction, or a neurologic disease, such as stroke or Parkinson's disease. Dysphagia can lead to aspiration and pneumonia.

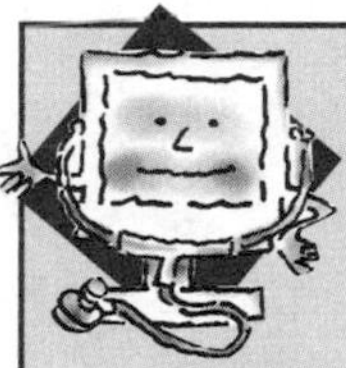

Interpretation station

GI abnormalities

This chart shows some common groups of findings for signs and symptoms of the GI system, along with their probable causes.

Sign or symptom and findings	Probable cause
Diarrhea	
• Soft, unformed stools or watery diarrhea that may be foul-smelling or grossly bloody • Abdominal pain, cramping, and tenderness • Fever	*Clostridium difficile* infection
• Diarrhea occurs within several hours of ingesting milk or milk products • Abdominal pain, cramping, and bloating • Borborygmi • Flatus	Lactose intolerance
• Recurrent bloody diarrhea with pus or mucus • Hyperactive bowel sounds • Occasional nausea and vomiting	Ulcerative colitis
Rectal bleeding	
• Moderate to severe rectal bleeding • Epistaxis • Purpura	Coagulation disorders
• Bright-red rectal bleeding with or without pain • Diarrhea or ribbon-shaped stools • Stools may be grossly bloody • Weakness and fatigue • Abdominal aching and dull cramps	Colon cancer
***Rectal bleeding** (continued)*	
• Chronic bleeding with defecation • Painful defecation	Hemorrhoids
Nausea and vomiting	
• Nausea and vomiting follow or accompany abdominal pain • Pain progresses rapidly to severe, stabbing pain in the right lower quadrant (McBurney's sign) • Abdominal rigidity and tenderness • Constipation or diarrhea • Tachycardia	Appendicitis
• Nausea and vomiting of undigested food • Diarrhea • Abdominal cramping • Hyperactive bowel sounds • Fever	Gastroenteritis
• Nausea and vomiting • Headache with severe, constant, throbbing pain • Fatigue • Photophobia • Light flashes • Increased noise sensitivity	Migraine headache

Skin color changes

A bluish umbilicus, called *Cullen's sign*, indicates intra-abdominal hemorrhage. Areas of abdominal redness may indicate inflammation. Bruising on the flank, or Turner's sign, indicates retroperitoneal hemorrhage. Dilated, tortuous, visible abdominal veins may indicate inferior vena cava obstruction. Cutaneous angiomas may signal liver disease.

Skin changes, such as Cullen's sign and Turner's sign, indicate hemorrhage.

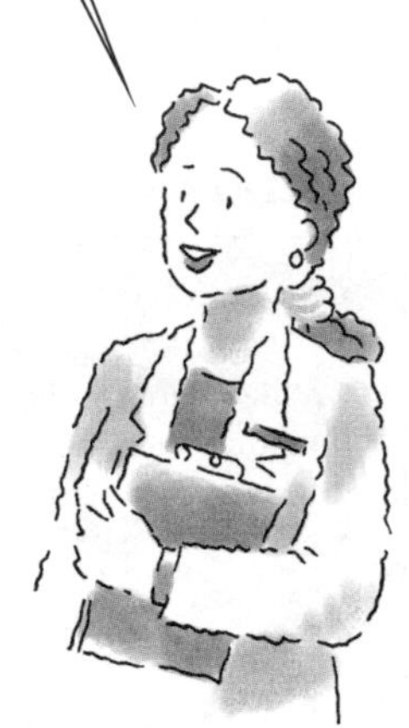

Constipation

Constipation can be caused by immobility, a sedentary lifestyle, and medications. The patient may complain of a dull ache in the abdomen, a full feeling, and hyperactive bowel sounds, which may be caused by irritable bowel syndrome. A patient with complete intestinal obstruction won't pass flatus or stool and won't have bowel sounds below the obstruction. Constipation occurs more commonly in older patients.

Diarrhea

Diarrhea may be caused by toxins, medications, or a GI condition such as Crohn's disease. Cramping, abdominal tenderness, anorexia, and hyperactive bowel sounds may accompany diarrhea. If fever occurs, the diarrhea may be caused by a toxin.

Distention

Distention may occur with gas, a tumor, or a colon filled with feces. It may also be caused by an incisional hernia, which may protrude when the patient lifts his head and shoulders.

Abnormal bowel sounds

Hyperactive bowel sounds indicate increased intestinal motility and have many causes, including laxative use, gastroenteritis, and life-threatening intestinal obstruction. Hypoactive bowel sounds can be caused by recent bowel surgery, a full colon, or paralytic ileus. (See *Abnormal abdominal sounds*.)

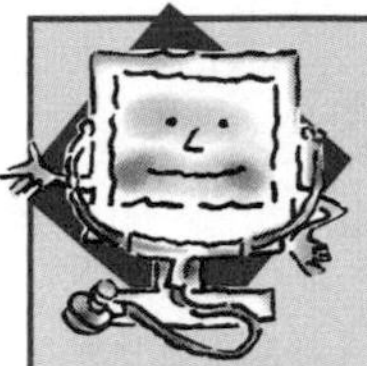

Interpretation station

Abnormal abdominal sounds

The chart below lists abnormal abdominal sounds that you may encounter. The characteristics and location of a sound can help you determine its possible cause.

Sound and description	Location	Possible cause
Abnormal bowel sounds		
Hyperactive sounds (unrelated to hunger)	Any quadrant	Diarrhea, laxative use, or early intestinal obstruction
Hypoactive, then absent sounds	Any quadrant	Paralytic ileus or peritonitis
High-pitched tinkling sounds	Any quadrant	Intestinal fluid and air under tension in a dilated bowel
High-pitched rushing sounds coinciding with abdominal cramps	Any quadrant	Intestinal obstruction
Systolic bruits		
Vascular blowing sounds resembling cardiac murmurs	Over abdominal aorta	Partial arterial obstruction or turbulent blood flow
	Over renal artery	Renal artery stenosis
	Over iliac artery	Hepatomegaly
	Over femoral artery	Arterial insufficiency in the legs
Venous hum (rare)		
Continuous, medium-pitched tone created by blood flow in a large engorged vascular organ such as the liver	Epigastric and umbilical regions	Increased collateral circulation between portal and systemic venous systems, as in cirrhosis
Friction rub (rare)		
Harsh, grating sound like two pieces of sandpaper rubbing together	Over liver and spleen	Inflammation of the peritoneal surface of the liver (as from a tumor) or of the spleen (as from an infarct)

Friction rubs and abdominal bruits

Friction rubs over the liver and spleen in the epigastric region may indicate splenic infarction or hepatic tumor. Abdominal bruits may be caused by aortic aneurysms or partial arterial obstruction.

Abdominal pain

Abdominal pain may result from ulcers, intestinal obstruction, appendicitis, cholecystitis, peritonitis, or other inflammatory disorders. A duodenal ulcer can cause gnawing abdominal pain in the midepigastrium 1½ to 3 hours after the patient has eaten. The pain may awaken the patient and be relieved by antacids or food. (See *Types of abdominal pain* and *Abdominal pain origins.*)

Tender situation

Rebound tenderness can be caused by peritonitis or appendicitis. Appendicitis may be accompanied by increased abdominal wall resistance and guarding. Not all patients have the classic right lower quadrant pain. Some older adults with appendicitis have less abdominal rigidity than younger patients.

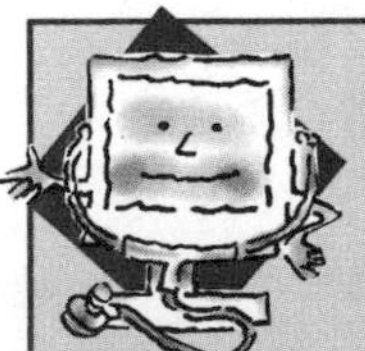

Interpretation station

Types of abdominal pain

If your patient complains of abdominal pain, ask him to describe the pain and ask how and when it started. This table will help you assess the pain and determine possible causes.

Type of pain	Possible cause
Burning	Peptic ulcer, gastroesophageal reflux disease
Cramping	Biliary colic, irritable bowel syndrome, diarrhea, constipation, flatulence
Severe cramping	Appendicitis, Crohn's disease, diverticulitis
Stabbing	Pancreatitis, cholecystitis

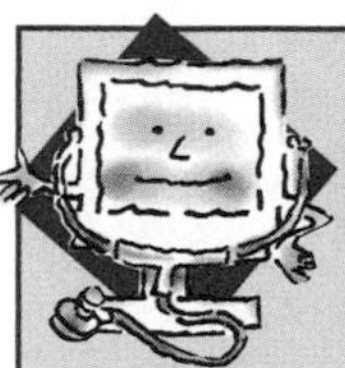

Interpretation station

Abdominal pain origins

What can you do to figure out which organ is affected if your patient has abdominal pain? Assess the location of his pain, and then look at this chart to get a quick idea of the most likely source of the pain.

Affected organ	Visceral pain	Parietal pain	Referred pain
Stomach	Midepigastrium	Midepigastrium and left upper quadrant	Shoulders
Small intestine	Periumbilical area	Over affected site	Midback (rare)
Appendix	Periumbilical area	Right lower quadrant	Right lower quadrant
Proximal colon	Periumbilical area and right flank for ascending colon	Over affected site	Right lower quadrant and back (rare)
Distal colon	Hypogastrium and left flank for descending colon	Over affected site	Left lower quadrant and back (rare)
Gallbladder	Midepigastrium	Right upper quadrant	Right subscapular area
Ureters	Costovertebral angle	Over affected site	Groin; scrotum in men, labia in women (rare)
Pancreas	Midepigastrium and left upper quadrant	Midepigastrium and left upper quadrant	Back and left shoulder
Ovaries, fallopian tubes, and uterus	Hypogastrium and groin	Over affected site	Inner thighs

Bloody stools

The passage of bloody stools, also known as *hematochezia*, usually indicates — and may be the first sign of — GI bleeding. It may also result from colorectal cancer, colitis, Crohn's disease, or an anal fissure or hemorrhoids.

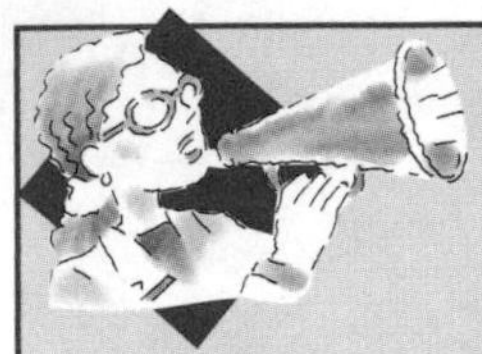

That's a wrap!

Gastrointestinal system review

Functions
- Ingestion and digestion of food
- Elimination of waste products

Structures

GI tract
- Mouth—responsible for chewing, salivation, and swallowing
- Pharynx—allows passage of food from the mouth to the esophagus
- Epiglottis—closes over larynx when food is swallowed to prevent aspiration into the airway
- Esophagus—moves food from the pharynx to the stomach
- Stomach—serves as a reservoir for food and secretes gastric juices that aid in digestion
- Small intestine—consists of the duodenum, the jejunum, and the ileum; absorbs end products of digestion into the bloodstream and digests carbohydrates, fats, and proteins
- Large intestine—consists of the cecum; the ascending, transverse, descending, and sigmoid colons; the rectum; and the anus; responsible for absorbing excess water and electrolytes, storing food residue, and eliminating waste products

Accessory organs
- Liver—metabolizes carbohydrates, fats, and proteins; detoxifies the blood; converts ammonia to urea; and synthesizes proteins and essential nutrients
- Gallbladder—stores bile from the liver until it's emptied into the duodenum
- Pancreas—releases insulin and glycogen into the bloodstream; secretes pancreatic enzymes that aid digestion
- Bile ducts—serve as passageways for bile from the liver to the intestines
- Abdominal aorta—supplies blood to the GI tract

Health history

Ask the patient about:
- past GI illnesses, surgery, and trauma
- medications, including laxative use
- current GI signs or symptoms
- family medical history, especially history of ulcerative colitis, colorectal cancer, peptic ulcers, and gastric cancer
- diet, exercise patterns, and alcohol, caffeine, and tobacco use.

Assessment

Mouth
- Inspect the mouth and jaw as well as the inner and outer lips, teeth, gums, and oral mucosa.
- Inspect the tongue.
- Palpate for areas of tenderness or lesions.

Abdomen
- Inspect the abdomen for symmetry, shape, and contour.
- Note abdominal movements and pulsations.
- Auscultate in each of the four abdominal quadrants to assess bowel sounds and over the abdominal arteries to check for bruits, venous hums, and friction rubs.
- Percuss the abdomen, listening for tympany over hollow organs (such as an empty stomach or intestine) and for dullness over solid organs (such as the liver) or feces-filled intestines.
- Palpate in all four quadrants of the abdomen, leaving painful areas for last.

Gastrointestinal system review *(continued)*

• Check for rebound tenderness if you suspect peritoneal inflammation; also check for ascites, a large accumulation of fluid in the peritoneal cavity.

Rectum and anus

• Inspect the perianal area.
• Palpate the rectum using a water-soluble lubricant on your gloved index finger.

Abnormal findings

• Nausea and vomiting—may be caused by existing illness or by certain medications
• Dysphagia—difficulty swallowing; has various causes; may lead to aspiration and pneumonia
• Cullen's sign—a bluish umbilicus; indicates intra-abdominal hemorrhage
• Turner's sign—bruising on the flank; indicates retroperitoneal hemorrhage
• Constipation—may occur with a dull abdominal ache, a full feeling, and hyperactive bowel sounds
• Diarrhea—may occur with cramping, abdominal tenderness, anorexia, and hyperactive bowel sounds
• Abdominal distention—may occur with gas, a tumor, or a colon filled with feces
• Abnormal bowels sounds—may be hyperactive (indicating increased intestinal motility) or hypoactive
• Friction rubs—may indicate splenic infarction or hepatic tumor
• Abdominal pain—may result from ulcers, intestinal obstruction, appendicitis, cholecystitis, peritonitis, or other inflammatory disorders

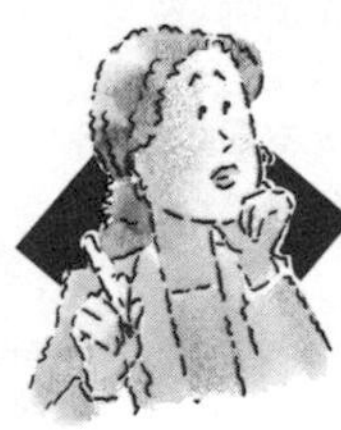

Quick quiz

1. When food is swallowed, the epiglottis:
A. opens.
B. closes.
C. opens or closes, depending on the type of food.
D. rotates.

Answer: B. The epiglottis, a thin flap of tissue over the larynx, closes during swallowing to prevent aspiration.

2. The correct sequence for an abdominal assessment is:
A. inspection, percussion, palpation, and auscultation.
B. percussion, auscultation, inspection, and palpation.
C. inspection, auscultation, percussion, and palpation.
D. auscultation, inspection, palpation, and percussion.

Answer: C. Percussion and palpation can increase intestinal motility and bowel sounds, so inspection and auscultation must be done first.

3. Hyperactive bowel sounds may be a sign of:
- A. ileus or bowel obstruction.
- B. peritonitis or opioid analgesic use.
- C. constipation, diarrhea, or laxative use.
- D. diminished peristalsis.

Answer: C. Hyperactive bowel sounds are a sign of constipation, diarrhea, or laxative use.

4. When you percuss over the liver, you should hear:
- A. dullness.
- B. resonance.
- C. tympany.
- D. hyperresonance.

Answer: A. Percussing over a solid organ, such as the liver or kidney, should create a dull sound.

5. To test a patient for rebound tenderness, position your hand at a:
- A. 30-degree angle to the abdomen.
- B. 45- to 60-degree angle to the abdomen.
- C. 90-degree angle to the abdomen.
- D. 120-degree angle to the abdomen.

Answer: C. Choosing a site away from the painful area, position your hand at a 90-degree angle to the abdomen. Push down slowly and deeply into the abdomen, and then withdraw your hand quickly.

Scoring

☆☆☆ If you answered all five questions correctly, congratulations! You effectively digested an abundance of facts concerning GI assessments.

☆☆ If you answered four questions correctly, super! Your ability to chew up the information in this chapter is truly impressive!

☆ If you answered fewer than four questions correctly, that's okay! All the information on GI assessments may have been a lot to swallow at one sitting. Why not go over it again?

Female genitourinary system

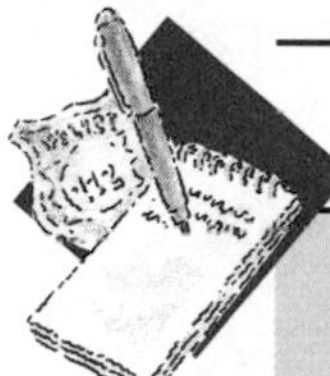

Just the facts

In this chapter, you'll learn:

- organs and structures that make up the female GU system
- methods to obtain a patient history
- techniques for performing a physical assessment of the female GU system
- abnormalities of the female GU system.

A look at the female GU system

The female genitourinary (GU) system encompasses the urinary tract and the reproductive organs and structures. Disorders of this system can have wide-ranging effects on other body systems. For example, ovarian dysfunction can alter hormonal balance. Kidney dysfunction can alter blood pressure, disrupt serum electrolytes, and affect production of the hormone erythropoietin, which regulates the production of red blood cells.

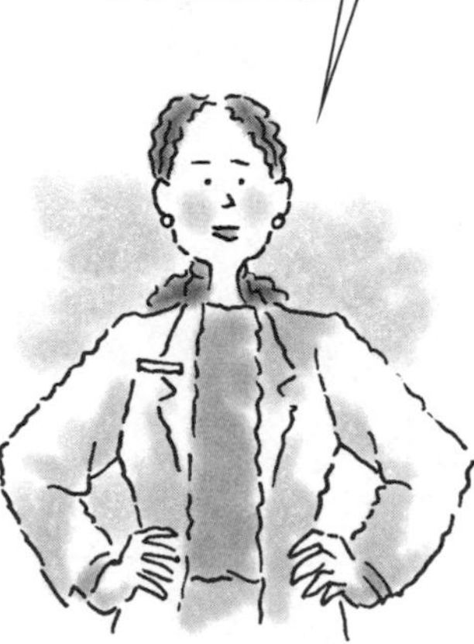

Subtle signs and symptoms

Assessing the female GU system can be a challenging task. Many patients with urinary disorders don't realize they're ill because they have only mild signs and symptoms or no symptoms at all. It's easy to overlook underlying problems.

Complex system

More women seek health care for reproductive disorders than for anything else. Assessing those problems can be difficult because the reproductive system is complex and its functions have far-reaching psychosocial implications.

Anatomy and physiology of the female GU system

To perform an accurate assessment, you'll need to have a firm grasp of the anatomy and physiology of the GU system. This section reviews the urinary system and the reproductive system.

Urinary system

The urinary system consists of the kidneys, ureters, bladder, and urethra. (See *Urinary system.*)

Kidneys

The essential functions of the urinary system — such as forming urine and maintaining the proper balance of fluids, minerals, and organic substances for homeostasis — take place in the highly vas-

Urinary system

This illustration shows the main structures of the urinary system.

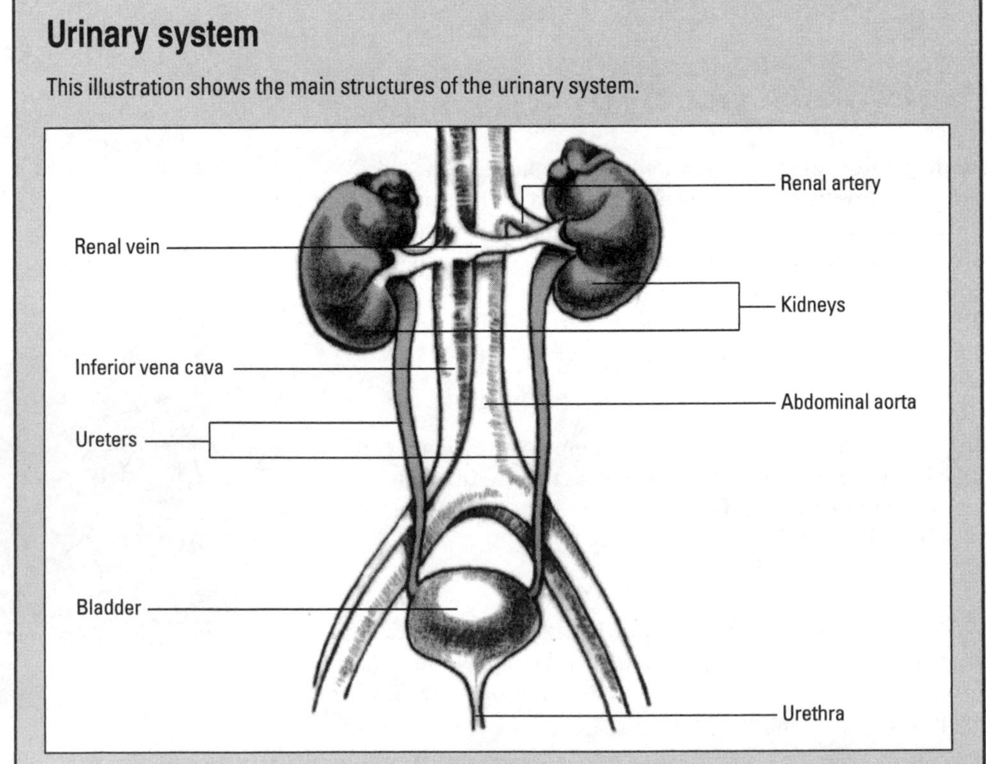

cular kidneys. These bean-shaped organs are 4½″ to 5″ (11.5 to 12.5 cm) long and 2½″ (6.4 cm) wide. Located retroperitoneally on either side of the lumbar vertebrae, the kidneys lie behind the abdominal organs and in front of the muscles attached to the vertebral column. The peritoneal fat layer protects them.

Makin' urine

Crowded by the liver, the right kidney extends slightly lower than does the left. Each kidney contains roughly one million nephrons. Urine gathers in the collecting tubules and ducts of the nephrons and eventually drains into the ureters, down into the bladder and, when urination occurs, out through the urethra.

Ureters

The ureters are 10″ to 12″ (25.5 to 30.5 cm) long. The left ureter is slightly longer than the right because of the left kidney's higher position. The diameter of each ureter varies from ⅛″ to ¼″ (3 to 6 mm), with the narrowest part at the ureteropelvic junction.

The rhythm of the flow

Located along the posterior abdominal wall, the ureters enter the bladder anteromedially. They carry urine from the kidneys to the bladder by peristaltic contractions that occur one to five times per minute.

Bladder

Located in the pelvis, the bladder is a hollow, muscular organ that serves as a container for urine collection. When the bladder is empty, it lies behind the pelvic bone; when it's full, it becomes displaced under the peritoneal cavity. Bladder capacity ranges from 500 to 1,000 ml in healthy adults. The bladders of children and elderly people have a lower capacity.

Urethra

The urethra is a small duct that carries urine from the bladder to the outside of the body. A woman's urethra is only 1″ to 2″ (2.5 to 5 cm) long and anterior to the vaginal opening.

The reproductive system is the source of most health complaints in women.

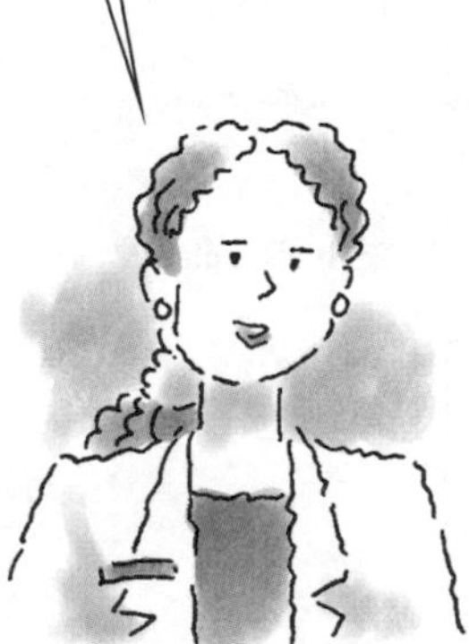

Reproductive system

The female reproductive system consists of external and internal genitalia. Let's start with external genitalia.

External genitalia

The external genitalia, collectively called the *vulva*, consist of the mons pubis, labia majora, labia minora, clitoris, vagina, urethra, and Skene's and Bartholin's glands. (See *External genitalia.*)

Mons pubis

The mons pubis is a mound of adipose tissue overlying the symphysis pubis. In adults, it's covered with pubic hair. Pubic hair first appears on average at age 10½. It may become sparse after menopause because of hormonal changes. Native Americans and Asians usually have less pubic hair than do people of other races.

Labia majora and minora

The outer vulval lips, or labia majora, are two rounded folds of adipose tissue that extend from the mons pubis to the perineum. The labia majora are covered with hair.

The inner vulval lips are called the *labia minora.* The anterolateral and medial parts join to form the prepuce or hood, the folds of skin that cap the clitoris. The posterior union of the labia minora is called the *fourchette* or *frenulum.*

External genitalia

This illustration shows the main parts of the external female genitalia.

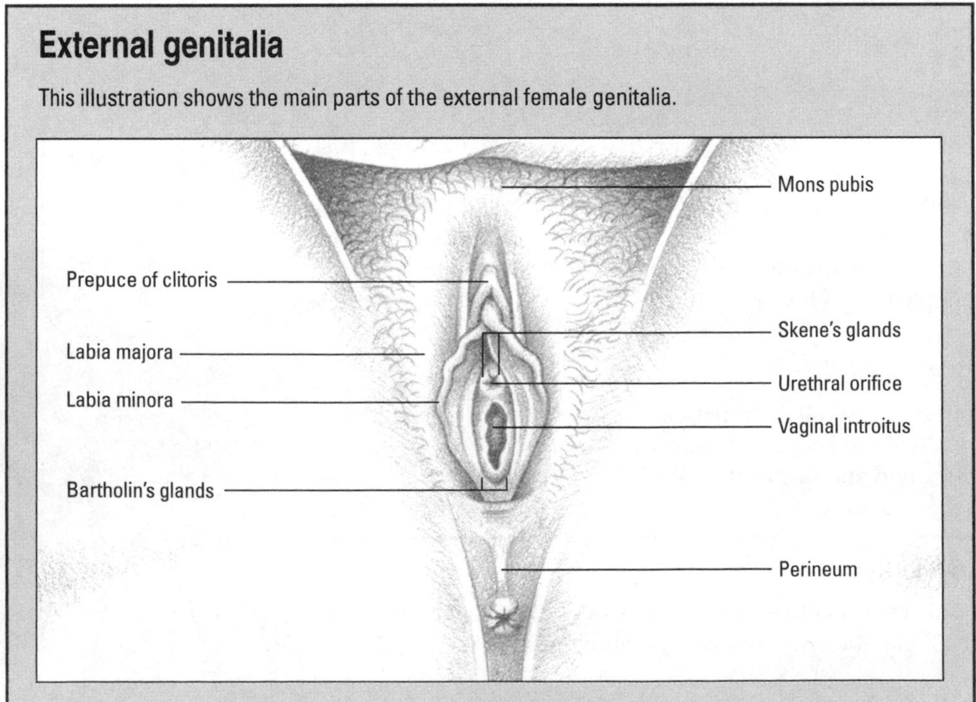

Clitoris, vestibule, and urethral opening

The clitoris is composed of erectile tissue and lies between the labia minora at the top of the vestibule, which contains the urethral and vaginal openings. The urethral opening is a slit below the clitoris.

Vaginal opening and perineum

The vaginal opening, or introitus, is posterior to the urethral orifice. This opening is a thin vertical slit in women who have intact hymens (the thin fold of mucous membrane that partially covers the vaginal opening). The opening is large with irregular edges in women whose hymens have been perforated. In some women, the hymen is absent.

The perineum is the area bordered anteriorly by the top of the labial fold and posteriorly by the anus.

Skene's and Bartholin's glands

Two kinds of glands have ducts that open into the vulva. Skene's glands are tiny structures just below the urethra, each containing 6 to 31 ducts. Bartholin's glands are found posterior to the vaginal opening. Neither of these glands can be seen, but they can be palpated if enlarged.

Fluid generators

Skene's and Bartholin's glands produce lubricating fluids important for the reproductive process. They can become infected, usually with organisms known to cause sexually transmitted diseases (STDs).

Internal genitalia

The internal genitalia include the vagina, uterus, ovaries, and fallopian tubes. (See *Internal genitalia*, page 256.)

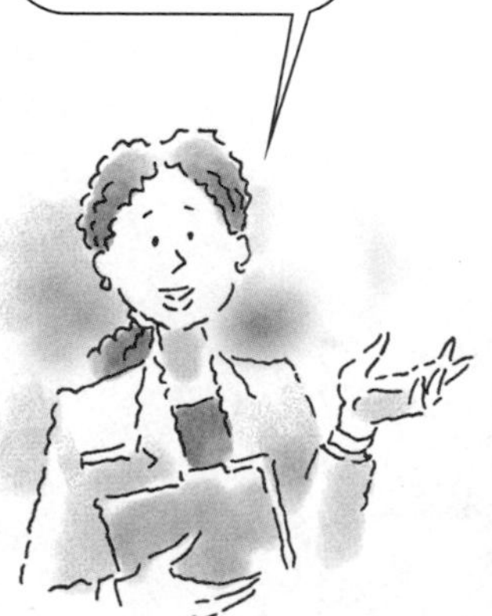

Vagina

A pink, hollow, collapsed tube, the vagina is located between the urethra and the rectum, extending up and back from the vulva to the uterus. It's the route of passage for childbirth and menstruation.

Uterus

The uterus is a hollow, pear-shaped, muscular organ that lies between the rectum and the bladder. It's divided into the fundus (the upper portion of the uterus) and the cervix, which protrudes into the vagina. The cervix contains mucus-secreting glands that help in reproduction and protect the uterus from pathogens. The func-

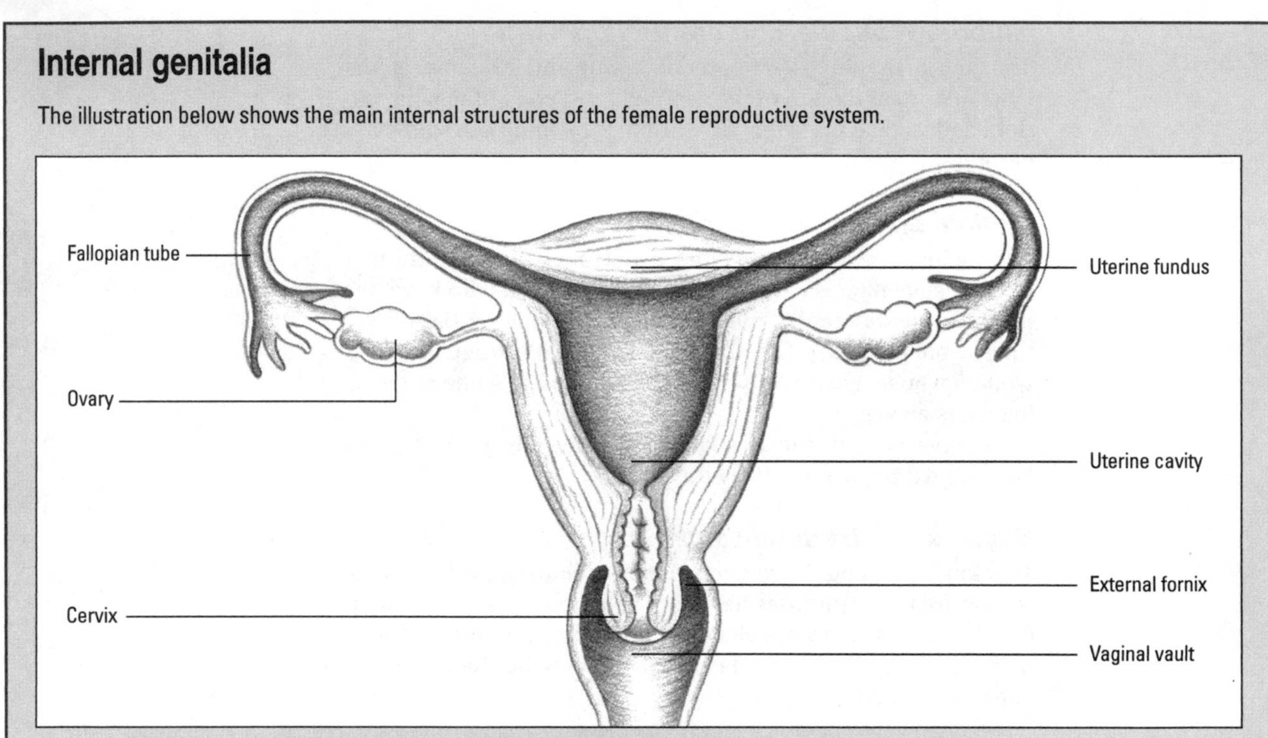

Internal genitalia

The illustration below shows the main internal structures of the female reproductive system.

tion of the uterus is to nurture and then expel the fetus during pregnancy.

Locations may vary

The position of the uterus in the pelvic cavity may vary, depending on bladder fullness. The uterus may also tilt in different directions.

Ovaries

A pair of oval glands about 1¼″ (3 cm) long, the ovaries are usually found in the lower abdominal cavity, one on each side of the uterus. They produce ova (or eggs) and release the hormones estrogen and progesterone. The ovaries become fully developed after puberty and shrink after menopause.

Fallopian tubes

Each approximately 4″ (10 cm) long, the two fallopian tubes extend from the ovaries into the upper portion of the uterus. Their funnel-shaped ends curve toward the ovaries and, during ovulation, help guide the ova to the uterus after expulsion from the ovaries. The fallopian tube is also the usual site of fertilization of the ova by the sperm.

Obtaining a health history

Because the urinary and reproductive systems are located so close together in women, you and your patient may have trouble differentiating signs and symptoms. Even if the patient's complaint seems minor, investigate it. Ask about its onset, duration, and severity and ask about measures taken to treat it. The information you gain will help you formulate a more appropriate care plan.

Asking about the urinary system

The most common complaints of the urinary system include output changes, such as polyuria, oliguria, and anuria; voiding pattern changes, such as hesitancy, frequency, urgency, nocturia, and incontinence; urine color changes; and pain.

Dredging up the past

Past illnesses and preexisting conditions can affect a patient's urinary tract health. For example, has the patient ever had a urinary tract infection (UTI), kidney trauma, or kidney stones? Kidney stones or trauma can alter the structure and function of the kidneys and bladder.

What's the problem?

Ask the patient about current problems and medications. Does she have diabetes, cardiovascular disease, or hypertension? Patients with diabetes have an increased risk of UTIs. Cardiovascular disease can alter kidney perfusion. Hypertension can contribute to renal failure and nephropathy.

Make sure "urine" the know about urination

Has she noticed a change in the color or odor of her urine? Does she have pain or burning during urination? Does she have problems with incontinence or frequency? Does she have allergies? Allergic reactions can cause tubular damage. A severe anaphylactic reaction can cause temporary renal failure and permanent tubular necrosis.

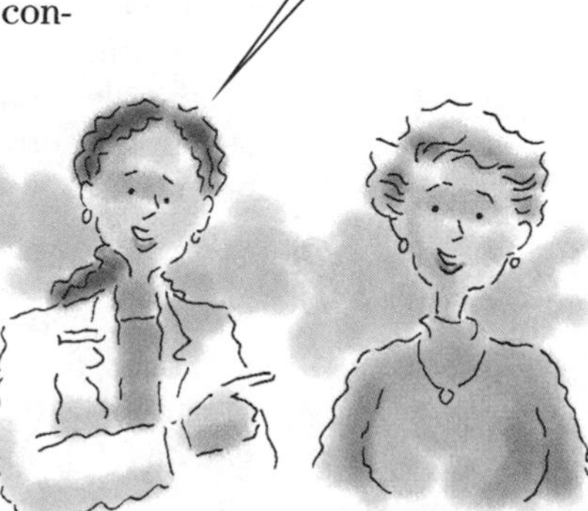

Discuss drugs

Make a list of all the prescribed medications, herbal preparations, and over-the-counter drugs the patient takes. Some drugs can affect the appearance of urine; nephrotoxic drugs can alter urinary function.

Familial factors

Also ask about the patient's family history to get information about her risk of developing kidney failure or kidney disease.

Asking about the reproductive system

The most common reproductive system complaints are pain, vaginal discharge, abnormal uterine bleeding, pruritus, and infertility. To obtain the most complete data about those problems, focus on the patient's current complaints, and then explore her reproductive, sexual-social, and family history. Ask her to describe symptoms in her own words, encouraging her to speak freely.

Ease into it

Many patients feel uncomfortable answering questions about their sexual health or reproductive system. Start with the less personal questions to establish rapport.

Go with the flow

Start by asking about her menstrual cycle. How old was she when she began to menstruate? How long does her menses usually last? How often does it occur? The normal cycle for menstruation is one menses every 21 to 38 days. The normal duration is 2 to 8 days. (See *Cultural influences on menstruation.*)

Does she have cramps, spotting, or an unusually heavy or light flow? Spotting between menses, or metrorrhagia, may be normal in patients taking low-dose hormonal contraceptives or progesterone; otherwise, spotting may indicate infection, cancer, or other abnormality.

In girls, menses generally starts by age 15. If it hasn't and if no secondary sex characteristics have developed, the patient should be evaluated by a doctor.

The sexual side

When the patient seems comfortable, ask her about her sexual practices, the number of sexual partners she currently has, whether she experiences pain with intercourse, if she has ever had an STD, and her human immunodeficiency virus status. When was her last Papanicolaou (Pap) test, and what was the result? Finally, ask if she has questions or concerns.

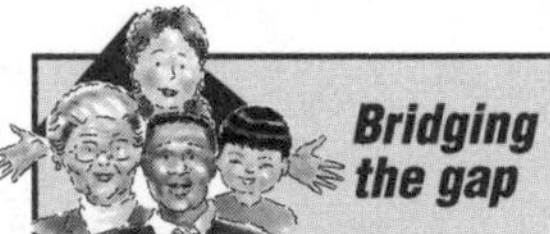

Bridging the gap

Cultural influences on menstruation

Studies have shown that a patient's ethnicity has a strong influence on the duration and heaviness of bleeding during menses. Black girls tend to have longer menses than White girls of the same age. They're also more likely to have a heavier menstrual blood flow than White girls. However, keep in mind that a girl's diet, exercise habits, and stress level may also influence the duration and heaviness of menstruation.

Past, present, and possible pregnancy

Ask the patient if she has ever been pregnant. If so, how many times has she been pregnant and how many times did she give birth? Has she had any miscarriages or therapeutic abortions? Did she have a vaginal or cesarean delivery? What kind of birth control, if any, does she use? If the patient is sexually active, talk to her about the importance of safer sex and the prevention of STDs.

Pause to reflect

If your patient is postmenopausal, ask for the date of her last menses. To find out more about her menopausal symptoms, ask her if she's having hot flashes, night sweats, mood swings, flushing, or vaginal dryness or itching.

Assessing the female GU system

To perform a physical assessment of the GU system, you'll use the techniques of inspection, percussion, and palpation.

Examining the urinary system

Before assessing specific structures of the urinary system, evaluate your patient's vital signs, weight, and mental status. These observations will provide clues about renal dysfunction.

For example, a patient's vital signs might reveal hypertension, which can cause renal dysfunction if it's uncontrolled. Be sure to check blood pressure in each arm. Weighing the patient can provide information about fluid status and is important for patients with urinary disorders or renal failure, especially those receiving dialysis.

Telltale behavior

Observing the patient's behavior can give you clues about her mental status. Does she have trouble concentrating, have memory loss, or seem disoriented? Kidney dysfunction can cause those symptoms. Progressive, chronic kidney failure can cause lethargy, confusion, disorientation, stupor, seizures, and coma.

Inspection

First, observe the color and shape of the area around the kidneys and bladder. The skin should be free from lesions, discolorations, inflammation, and swelling.

Check blood pressure in each arm because hypertension can lead to renal dysfunction.

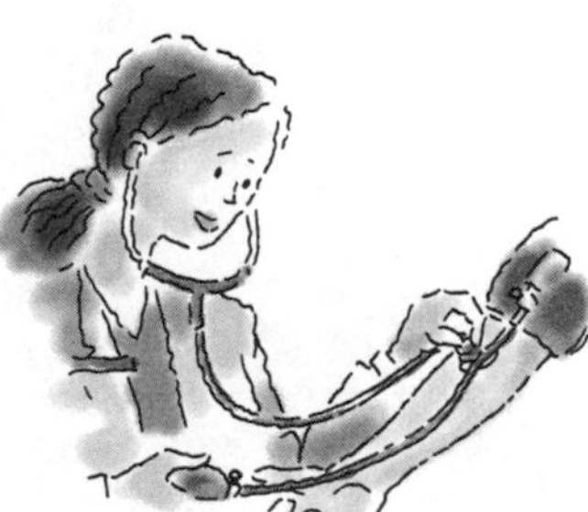

Percussion

Kidney percussion checks for costovertebral angle tenderness that occurs with inflammation. To percuss over the kidneys, have the patient sit up. Place the ball of your nondominant hand on her back at the costovertebral angle of the 12th rib. Strike the ball of that hand with the ulnar surface of your other hand. Use just enough force to cause a painless but perceptible thud.

The bladder matters

To percuss the bladder, first ask the patient to empty it. Then have her lie in the supine position. Start at the symphysis pubis and percuss upward toward the bladder and over it. You should hear tympany. A dull sound signals retained urine.

Palpation

Because the kidneys lie behind other organs and are protected by muscle, they normally aren't palpable unless they're enlarged. However, in very thin patients, you may be able to feel the lower end of the right kidney as a smooth round mass that drops on inspiration. (See *Palpating the kidneys.*)

In elderly patients, you may be able to palpate both kidneys because of decreased muscle tone and elasticity. If the kidneys feel enlarged, the patient may have hydronephrosis, cysts, or tumors.

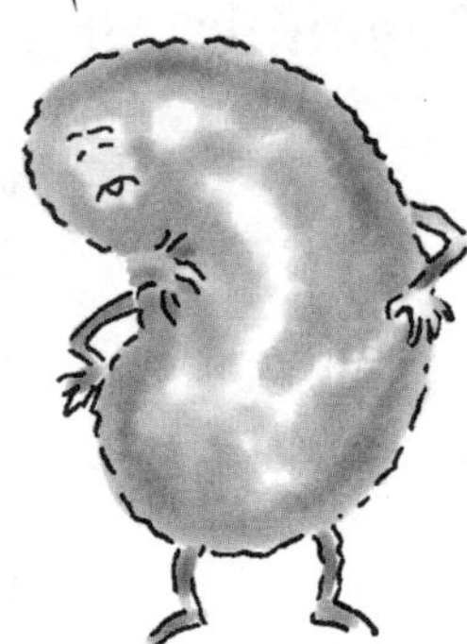

If the bladder is full, you'll feel it

You won't be able to palpate the bladder unless it's distended. With the patient in a supine position, use the fingers of one hand to palpate the lower abdomen in a light dipping motion. A distended bladder will feel firm and relatively smooth, extending above the symphysis pubis. If the patient is 12 or more weeks pregnant, you might actually be feeling the fundus of the uterus, palpable just above the symphysis pubis.

Examining the reproductive system

Before the examination, ask the patient to void to prevent discomfort and inaccurate findings during palpation. Have her disrobe and put on an examination gown. Help her into the dorsal lithotomy position, and drape all areas not being examined. Make sure you explain the procedure to her before the examination.

You'll begin by examining her external genitalia and then her internal genitalia.

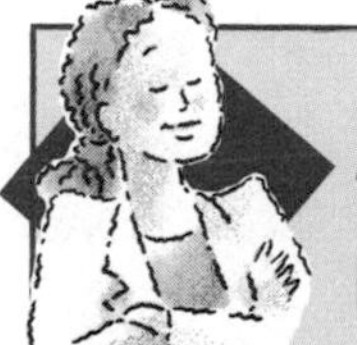

Peak technique

Palpating the kidneys

To palpate the kidneys, first have the patient lie in a supine position. To palpate the right kidney, stand on her right side. Place your left hand under her back and your right hand on her abdomen.

Instruct the patient to inhale deeply, so her kidney moves downward. As she inhales, press up with your left hand and down with your right, as shown at right.

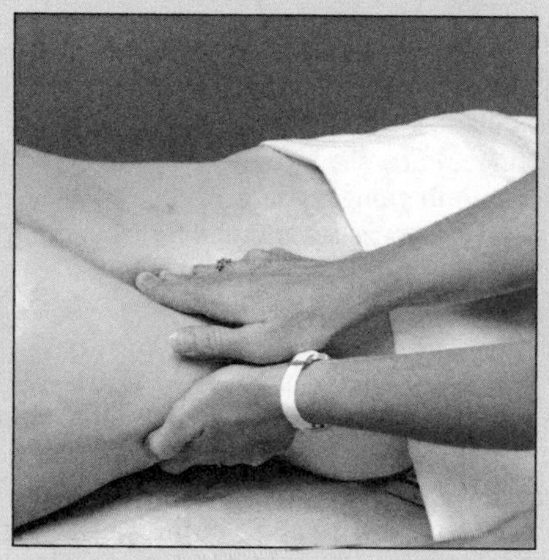

To palpate the left kidney, reach across the patient's abdomen, placing your left hand behind her left flank. Place your right hand over the area of the left kidney. Ask the patient to inhale deeply again. As she does so, pull up with your left hand and press down with your right.

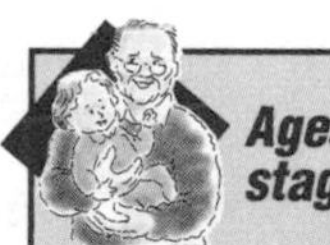

Ages and stages

Pubic hair development

Pubic hair changes in density, color, and texture throughout a woman's life. Before adolescence, the pubic area is covered only with body hair. In adolescence, this body hair grows thicker, darker, coarser, and curlier. In full maturity, it spreads over the symphysis pubis and inner thighs. In later years, the hair grows thin, gray, and brittle.

Inspecting the external genitalia

First, put on a pair of gloves. Spread the labia and locate the urethral meatus. It should be a pink, irregular, slitlike opening at the midline, just above the vagina. Note the presence of discharge (a sign of urethral infection) or ulcerations (a sign of an STD). Inspect the external genitalia and pubic hair to assess sexual maturity. (See *Pubic hair development.*)

A look at the labia

Using your index finger and thumb, gently spread the labia majora and minora. They should be moist and free from lesions. You may detect a normal discharge that varies from clear and stretchy before ovulation to white and opaque after ovulation. The discharge should be odorless and nonirritating to the mucosa.

View the vestibule

Examine the vestibule, especially the area around the Bartholin's and Skene's glands. Check for swelling, redness, lesions, discharge, and unusual odor. If you detect any of these conditions, notify the doctor and obtain a specimen for culture. Finally, inspect the vaginal opening, noting whether the hymen is intact or perforated.

Palpating the external genitalia

Spread the labia with one hand and palpate with the other. The labia should feel soft and the patient shouldn't feel any pain. Note swelling, hardness, or tenderness. If you detect a mass or lesion, palpate it to determine its size, shape, and consistency.

A gentle touch

If you find swelling or tenderness, see if you can palpate Bartholin's glands, which normally aren't palpable. To do this, insert your finger carefully into the patient's posterior introitus, and place your thumb along the lateral edge of the swollen or tender labium. Gently squeeze the labium. If discharge from the duct results, culture it.

Under fire

If the urethra is inflamed, milk it and the area of Skene's glands. First, moisten your gloved index finger with water. Then separate the labia with your other hand, and insert your index finger about 1¼″ (3 cm) into the anterior vagina. With the pad of your finger, gently press and pull outward. Continue palpating down to the introitus. This procedure shouldn't cause the patient discomfort. Culture the discharge.

Inspecting the internal genitalia

Nurses don't routinely inspect internal genitalia unless they're in advanced practice. However, you may be asked to assist with this examination. To start, select an appropriate speculum for your patient. (See *Speculum types.*)

Warm welcome

Hold the speculum under warm, running water to lubricate and warm the blades. Don't use other lubricants; many of them are bacteriostatic and can alter Pap test results.

Tell her about it

Sit or stand at the foot of the examination table. Tell the patient she'll feel internal pressure and possibly some slight, transient discomfort as you insert and open the speculum.

Just relax

Using your dominant hand, hold the speculum by the base with the blades anchored between your index and middle fingers. This causes less discomfort and keeps the blades from accidentally opening during insertion. Encourage the patient to take slow, deep

Encourage the patient to take slow, deep breaths to promote relaxation and minimize discomfort. Helping the patient relax will also help ensure accurate examination results.

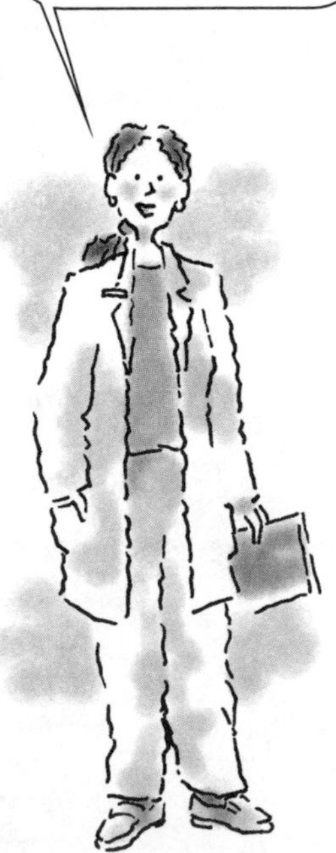

Speculum types

Specula come in various shapes and sizes. Choose an appropriate one for your patient. A Graves' speculum is usually used. However, if the patient has an intact hymen, has never given birth through the vaginal canal, or has a contracted introitus from menopause, use a Pederson speculum, which has narrower blades. The illustrations here show the parts of a typical speculum and three types of specula available.

Parts of a speculum

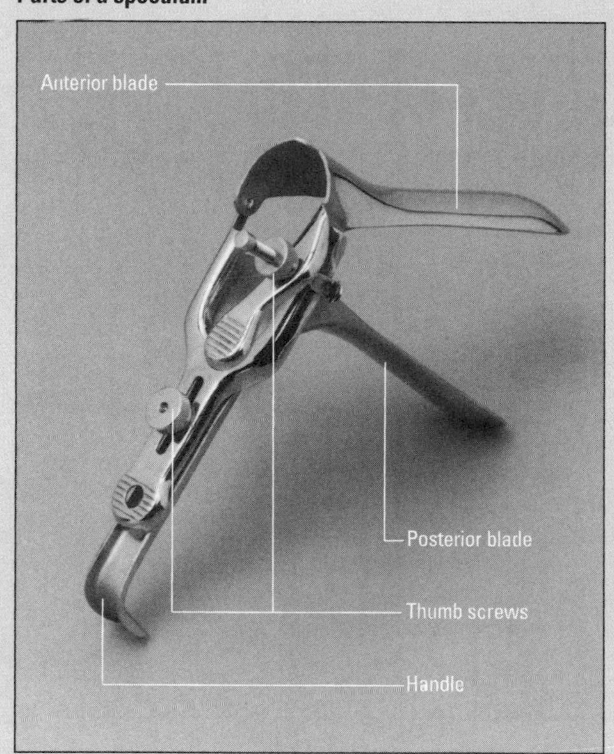

Types of specula

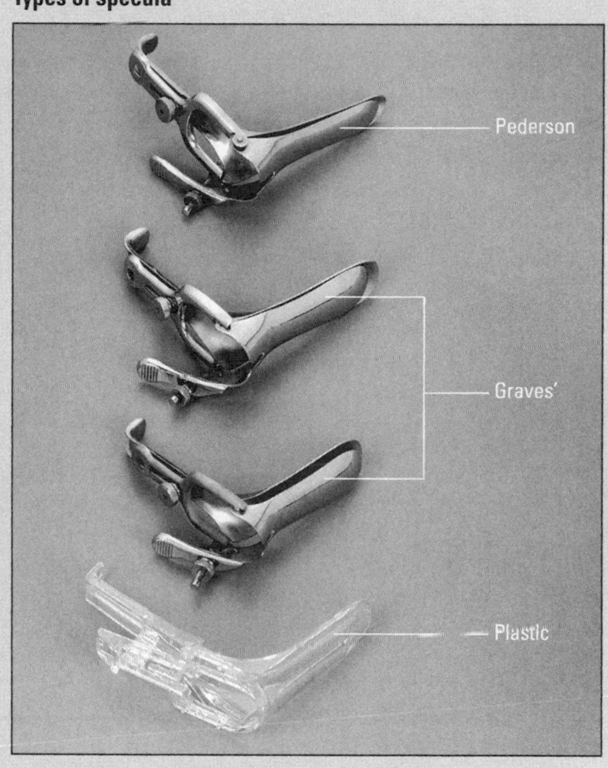

breaths during insertion to relax her abdominal muscles. (See *Inserting a speculum*, page 264.)

A look inside

After inserting the speculum, observe the color, texture, and integrity of the vaginal lining. A thin, white, odorless discharge on the vaginal walls is normal. Using the thumb of the hand holding the speculum, press the lower lever to open the blades. Lock them in the open position by tightening the thumb screw above the lever.

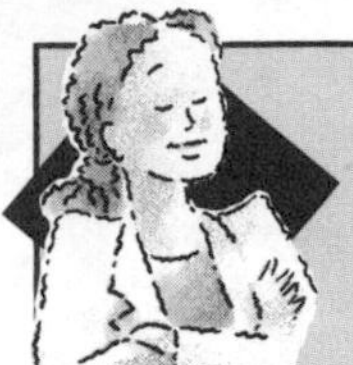

Peak technique

Inserting a speculum

Proper positioning and insertion of the speculum are important for the comfort of the patient and for the proper visualization of internal structures.

Initial insertion
Place the index and middle fingers of your nondominant hand about 1″ (2.5 cm) into the vagina and spread the fingers to exert pressure on the posterior vagina. Hold the speculum in your dominant hand, and insert the blades between your fingers, as shown below.

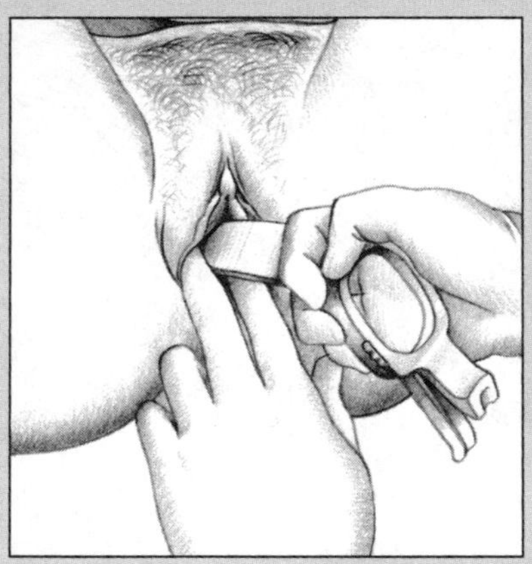

Deeper insertion
Ask the patient to bear down to open the introitus and relax the perineal muscles. Point the speculum slightly downward, and insert the blades until the base of the speculum touches your fingers, inside the vagina.

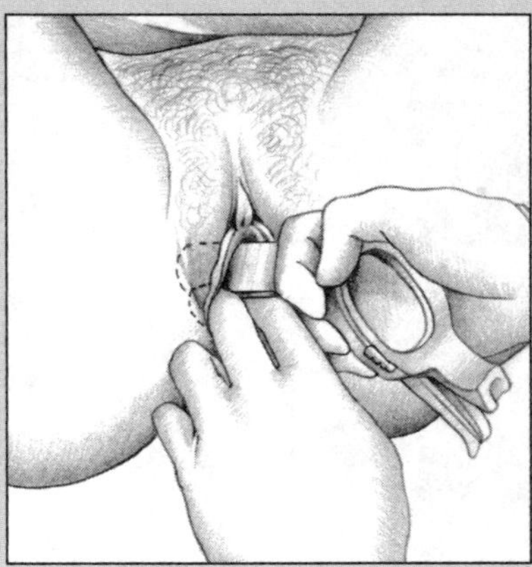

Rotate and open
Rotate the speculum in the same plane as the vagina, and withdraw your fingers. Open the blades as far as possible and lock them. You should now be able to view the cervix clearly.

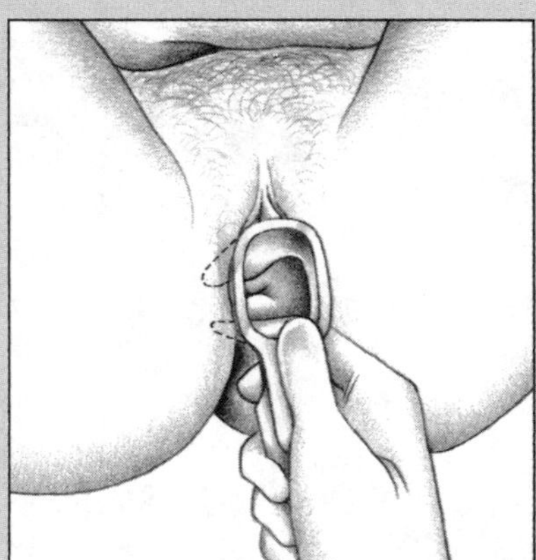

The typical view

Examine the cervix for color, position, size, shape, mucosal integrity, and discharge. It should be smooth and round. The central cervical opening, or cervical os, is circular in a woman who hasn't given birth vaginally and a horizontal slit in a woman who has. Expect to see a clear, watery cervical discharge during ovulation and a slightly bloody discharge just before menstruation. (See *The normal os.*)

Use the speculum to obtain a specimen for a Pap test. Finally, unlock and close the blades and withdraw the speculum.

The normal os

These illustrations show the difference between the os of a woman who has never given birth vaginally (is nulliparous) and the os of a woman who has (is parous).

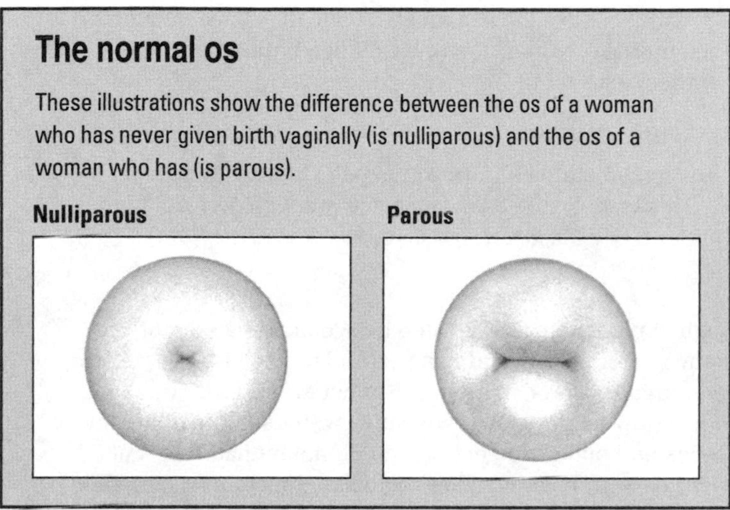

Palpating the internal genitalia

To palpate the internal genitalia, lubricate the index and middle fingers of your gloved dominant hand. Stand at the foot of the examination table and position the hand for insertion into the vagina by extending your thumb, index, and middle fingers and curling your ring and little finger toward your palm.

Use the thumb and index finger of your other hand to spread the labia majora. Insert your two lubricated fingers into the vagina, exerting pressure posteriorly to avoid irritating the anterior wall and urethra.

Probing the issue

When your fingers are fully inserted, note tenderness or nodularity in the vaginal wall. Ask the patient to bear down so you can assess the support of the vaginal outlet. Bulging of the vaginal wall may indicate a cystocele or a rectocele.

Making a clean sweep

To palpate the cervix, sweep your fingers from side to side across the cervix and around the os. The cervix should be smooth and firm and protrude ¼″ to 1¼″ (0.5 to 3 cm) into the vagina. If you palpate nodules or irregularities, the patient may have cysts, tumors, or other lesions.

Movin' right along

Next, place your fingers into the recessed area around the cervix. The cervix should move in all directions. If the patient reports pain during this part of the examination, she may have inflammation of the uterus or adnexa (ovaries, fallopian tubes, and ligaments of the uterus).

If the patient experiences pain when the cervix is palpated, she may have inflammation of the uterus or adnexa.

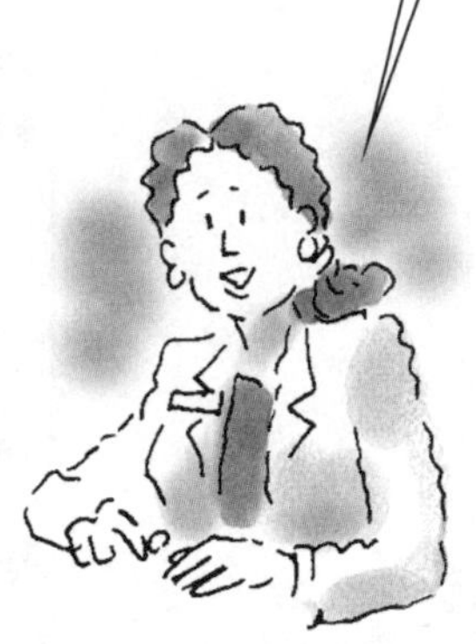

Two hands are better than one

A bimanual examination allows you to palpate the uterus and ovaries. Usually, only nurses in advanced practice perform bimanual palpation. (See *Performing a bimanual examination.*)

The last step

Rectovaginal palpation, the last step in a genital assessment, examines the posterior part of the uterus and the pelvic cavity. Warn the patient that this procedure may be uncomfortable.

Put on a new pair of gloves and apply water-soluble lubricant to the index and middle fingers of your dominant hand. Instruct the patient to bear down with her vaginal and rectal muscles; then insert your index finger a short way into her vagina and your middle finger into her rectum.

Testing the tone

Use your middle finger to assess rectal muscle and sphincter tone. Insert your finger deeper into the rectum, and palpate the rectal wall with your middle finger. Sweep the rectum with your fingers, assessing for masses or nodules.

Palpate the posterior wall of the uterus through the anterior wall of the rectum, evaluating the uterus for size, shape, tenderness, and masses. The rectovaginal septum, the wall between the rectum and the vagina, should feel smooth and springy.

On the edge of discovery

Place your nondominant hand on the patient's abdomen at the symphysis pubis. With your index finger in the vagina, palpate deeply to feel the posterior edge of the cervix and the lower posterior wall of the uterus.

When you're finished, discard the gloves and wash your hands. Help the patient to a sitting position, and provide privacy for dressing and personal hygiene.

Abnormal findings

This section discusses common abnormalities of the GU system. (See *Female GU abnormalities*, pages 268 and 269.)

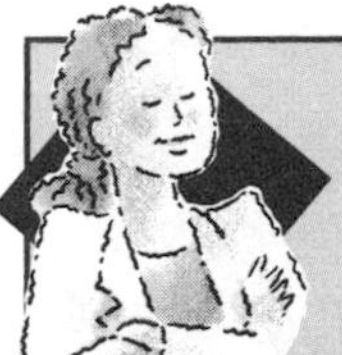

Peak technique

Performing a bimanual examination

During a bimanual examination, palpate the uterus and ovaries from the inside and the outside simultaneously. The illustrations here show how to perform such an examination.

1. Proper position

After putting on gloves, place the index and third fingers of your dominant hand in the patient's vagina and move them up to the cervix. Place the fingers of your other hand on the patient's abdomen between the umbilicus and the symphysis pubis, as shown below.

Elevate the cervix and uterus by pressing upward with the two fingers inside the vagina. At the same time, press down and in with the hand on the abdomen. Try to grasp the uterus between your hands.

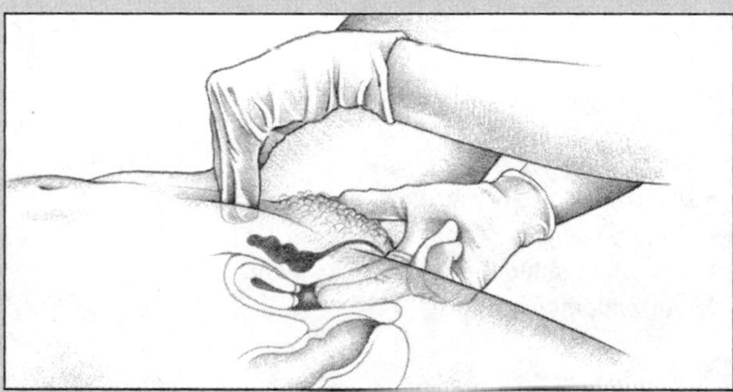

2. Note the position

Next, move your fingers into the posterior fornix, pressing upward and forward to bring the anterior uterine wall up to your nondominant hand. Use your dominant hand to palpate the lower portion of the uterine wall. Note the position of the uterus.

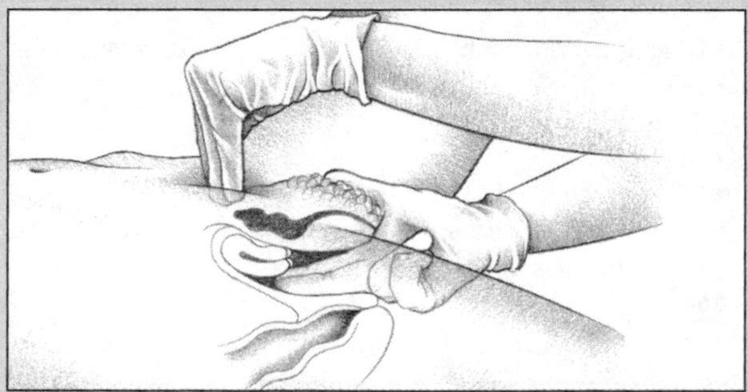

3. Palpate the walls

Slide your fingers farther into the anterior section of the fornix, the space between the uterus and cervix. You should feel part of the posterior uterine wall with this hand. You should feel part of the anterior uterine wall with the fingertips of your nondominant hand. Note the size, shape, surface characteristics, consistency, and mobility of the uterus as well as tenderness.

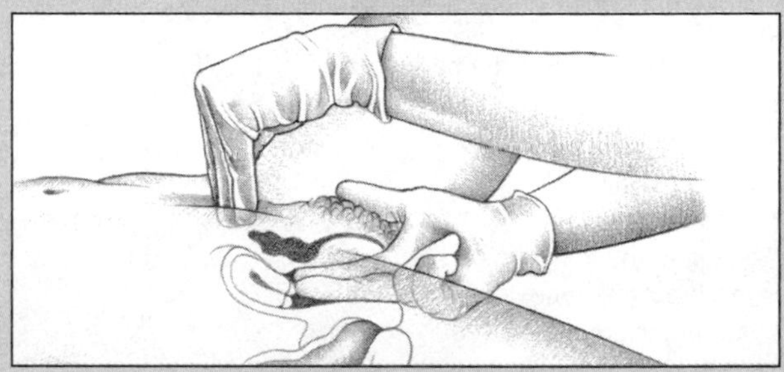

4. Palpate the ovaries

After palpating the anterior and posterior walls of the uterus, move your nondominant hand toward the right lower quadrant of the abdomen. Slip the fingers of your dominant hand into the right fornix and palpate the right ovary. Then palpate the left ovary. Note the size, shape, and contour of each ovary. The ovaries may not be palpable in women who aren't relaxed or who are obese. They shouldn't be palpable in postmenopausal women. Remove your hand from the patient's abdomen and your fingers from her vagina, and discard your gloves.

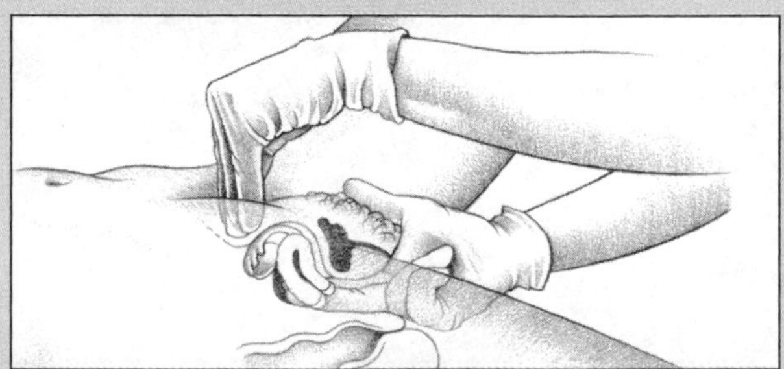

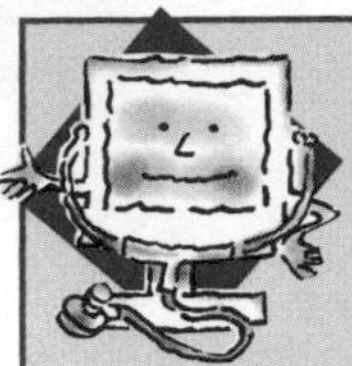

Interpretation station

Female GU abnormalities

This chart shows some common groups of findings for disorders of the female genitourinary (GU) system, along with their probable causes.

Sign or symptom and findings	Probable cause
Dysmenorrhea	
• Steady, aching pain that begins before menses and peaks at the height of menstrual flow; may occur between menses • Pain may radiate to the perineum or rectum • Premenstrual spotting • Dyspareunia • Infertility • Nausea and vomiting • Tender, fixed adnexal mass palpable on bimanual examination	Endometriosis
• Severe abdominal pain • Fever • Malaise • Foul-smelling, purulent vaginal discharge • Menorrhagia • Cervical motion tenderness and bilateral adnexal tenderness or pelvic examination	Pelvic inflammatory disease
• Cramping pain that begins with menstrual flow and diminishes with decreasing flow • Abdominal bloating • Breast tenderness • Depression • Irritability • Headache • Diarrhea	Premenstrual syndrome

Sign or symptom and findings	Probable cause
Dysuria	
• Urinary frequency • Nocturia • Straining to void • Hematuria • Perineal or low-back pain • Fatigue • Low-grade fever	Cystitis
• Dysuria throughout voiding • Bladder distention • Diminished urinary stream • Urinary frequency and urgency • Sensation of bloating or fullness in the lower abdomen or groin	Urinary system obstruction
• Urinary urgency • Hematuria • Bladder spasms • Feeling of warmth or burring during urination	Urinary tract infection
Urinary incontinence	
• Urge or overflow incontinence • Hematuria • Dysuria • Nocturia • Urinary frequency • Suprapubic pain from bladder spasms • Palpable mass on bimanual examination	Bladder cancer

Female GU abnormalities *(continued)*

Sign or symptom and findings	Probable cause
Urinary incontinence *(continued)*	
• Overflow incontinence • Painless bladder distention • Episodic diarrhea or constipation • Orthostatic hypotension • Syncope • Dysphagia	Diabetic neuropathy
• Urinary urgency and frequency • Visual problems • Sensory impairment • Constipation • Muscle weakness • Emotional lability	Multiple sclerosis
Vaginal discharge	
• Profuse, white, curdlike discharge with a yeasty, sweet odor • Exudate may be lightly attached to the labia and vaginal walls • Vulvar redness and edema • Intense labial itching and burning • External dysuria	Candidiasis
Vaginal discharge *(continued)*	
• Yellow, mucopurulent, odorless, or acrid discharge • Dysuria • Dyspareunia • Vaginal bleeding after douching or coitus	*Chlamydia* infection
• Yellow or green, foul-smelling discharge that can be expressed from the Bartholin's or Skene's ducts • Dysuria • Urinary frequency and incontinence • Vaginal redness and swelling	Gonorrhea

Urinary abnormalities

Common abnormal findings in the female urinary system include polyuria; hematuria; urinary frequency, urgency, and hesitancy; nocturia; urinary incontinence; and dysuria.

Polyuria

A fairly common finding, polyuria is the production and excretion of more than 2,500 ml of urine daily. It usually results from diabetes insipidus, diabetes mellitus, or diuretic use.

Plenty of polyuria causes

Other causes of polyuria include psychological, neurologic, or renal disorders. Urologic disorders, such as pyelonephritis and postobstructive uropathy, can also cause polyuria. Patients with polyuria are at risk for developing hypovolemia.

Hematuria

Hematuria, the presence of blood in the urine, causes brown or bright red urine. The timing of hematuria suggests the location of the underlying problem. Bleeding at the start of urination is caused by a disorder of the urethra; bleeding at the end of urination signifies a disorder of the bladder neck.

Above or below the neck

Bleeding that occurs throughout urination indicates a disorder located above the bladder neck. Hematuria can also be caused by GI, vaginal, or certain coagulation disorders.

Urinary frequency, urgency, and hesitancy

Urinary frequency, abnormally frequent urination, commonly results from decreased bladder capacity and is a classic symptom of a UTI. Frequency also occurs with urethral stricture, neurologic disorders, pregnancy, and uterine tumors.

It's a pain

In many cases, the sudden urge to urinate, or urinary urgency, is accompanied by bladder pain and is another symptom of a UTI. Even small amounts of urine in the bladder can cause pain because inflammation decreases bladder capacity. Urgency without pain may be a symptom of an upper motor neuron lesion that affects bladder control.

Trouble starting up

Difficulty starting a urine stream, or urinary hesitancy, can occur with a UTI, a partial obstruction of the lower urinary tract, neuromuscular disorders, or the use of certain drugs.

Nocturia

Excessive urination at night, or nocturia, is a common sign of kidney or lower urinary tract disorders. It can result from a disruption of the normal urine patterns or from overstimulation of the nerves and muscles that control urination. It may also be caused by cardiovascular, endocrine, or metabolic disorders and is a common adverse effect of diuretics.

Urinary incontinence

Urinary incontinence is a common complaint that may be transient or permanent. The amount of urine released may be small or large. Possible causes include stress incontinence, tumor, bladder cancer and calculi, and neurologic disorders such as Guillain-Barré syndrome, multiple sclerosis, and spinal cord injury.

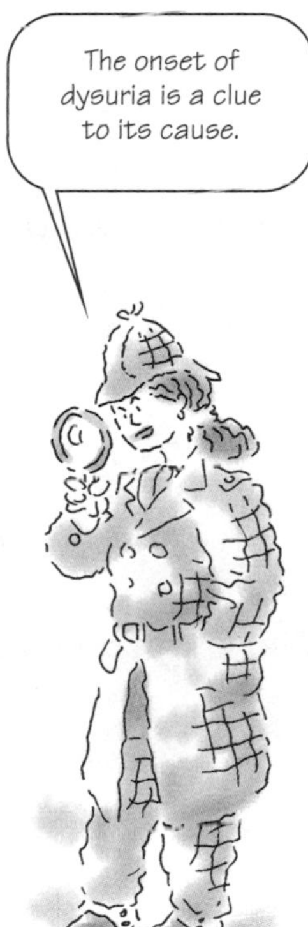

Dysuria

Dysuria, or pain during urination, signals a lower UTI. The onset of pain suggests the cause of dysuria. For example, pain just before urination indicates bladder irritation or distention. Pain at the start of urination usually signals a bladder outlet obstruction. Pain at the end of urination can be a sign of bladder spasm, and pain throughout urination may indicate pyelonephrosis, especially when fever, chills, hematuria, and flank pain are also present.

Genital abnormalities

Common female genital abnormalities include genital lesions, vaginal inflammation and discharge, cervical lesions and polyps, vaginal and uterine prolapse, and rectocele.

Genital lesions

In the early stages, syphilitic chancre causes a red, painless, eroding lesion with a raised, indurated border. The lesion usually appears inside the vagina but may also appear on the external genitalia.

Watch those warts

Genital warts, an STD caused by human papillomavirus, produce painless warts on the vulva, vagina, cervix, or anus. Warts start as tiny red or pink swellings that grow and develop stemlike structures. Multiple swellings with a cauliflower appearance are common.

Herpes breakdown

Genital herpes produces multiple, shallow vesicles, lesions, or crusts inside the vagina, on the external genitalia, on the buttocks and, sometimes, on the thighs. Dysuria, regional lymph node inflammation, pain, edema, and fever may be present. A Pap test reveals multinucleated giant cells with intranuclear inclusion bodies.

Vaginal inflammation and discharge

Vaginitis usually results from an overgrowth of infectious organisms. It causes redness, itching, dyspareunia (painful intercourse), dysuria, and a malodorous discharge. Bacterial vaginosis causes a fishy odor and a thin, grayish white discharge. *Candida albicans*, a fungal infection, causes pruritus and a thick, white, curdlike discharge that appears in patches on the cervix and vaginal walls. The discharge has a yeastlike odor.

Strawberry signs

Trichomoniasis may cause an abundant malodorous discharge that's either yellow or green and frothy or watery. In addition to redness, you may note red papules on the cervix and vaginal walls, giving the tissue a "strawberry" appearance.

STD with subtlety

A common but in many cases subtle STD, *Chlamydia trachomatis* causes a mucopurulent cervical discharge and cystitis. However, 75% of women with chlamydia are asymptomatic.

Getting to know gonorrhea

Gonorrhea commonly produces no symptoms, but it may cause a purulent green-yellow discharge and cystitis.

Cervical lesions and polyps

During a speculum examination, you may detect late-stage cervical cancer as hard, granular, friable lesions; in the early stages, the cervix looks normal. Cervical polyps are bright red, soft, and fragile. They're usually benign, but they may bleed. They usually arise from the endocervical canal.

Cervical cyanosis

Cervical cyanosis may accompany any disorder that causes systemic hypoxia or venous congestion in the cervix. It's also common during pregnancy and may be observed in women using hormonal contraceptives.

Vaginal and uterine prolapse

Also called *cystocele*, vaginal prolapse occurs when the anterior vaginal wall and bladder prolapse into the vagina. During speculum examination, you'll see a pouch or bulging on the anterior wall as the patient bears down. The uterus may also prolapse into the vagina and even be visible outside the body.

Rectocele

Rectocele is the herniation of the rectum through the posterior vaginal wall. On examination, you'll see a pouch or bulging on the posterior wall as the patient bears down.

Menstrual abnormalities

Common menstrual abnormalities include dysmenorrhea and amenorrhea.

Dysmenorrhea

Dysmenorrhea — painful menstruation — affects more than 50% of menstruating women; in fact, it's the leading cause of lost time from school and work among women of childbearing age. It's usually characterized by mild to severe cramping or colicky pain in the pelvis or lower abdomen that may radiate to the thighs and lower sacrum. The pain gradually subsides as bleeding tapers off.

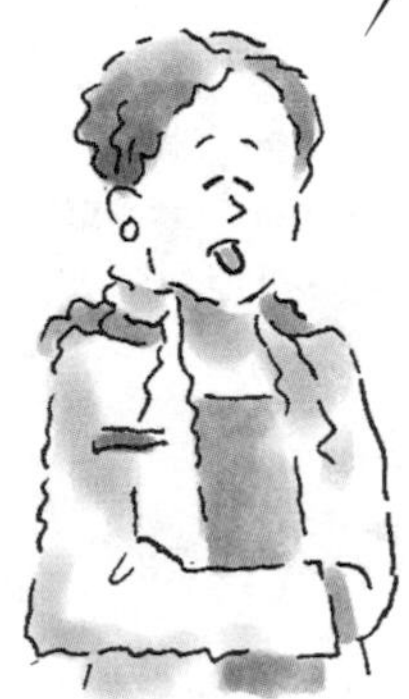

Amenorrhea

The absence of menstrual flow, amenorrhea, can be classified as primary or secondary. With primary amenorrhea, menstruation fails to begin before age 16. With secondary amenorrhea, menstruation begins at an appropriate age but later ceases for 3 or more months in the absence of normal physiologic causes, such as pregnancy, lactation, or menopause. Amenorrhea may result from anovulation or physical obstruction to menstrual outflow, such as from an imperforate hymen, cervical stenosis, or intrauterine adhesions. It may also result from drug or hormonal treatments.

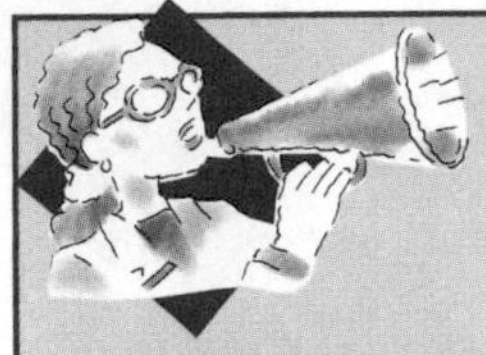

That's a wrap!

Female genitourinary system review

Structures of the urinary system

- Kidneys—form urine; maintain homeostasis; contain nephrons
- Ureters—carry urine from the kidneys to the bladder
- Bladder—container for urine collection
- Urethra—carries urine from the bladder to outside of the body

Structures of the internal genitalia

- Vagina—route of passage for childbirth and menstruation
- Uterus—nurtures and then expels the fetus during pregnancy; divided into the fundus and cervix
- Ovaries—produce ova and release the hormones estrogen and progesterone
- Fallopian tubes—the usual site of fertilization of the ova by the sperm; help to guide the ova to the uterus after expulsion from the ovaries

Health history

Ask about:

- urinary tract infections, kidney disease or kidney stones, and past medical history
- menstruation and sexual practices
- pregnancy and birth control
- menopause.

Assessment

Urinary system

- Inspect the areas over the kidneys and bladder.
- Percuss the kidneys (to check for costovertebral angle tenderness) and bladder.
- Attempt to palpate the kidneys and bladder, although they aren't normally palpable unless the kidneys are enlarged or the bladder is distended.

Reproductive system

- Inspect the external genitalia; note the appearance of pubic hair to determine sexual maturity.
- Palpate the external genitalia—this should be pain-free for the patient.
- Inspect internal genitalia using a speculum lubricated with warm water.
- Examine the vaginal wall for color, texture, and integrity, and the cervix for color, position, size, shape, mucosal integrity, and discharge.
- Palpate the internal genitalia, including bimanual palpation and rectovaginal palpation.

Abnormal findings

Urinary system

- Polyuria—overproduction of urine
- Hematuria—blood in the urine, causing urine to turn brown or bright red
- Urinary frequency—abnormally frequent urination
- Urinary urgency—sudden urge to urinate
- Urinary hesitance—difficulty starting urine stream
- Nocturia—excessive urination at night
- Urinary incontinence—involuntary release of urine
- Dysuria—painful urination

Reproductive system

- Genital lesions—may result from syphilis (red, painless, eroding lesion with a raised, indurated border); genital warts (painless tiny red or pink swellings that develop stemlike structures); or genital herpes (multiple, shallow vesicles, lesions, or crusts)

Female genitourinary system review *(continued)*

- Vaginal discharge—may result from bacterial vaginosis (thin, grayish white discharge); *Candida albicans* (thick, white, curdlike discharge); trichomoniasis (malodorous, yellow or green, and watery or frothy discharge); chlamydia (mucopurulent discharge); or gonorrhea (purulent green-yellow discharge)
- Cervical polyps—bright, red, soft, and fragile lesions
- Vaginal and uterine prolapse—anterior vaginal wall and bladder prolapse into the vagina
- Rectocele—herniation of the rectum through the posterior vaginal wall
- Dysmenorrhea—painful menstruation
- Amenorrhea—the absence of menstrual flow

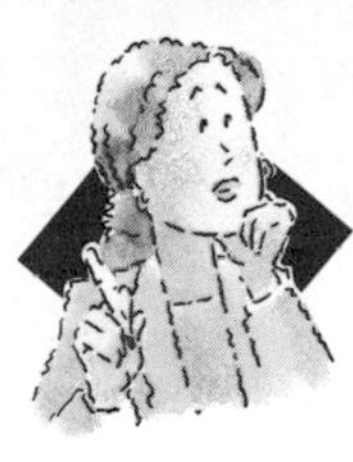

Quick quiz

1. Using commercial lubricants on speculum blades before inserting them into the vagina should be avoided because:

A. lubricants can alter test results.
B. additional lubrication is unnecessary.
C. many patients are hypersensitive to lubricants.
D. lubricants can discolor the vaginal tissue.

Answer: A. Most commercial lubricants are bacteriostatic and can alter test and culture results. Hold the speculum blades under warm running water to lubricate them.

2. Your patient complains of lower abdominal pressure, and you note a firm mass extending above the symphysis pubis. You suspect:

A. a distended bladder.
B. an enlarged kidney.
C. a UTI.
D. an inflamed ovary.

Answer: A. The bladder is usually nonpalpable unless it's distended. The feeling of pressure is usually relieved with urination.

3. The ducts of Skene's glands open into the:

A. perianal area.
B. clitoris.
C. urethra.
D. vulva.

Answer: D. Skene's glands are multiple, tiny structures located just below the urethra, each containing 6 to 31 ducts that empty into the vulva.

4. Your patient reports a 32-day menstrual cycle. You know this cycle is probably:

A. a normal variation.
B. a sign of metrorrhagia.
C. a precursor to uterine cancer.
D. a precursor to menopause.

Answer: A. The menstrual cycle varies from woman to woman. If a woman's pattern changes, she should be evaluated further.

5. Your patient complains of a thick, white vaginal discharge and vaginal itch. You suspect:

A. gonorrhea.
B. *Candida albicans.*
C. bacterial vaginosis.
D. trichomoniasis.

Answer: B. *Candida albicans*, or yeast infection, causes pruritus and a thick, white, curdlike discharge with a yeastlike odor that appears in patches on the cervix and vaginal walls.

6. Your teenage patient complains of a perineal sore. You suspect:

A. gonorrhea.
B. chlamydia.
C. herpes.
D. cervical polyps.

Answer: C. Herpes causes multiple shallow vesicles, lesions, or crusts inside the vagina, on the external genitalia, on the buttocks, and sometimes on the thighs.

Scoring

☆☆☆ If you answered all six questions correctly, fantastic! Your ability to flow through this information is most impressive.

☆☆ If you answered four or five questions correctly, excellent! Your study of this chapter has "reproduced" wonderful results.

☆ If you answered fewer than four questions correctly, don't despair. Why not cycle through the chapter again?

Male genitourinary system

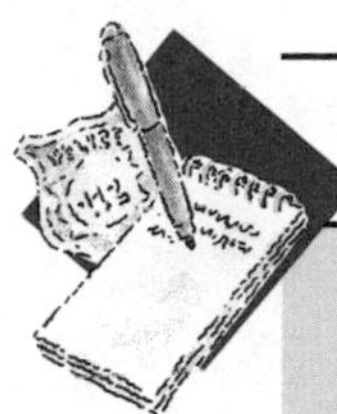

Just the facts

In this chapter, you'll learn:

- characteristics of the organs and structures of the male genitourinary (GU) system
- methods to obtain a patient history about the male GU system
- techniques to conduct a physical assessment of the male GU system
- causes of male GU system abnormalities and how to recognize them.

A look at the male GU system

A disorder of the male urinary or reproductive system can have far-reaching consequences. In addition to affecting the system itself, such a disorder can trigger problems in other body systems. It can also affect the patient's quality of life, self-esteem, and sense of well-being.

Despite these consequences, many men are reluctant to discuss their problems with a nurse or have intimate areas of their bodies examined. Your challenge, then, is to perform an assessment that's both skilled and sensitive. To do so, you must be aware of your own feelings about sexuality. If you appear comfortable discussing the patient's problem, he'll be encouraged to talk openly too.

To thoroughly and accurately assess your patient's GU system, you'll need to know the organs and structures of the urinary and reproductive systems and how they work.

Remember, your patient will take his cue from you. If you're comfortable discussing his problem, he'll be encouraged to talk openly.

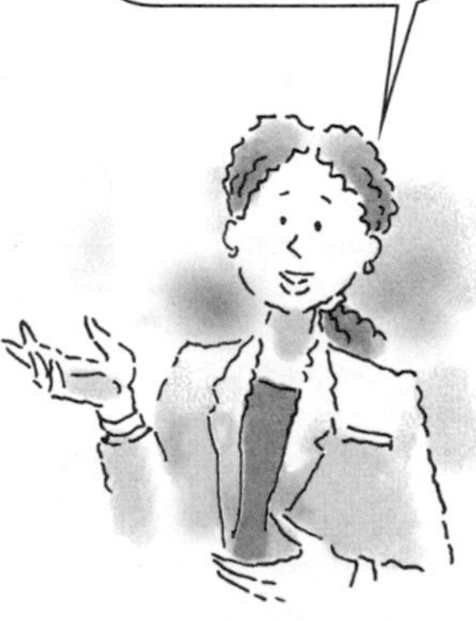

Urinary system

The urinary system helps maintain homeostasis by regulating fluid and electrolyte balance. It consists of the kidneys, ureters, bladder, and urethra. The essential functions of the system, such as forming urine and maintaining homeostasis, occur in the highly vascular kidneys.

Although the male and female urinary systems function in the same way, a man's urethra is 6″ (15.2 cm) longer than is a woman's. That's because it must pass through the erectile tissue of the penis.

Reproductive system

In men, the urethra is also part of the reproductive system because it carries semen as well as urine. The male reproductive sys-

Male reproductive system

This illustration shows the important structures of the male reproductive system.

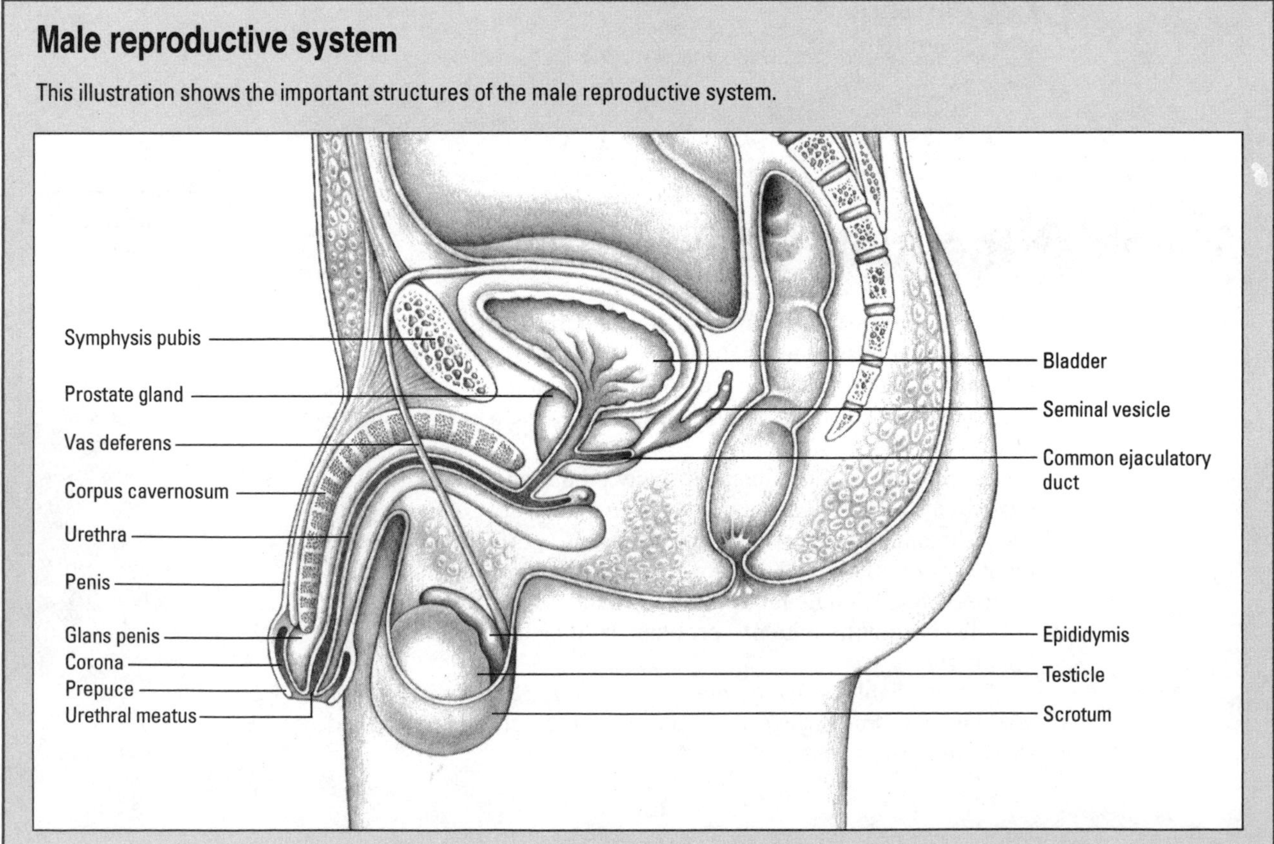

tem also includes the penis, scrotum, testicles, epididymis, vas deferens, seminal vesicles, and prostate gland. (See *Male reproductive system.*)

Penis

The penis consists of the shaft, glans, urethral meatus, corona, and prepuce. The skin of the penis is hairless and usually is darker than the skin on other parts of the body.

The shaft contains three columns of vascular erectile tissue. The glans is located at the end of the penis. The urethral meatus, which is a slitlike opening, is located ventrally at the tip of the glans. The corona is formed by the junction of the glans and the shaft. The prepuce (or foreskin), the loose skin covering the glans, is commonly removed shortly after birth in a surgical procedure called *circumcision.* (See *Circumcision as a religious practice.*)

When the penile tissues are engorged with blood, the erect penis can discharge sperm. During sexual activity, sperm and semen are forcefully ejaculated from the urethral meatus.

Scrotum

A loose, wrinkled, deeply pigmented sac that consists of a muscle layer covered by skin, the scrotum is located at the base of the penis. Each of its two compartments contains a testicle, an epididymis, and portions of the spermatic cord. The left side of the scrotum is usually lower than the right because the left spermatic cord is longer.

Testicles

The testicles are oval, rubbery structures suspended vertically and slightly forward in the scrotum. They produce testosterone and sperm.

Where it all begins

Testosterone stimulates the changes that occur during puberty, which starts between ages 9½ and 13½. The testicles enlarge (the first sign of pubertal changes), pubic hair grows, and penis size increases. Secondary sex characteristics appear, such as facial and body hair, muscle development, and voice changes.

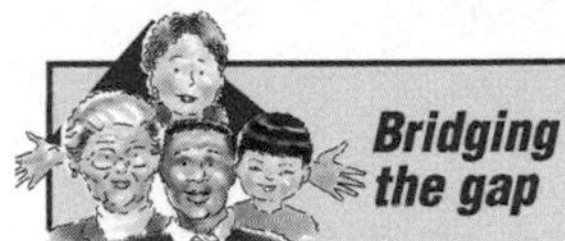

Circumcision as a religious practice

In some religions, such as Judaism and Islam, circumcision is a religious practice. In Judaism, circumcision signifies a covenant between God and the Jewish people. All Jewish males are circumcised when they're 8 days old during a ritual called a *brit milah,* or *bris.* The circumcision may be performed by a mohel (a Jew with special training) or by the neonate's father.

In the Islamic religion, circumcision is considered a rule of cleanliness. Islamic boys may be circumcised from the time they're 7 days old until they become 7 years old, although there's no fixed age. Adult males converting to Islam may choose to be circumcised; however, it isn't required.

Epididymis

The epididymis is a reservoir for maturing sperm. It curves over the posterolateral surface of each testicle, creating a visible bulge on the surface. In a small number of men, the epididymis is located anteriorly.

Vas deferens

The vas deferens — a storage site and the pathway for sperm — begins at the lower end of the epididymis, climbs the spermatic cord, travels through the inguinal canal, and ends in the abdominal cavity, where it rests on the fundus of the bladder.

Seminal vesicles

A pair of saclike glands, the seminal vesicles are found on the lower posterior surface of the bladder in front of the rectum. Secretions from the seminal vesicles help form seminal fluid.

Prostate gland

About 2½″ (6 cm) long, the prostate surrounds the urethra just below the bladder. It produces a thin, milky, alkaline fluid that mixes with seminal fluid during ejaculation to enhance sperm activity.

Obtaining a health history

Common complaints about the urinary system include pain during urination and changes in voiding pattern and urine color and output. The most common complaints about the reproductive system are penile discharge, erectile dysfunction, infertility, and scrotal or inguinal masses, pain, and tenderness. As you obtain a history, remember that the patient may feel uncomfortable discussing urinary or reproductive problems. (See *Putting your patient at ease.*)

Asking about past health and family health

Ask the patient about his medical history, especially the presence of diabetes or hypertension. Has he ever had a kidney or bladder infection or an infection of the reproductive system? How about kidney or bladder trauma or kidney stones? Has he ever been catheterized? (See *Assessing urine appearance.*) Also inquire about his family's health to get information on his risk of developing renal failure or kidney disease.

Assessing urine appearance

How your patient's urine looks can provide clues about his general health and the source of his genitourinary problem. During the health history, ask whether he has noticed any change in color. If he has, use this list to help interpret the changes:

- Pale and diluted — diabetes insipidus, diuretic therapy, excessive fluid intake
- Dark yellow or amber and concentrated — acute febrile disease, inadequate fluid intake, severe diarrhea or vomiting
- Blue-green — methylene blue ingestion
- Green-brown — bile duct obstruction
- Dark brown or black — acute glomerulonephritis, intake of such drugs as chlorpromazine
- Orange-red or orange-brown — obstructive jaundice, urobilinuria, intake of such drugs as rifampin or phenazopyridine
- Red or red-brown — hemorrhage, porphyria, intake of such drugs as phenazopyridine.

Putting your patient at ease

Here are some tips for helping your patient feel more comfortable during the health history:

- Make sure that the room is private and that you won't be interrupted.
- Tell the patient that his answers will remain confidential, and phrase your questions tactfully.
- Start with less sensitive areas and work up to more sensitive areas such as sexual function.
- Don't rush or omit important facts because the patient seems embarrassed.
- Be especially tactful with older men, who may see a normal decrease in sexual prowess as a sign of declining health and may be less willing to talk about sexual problems than younger men are.
- When asking questions, keep in mind that many men view sexual problems as a sign of diminished masculinity. Phrase your questions carefully, and offer reassurance as needed.
- Consider the patient's educational and cultural background. If he uses slang or euphemisms to talk about his sexual organs or function, make sure you're both talking about the same thing.

Asking about current health

Ask the patient whether he's circumcised. If he isn't, ask if he can retract and replace the prepuce (foreskin) easily? An inability to retract the prepuce is called *phimosis;* an inability to replace it is called *paraphimosis.* Untreated, these conditions can impair local circulation and lead to edema and even gangrene.

Inquire whether the patient has noticed sores, lumps, or ulcers on his penis. These can signal a sexually transmitted disease (STD). Does he have scrotal swelling? This can indicate an inguinal hernia, a hematocele, epididymitis, or a testicular tumor. Also ask whether he has penile discharge or bleeding.

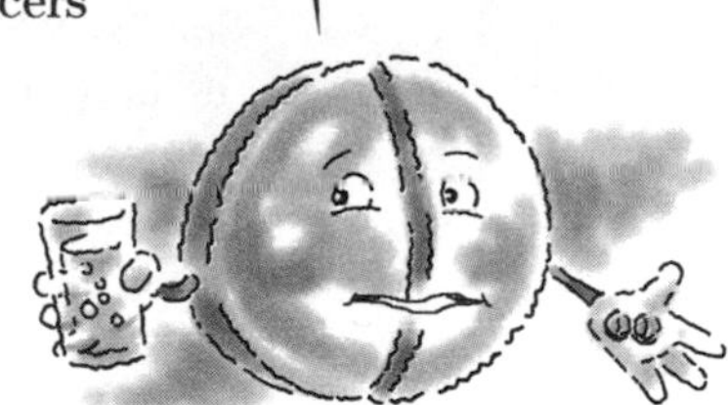

Drug connection

Ask what medications the patient regularly takes, including over-the-counter, prescription, herbal, and illicit drugs. Some drugs can affect the appearance of urine or alter GU function.

Asking about sexual health and practices

Finally, ask the patient about his sexual preference and practices so that you can assess risk-taking behaviors. How many sexual partners does he currently have? How many has he had in the past? Has he ever had an STD? If so, did he receive treatment? What precautions does he take to prevent contracting STDs? What's his human immunodeficiency virus status? Also ask about birth control measures. Has he had a vasectomy? (See *Don't forget to ask elderly patients*, page 282.)

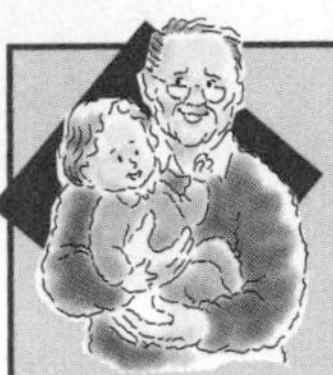

Ages and stages

Don't forget to ask elderly patients

Most people erroneously believe that sexual performance normally declines with age. Many also believe—also erroneously—that elderly people are incapable of having sex, that they aren't interested in sex, or that they can't find elderly partners who are interested in sex.

Harboring these beliefs could prevent you from asking your elderly male patients about their sexual health. The truth is, your patient may be experiencing a sexual problem that he's too embarrassed to bring up on his own. Therefore, be sure to ask elderly patients about their sexual health and provide support as needed. If the patient is dissatisfied with his sexual performance, bring this to the attention of the doctor. The doctor can then investigate the cause of the problem and initiate treatment as needed. Be aware that organic disease must be ruled out before counseling to improve sexual performance can start.

Taking precautions

Also ask the patient about his sexual health. Has he ever had trauma to his penis or scrotum? Was he ever diagnosed with an undescended testicle? Has he ever been diagnosed with a low sperm count? If so, caution him that hot baths, frequent bicycle or motorcycle riding, and tight underwear or athletic supporters can elevate scrotal temperature and temporarily decrease sperm count. If he participates in sports, ask how he protects himself from possible genital injuries. This is also a good time to ask him whether he knows how to examine his testicles for signs of testicular cancer. (See *Testicular self-examination.*)

Testicular self-examination

During the patient history, ask your patient whether he performs monthly testicular self-examinations. If he doesn't, explain that testicular cancer, the most common cancer in men ages 20 to 35, can be treated successfully when it's detected early.

Teaching the technique
To do this examination, the patient should hold his penis out of the way with one hand, then roll each testicle between the thumb and first two fingers of his other hand. A normal testicle should have no lumps, move freely in the scrotal sac, and feel firm, smooth, and rubbery. Both testicles should be the same size, although the left one is usually lower than the right because the left spermatic cord is longer.

If the patient finds any abnormalities, he should notify his doctor immediately.

Assessing the male GU system

To perform a physical assessment of the male GU system, use the techniques of inspection, percussion, palpation, and auscultation. Assessment of the urinary system may be done with assessment of the GU system or as part of the GI assessment.

Examining the urinary system

In many ways, assessing the male urinary system is similar to assessing the female urinary system. Before examining specific structures, check the patient's blood pressure and weight.

Scan the skin

Also, observe the patient's skin. A person with decreased renal function may be pale because of a low hemoglobin level or may even have uremic frost—snowlike crystals on the skin from metabolic wastes. Also look for signs of fluid imbalance, such as dry mucous membranes, sunken eyeballs, edema, or ascites.

Before performing an assessment, ask the patient to urinate; then help him into the supine position with his arms at his sides. As you proceed, expose only the areas being examined.

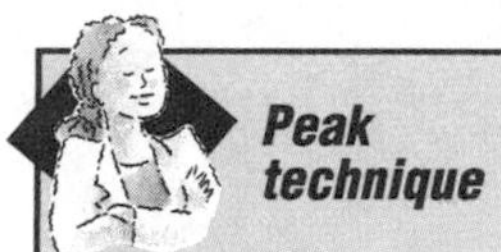

Performing fist percussion

To assess the kidneys by indirect fist percussion, ask the patient to sit up with his back to you. Warn him that you'll be gently striking his back. Then place one hand at the costovertebral angle and strike it with the ulnar surface of your other hand, as shown below.

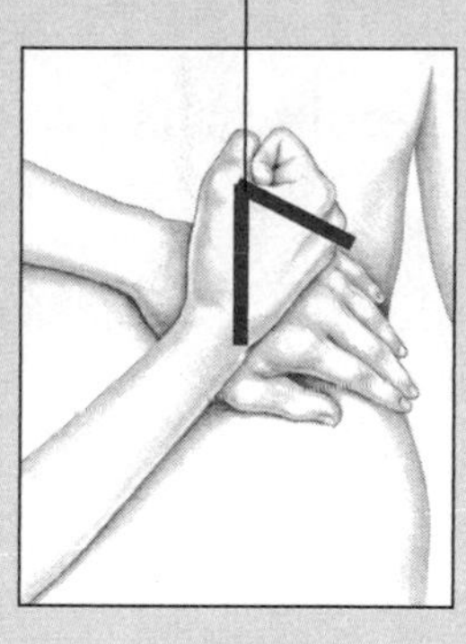

Inspection

First, inspect the patient's abdomen. When he's supine, his abdomen should be symmetrical and smooth, flat, or concave. The skin should be free from lesions, bruises, discolorations, and prominent veins.

Silvery streaks of striae

Watch for abdominal distention with tight, glistening skin and striae (silvery streaks caused by rapidly developing skin tension). These are signs of ascites, which may accompany nephrotic syndrome. This syndrome is characterized by edema, increased urine protein levels, and decreased serum albumin levels.

Percussion and palpation

First, tell the patient what you're going to do; otherwise, he may be startled and you could mistake his reaction for a feeling of acute tenderness. Percuss the kidneys, checking for pain or tenderness, which suggests a kidney infection. Remember to percuss both sides of the body to assess both kidneys. Then percuss the bladder to elicit tympany or dullness. (See *Performing fist percussion.*)

Dullness = retention

A dull sound instead of the normal tympany may indicate retained urine in the bladder caused by bladder dysfunction or infection. You can also palpate the bladder to check for distention. Because the kidneys aren't usually palpable, detecting an enlarged kidney may prove important. Kidney enlargement may accompany hydronephrosis, a cyst, or a tumor.

Auscultation

Auscultate the renal arteries to rule out bruits, which signal renal artery stenosis. You can do this during assessment of the GU system or as part of an abdominal assessment.

Examining the reproductive system

Before examining the reproductive system, put on gloves. Make the patient as comfortable as possible, and explain what you're doing every step of the way. Make sure that the privacy curtain is fully drawn or that the door is closed to help the patient feel less embarrassed.

Inspection

Inspect the penis, scrotum, and testicles as well as the inguinal and femoral areas.

Penis

Start by examining the penis. Penis size depends on the patient's age and overall development. The penile skin should be slightly wrinkled and pink to light brown in white patients and light brown to dark brown in black patients. Check the penile shaft and glans for lesions, nodules, inflammations, and swelling. Inspect the glans of an uncircumcised penis by retracting the prepuce. Also check the glans for smegma, a cheesy secretion commonly found beneath the prepuce.

Pressing the point

Then gently compress the tip of the glans to open the urethral meatus. It should be located in the center of the glans and be pink and smooth. Inspect it for swelling, discharge, lesions, inflammation and, especially, genital warts. If you note discharge, obtain a culture specimen. (See *Examining the urethral meatus.*)

Peak technique

Examining the urethral meatus

To inspect the urethral meatus, compress the tip of the glans, as shown below.

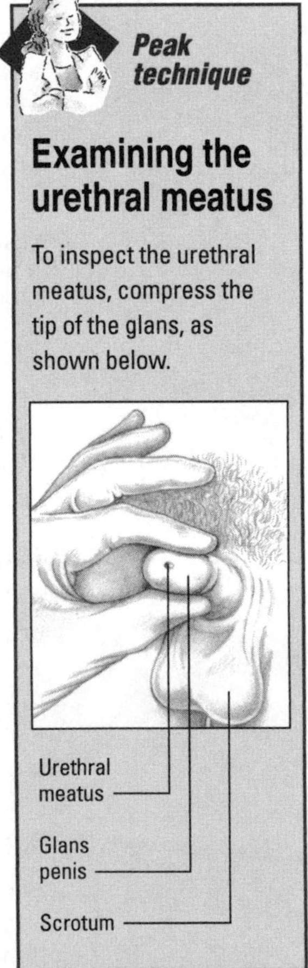

Scrotum and testicles

Have the patient hold his penis away from his scrotum so you can observe the scrotum's general size and appearance. The skin here is darker than on the rest of the body. Spread the surface of the scrotum, and examine the skin for swelling, nodules, redness, ulceration, and distended veins.

It's perfectly normal!

Sebaceous cysts — firm, white to yellow, nontender cutaneous lesions — are a normal finding. Also check for pitting edema, a sign of cardiovascular disease. Spread the pubic hair and check the skin for lesions and parasites. If the patient is a child, check especially for penile enlargement. (See *Assessing pediatric patients.*)

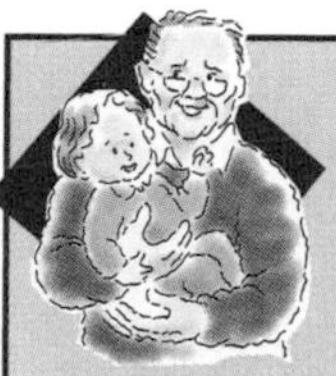

Ages and stages

Assessing pediatric patients

Before palpating a boy's scrotum for a testicular examination, explain what you'll be doing and why. A younger child may want his parent present for comfort; however, an older boy will probably want privacy. Make sure he's comfortably warm and as relaxed as possible. Cold and anxiety may cause his testicles to retract so that you can't palpate them.

Hernia and hydroceles

If you see an enlarged scrotum in a boy younger than age 2, suspect a scrotal extension of an inguinal hernia, a hydrocele, or both. Hydroceles, usually associated with inguinal hernias, are common in children of this age-group. To differentiate between the two, remember that hydroceles transilluminate and aren't tender or reducible.

Obesity

An adolescent boy who's obese may appear to have an abnormally small penis. You may have to retract the fat pad over the symphysis pubis to properly assess penis size.

Inguinal and femoral areas

Have the patient stand. Then ask him to hold his breath and bear down while you inspect the inguinal and femoral areas for bulges or hernias. A hernia is a loop of bowel that comes through a muscle wall.

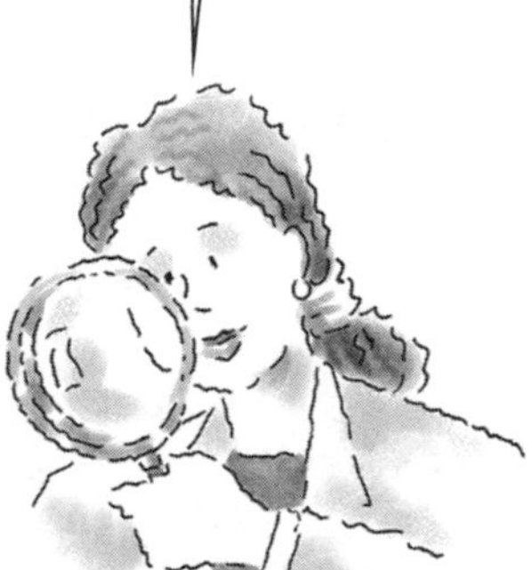

Palpation

Palpate the penis, testicles, epididymides, spermatic cords, inguinal and femoral areas, and prostate gland.

Penis

Use your thumb and forefinger to palpate the entire penile shaft. It should be somewhat firm, and the skin should be smooth and movable. Note swelling, nodules, or indurations.

Testicles

Gently palpate both testicles between your thumb and first two fingers. Assess their size, shape, and response to pressure. A normal response is a deep visceral pain. The testicles should be equal in size, move freely in the scrotal sac, and feel firm, smooth, and rubbery.

The shadow knows

If you note hard, irregular areas or lumps, transilluminate them by darkening the room and pressing the head of a flashlight against the scrotum, behind the lump. The testicle and any lumps, masses, warts, or blood-filled areas will appear as opaque shadows.

Transilluminate the other testicle to compare your findings. This is also a good time to reinforce the methods for and importance of doing a monthly testicular self-examination.

Epididymides

Next, palpate the epididymides, which are usually located in the posterolateral area of the testicles. They should be smooth, discrete, nontender, and free from swelling and induration.

Spermatic cords

Palpate both spermatic cords, which are located above each testicle. Palpate from the base of the epididymis to the inguinal canal. The vas deferens is a smooth, movable cord inside the spermatic cord.

It's a "no glow"

If you feel swelling, irregularity, or nodules, transilluminate the problem area, as described above. If serous fluid is present, you won't see a glow.

Inguinal area

To assess the patient for a direct inguinal hernia, place two fingers over each external inguinal ring and ask the patient to bear down. If he has a hernia, you'll feel a bulge.

Stand up, please!

To assess the patient for an indirect inguinal hernia, examine him while he's standing and then while he's in a supine position with his knee flexed on the side you're examining. (See *Palpating for an indirect inguinal hernia.*)

Place your index finger on the neck of the scrotum and gently push upward into the inguinal canal. When you've inserted your finger as far as possible, ask the patient to bear down or cough. A hernia feels like a mass of tissue that withdraws when it meets the finger.

Femoral area

Although you can't palpate the femoral canal, you can estimate its location to help detect a femoral hernia. Place your right index finger on the right femoral artery with your finger pointing toward

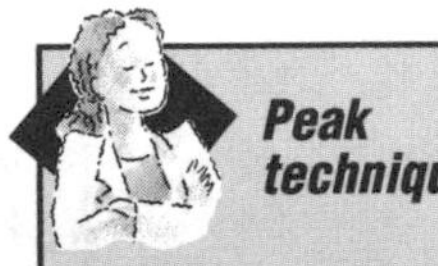

Palpating for an indirect inguinal hernia

To palpate for an indirect inguinal hernia, place your gloved finger on the neck of the scrotum and insert it into the inguinal canal, as shown below. Then ask the patient to bear down. If the patient has a hernia, you'll feel a soft mass at your fingertip.

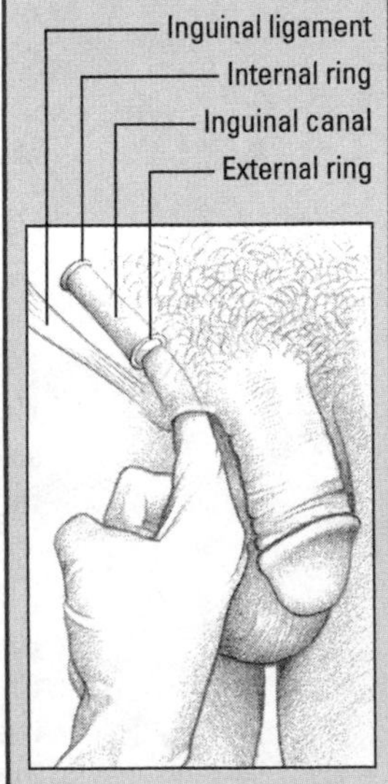

the patient's head. Keep your other fingers close together. Your middle finger will rest on the femoral vein, and your ring finger on the femoral canal. Note tenderness or masses. Use your left hand to check the patient's left side.

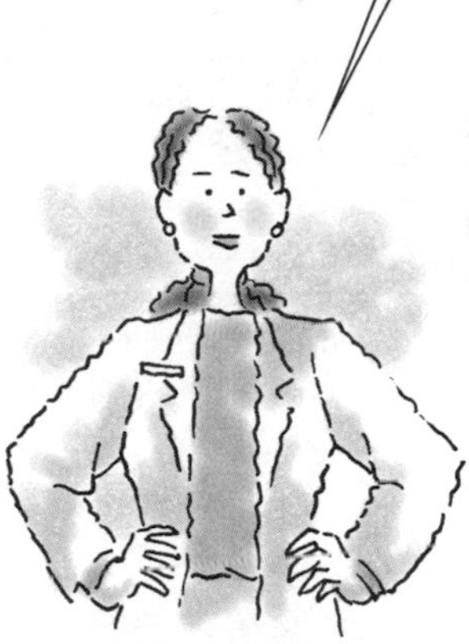

Prostate gland

Tell the patient that you need to place your finger in his rectum to examine his prostate gland, and warn him that he'll feel some pressure or urgency during the examination. Have him stand and lean over the examination table. If he can't do this, have him lie on his left side, with his right knee and hip flexed or with both knees drawn toward his chest. Inspect the skin of the perineal, anal, and posterior scrotal areas. It should be smooth and unbroken, with no protruding masses.

Probing the issue

Then lubricate the gloved index finger of your dominant hand and insert it into the rectum. Tell the patient to relax to ease the passage of the finger through the anal sphincter. If he's having difficulty relaxing the anal sphincter, ask him to bear down as if having a bowel movement while you gently insert your finger. With your finger pad, palpate the prostate gland on the anterior rectal wall just past the anorectal ring. The gland should feel smooth, rubbery, and about the size of a walnut. (See *Palpating the prostate gland.*)

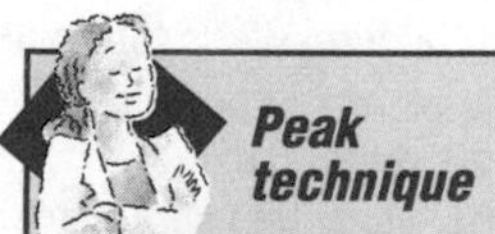

Palpating the prostate gland

To palpate the prostate gland, insert a lubricated, gloved index finger into the rectum. Palpate the prostate on the anterior rectal wall, just past the anorectal ring.

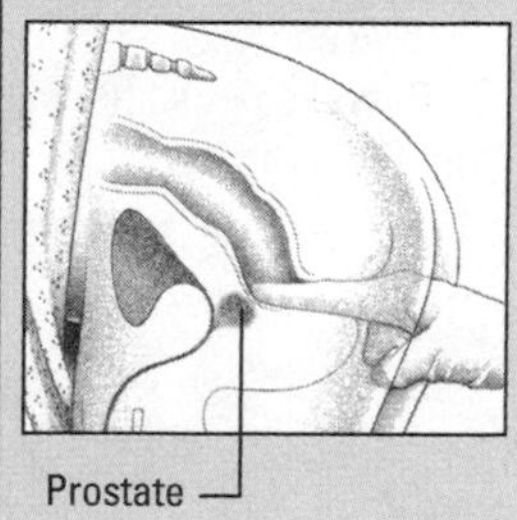

A growing problem

If the prostate gland protrudes into the rectal lumen, it's probably enlarged. An enlarged prostate gland is classified from grade 1 (protruding less than ⅜″ [1 cm] into the rectal lumen) to grade 4 (protruding more than 1¼″ [3.2 cm] into the rectal lumen). Also note tenderness or nodules.

Abnormal findings

Your assessment may uncover abnormalities of the GU system. Although the urinary problems discussed below also occur in women, the causes described are unique to men. (See *Male GU abnormalities*, pages 288 and 289.)

Urinary problems

Possible urinary problems include hematuria; urinary frequency, urgency, and hesitancy; nocturia; and urinary incontinence.

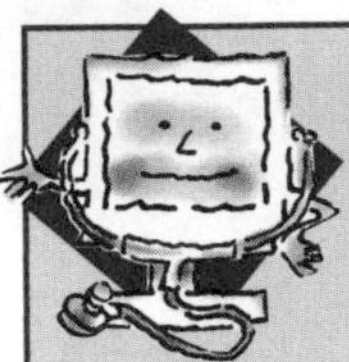

Interpretation station

Male GU abnormalities

After you assess the patient, a group of findings may lead you to suspect a particular disorder. The chart below shows common groups of findings for the male genitourinary (GU) system, along with their signs and symptoms and probable causes.

Sign or symptom and findings	Probable cause
Penile lesions	
• Fluid-filled vesicles on the glans penis, prepuce (foreskin), or penile shaft • Painful ulcers • Tender inguinal lymph nodes • Fever • Malaise • Dysuria	Genital herpes
• Painless warts (tiny pink swellings that grow and become pedunculated) near the urethral meatus • Lesions that spread to the perineum and the perianal area • Cauliflower appearance of multiple swellings	Genital warts
• Sharply defined, slightly raised, scaling patches on the inner thigh or groin (bilaterally) or on the scrotum or penis • Severe pruritus	Tinea cruris (jock itch)
Scrotal swelling	
• Swollen scrotum that's soft or unusually firm • Bowel sounds that may be auscultated in the scrotum	Hernia

Sign or symptom and findings	Probable cause
***Scrotal swelling** (continued)*	
• Gradual scrotal swelling • Scrotum that's soft and cystic or firm and tense • Painless • Round, nontender scrotal mass on palpation • Glowing when transilluminated	Hydrocele
• Scrotal swelling with sudden and severe pain • Unilateral elevation of the affected testicle • Nausea and vomiting	Testicular torsion
Penile discharge	
• Purulent or milky urethral discharge • Sudden fever and chills • Lower back pain • Myalgia • Perineal fullness • Arthralgia • Urinary frequency and urgency • Cloudy urine • Dysuria • Tense, boggy, very tender, warm prostate palpated on digital rectal examination	Prostatitis
• Opaque, gray, yellowish, or blood-tinged discharge that's painless • Dysuria • Eventual anuria	Urethral neoplasm

Male GU abnormalities *(continued)*

Sign or symptom and findings	Probable cause
Penile discharge *(continued)*	
• Scant or profuse urethral discharge that's thin and clear, mucoid, or thick and purulent • Urinary hesitancy, frequency, and urgency • Dysuria • Itching and burning around the meatus	Urethritis
Urinary hesitancy	
• Reduced caliber and force of urinary stream • Perineal pain • Feeling of incomplete voiding • Inability to stop urine stream • Urinary frequency • Urinary incontinence • Bladder distention	Benign prostatic hyperplasia
Urinary hesitancy *(continued)*	
• Urinary frequency and dribbling • Nocturia • Dysuria • Bladder distention • Perineal pain • Constipation • Hard, nodular prostate palpated on digital rectal examination	Prostatic cancer
• Dysuria • Urinary frequency and urgency • Hematuria • Cloudy urine • Bladder spasms • Costovertebral angle tenderness • Suprapubic, low back, pelvic, or flank pain • Urethral discharge	Urinary tract infection

Hematuria

Hematuria (presence of blood in the urine) may indicate urinary tract infection (UTI), renal calculi, or trauma to the urinary mucosa. It may be a temporary condition after urinary tract or prostate surgery or after urethral catheterization.

A red flag

A patient with hematuria may have brown or bright red urine. Bleeding at the end of urination signals a disorder of the bladder neck, urethra, or prostate gland.

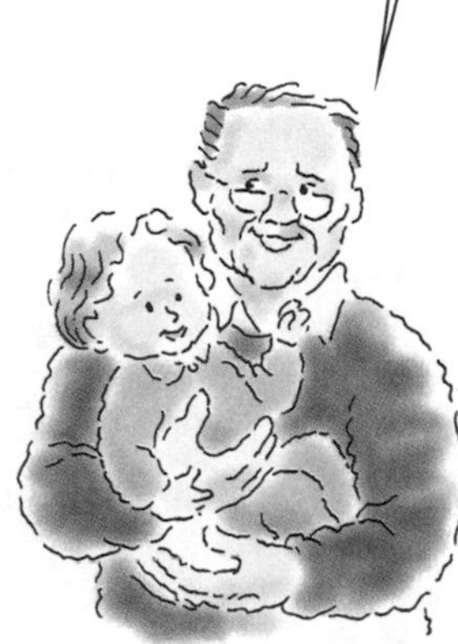

Thanks to my enlarged prostate, we have opposite problems — he goes all the time, and I can't go at all!

Urinary frequency, urgency, and hesitancy

Urinary frequency (abnormally frequent urination) and urgency (intense and immediate desire to urinate) are classic symptoms of a UTI. Urinary frequency also occurs with benign prostatic hyperplasia, urethral stricture, and a prostate tumor, which can put pressure on the bladder.

Incomplete passage

Urinary hesitancy (hesitancy in beginning the urine stream) is most common in the older patient who has an enlarged prostate gland, which can cause partial obstruction of the urethra.

Nocturia

Excessive urination at night, or nocturia, is a common sign of renal or lower urinary tract disorders. It can result from benign prostatic hyperplasia, when significant urethral obstruction develops, or from prostate cancer. It may also result from increased fluid intake or diuretic medications.

Urinary incontinence

Urinary incontinence (involuntary release of urine) may be caused by benign prostatic hyperplasia, prostate infection, or prostate cancer.

Reproductive system problems

A number of reproductive system problems may occur, many of which are discussed below.

Penile lesions

Lesions on the penis can vary in appearance. A hard, nontender nodule, especially in the glans or inner lip of the prepuce, may indicate penile cancer. (See *Male genital lesions.*)

Penile discharge

A profuse, yellow discharge from the penis suggests gonococcal urethritis. Other symptoms may include urinary frequency, burning, and urgency. Without treatment, the prostate gland, epididymis, and periurethral glands become inflamed. A copious, watery, purulent urethral discharge may indicate chlamydial infection; a bloody discharge may indicate infection or cancer in the urinary or reproductive tract.

Paraphimosis

In paraphimosis, the prepuce is so tight that, when retracted, it gets caught behind the glans and can't be replaced. Edema can result.

Male genital lesions

Several types of lesions may affect the male genitalia. Some of the more common types are described here.

Penile cancer
Penile cancer causes a painless, ulcerative lesion on the glans or prepuce (foreskin), possibly accompanied by discharge.

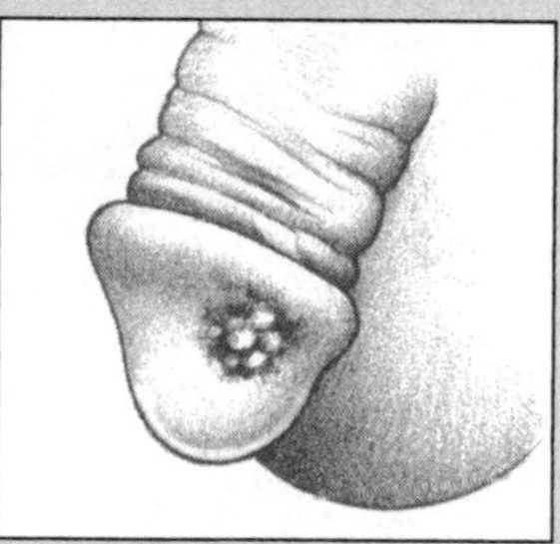

Genital herpes
Genital herpes causes a painful, reddened group of small vesicles or blisters on the prepuce, shaft, or glans. Lesions eventually disappear but tend to recur.

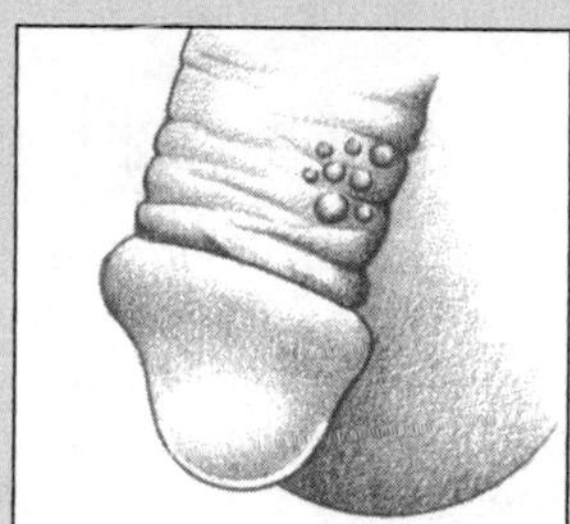

Genital warts
Genital warts are flesh-colored, soft, moist papillary growths that occur singly or in cauliflower-like clusters. They may be barely visible or several inches in diameter.

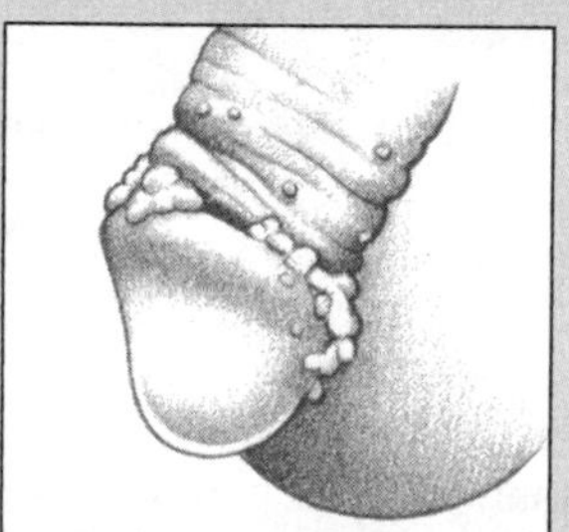

Syphilis
Syphilis causes a hard, round papule on the penis. When palpated, this syphilitic chancre may feel like a button. Eventually, the papule erodes into an ulcer. You may also note swollen lymph nodes in the inguinal area.

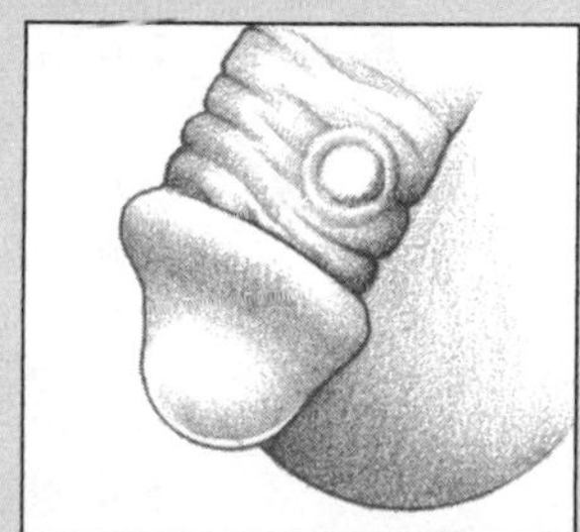

Cleaning up

Instruct uncircumcised men to retract the prepuce each time they clean the glans and then to replace it afterward. Frequent retraction and cleaning of the prepuce prevents excessive tightness, which in turn prevents the prepuce from closing off the urinary meatus and constricting the glans.

Displacement of the urethral meatus

When the urethral meatus is located on the underside of the penis, the condition is called hypospadias. When the urethral meatus is located on the top of the penis, it's called epispadias. Both conditions are congenital and may contribute to infertility.

Testicular tumor

A painless scrotal nodule that can't be transilluminated may be a testicular tumor. This disorder occurs most commonly in men ages 20 to 35. The tumor can grow, enlarging the testicle.

Scrotal swelling

Scrotal swelling occurs when a condition affecting the testicles, epididymis, or scrotal skin produces edema or a mass. It commonly results from a hydrocele or hernia.

Checking the fluid level

An enlarged scrotum may be a sign of hydrocele, or a collection of fluid in the testicle. Hydrocele is associated with conditions that cause poor fluid reabsorption, such as cirrhosis, heart failure, and testicular tumor. A hydrocele can be transilluminated.

Butting in

A hernia is a protrusion of an organ through an abnormal opening in the muscle wall. It may be direct or indirect, inguinal or femoral.

A direct inguinal hernia emerges from behind the external inguinal ring and protrudes through it. This type of hernia seldom descends into the scrotum and usually affects men older than age 40.

An indirect inguinal hernia is the most common type of hernia; it occurs in men of all ages. It can be palpated in the internal inguinal canal with its tip in or beyond the canal, or the hernia may descend into the scrotum.

A femoral hernia feels like a soft tumor below the inguinal ligament in the femoral area. It may be difficult to distinguish from a lymph node and is uncommon in men.

Prostate gland enlargement

A smooth, firm, symmetrical enlargement of the prostate gland indicates benign prostatic hyperplasia, which typically starts after age 50. This finding may be associated with nocturia, urinary hesitancy and frequency, and recurring UTIs.

In acute prostatitis, the prostate gland is firm, warm, and extremely tender and swollen. Because bacterial infection causes the condition, the patient usually has a fever.

Prostate gland lesions

Hard, irregular, fixed lesions that make the prostate feel asymmetrical suggest prostate cancer. Palpation may be painful. This condition also causes urinary dysfunction. Back and leg pain may occur with bone metastases in advanced stages.

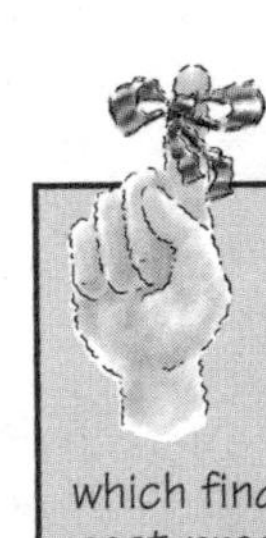

Memory jogger

To help you remember which findings suggest prostate cancer, think of the mnemonic **PAINS:**

Prostate cancer

Asymmetric

Irregular

Nodules

Stony (hard) and fixed.

Erectile dysfunction

Erectile dysfunction is the inability to achieve and maintain penile erection sufficient to complete satisfactory sexual intercourse; ejaculation may or may not be affected. Erectile dysfunction varies from occasional and minimal to permanent and complete. It may result from psychological, vascular, neurologic, or hormonal disorders or malfunctions. Fatigue, poor health, age, and drugs can also disrupt normal sexual function.

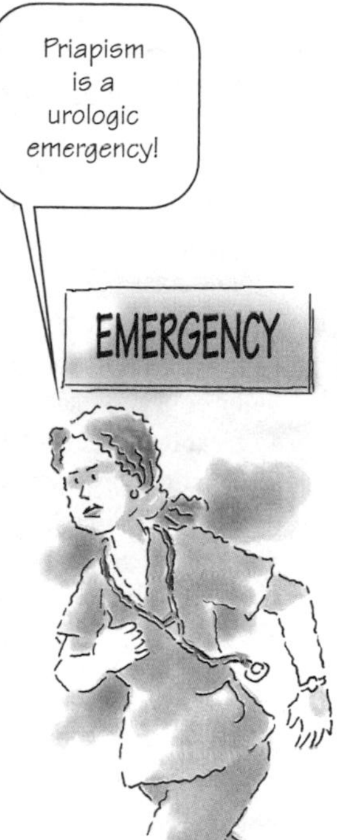

Priapism

A urologic emergency, priapism is a persistent, painful erection that's unrelated to sexual excitation. It may last for several hours or days and is usually accompanied by a severe, constant, dull aching in the penis. Unfortunately, the patient may be too embarrassed to seek medical help right away. Lack of prompt treatment can cause penile ischemia and thrombosis. Priapism may result from a blood disorder (such as sickle cell anemia), a neoplasm, trauma, or the use of certain drugs.

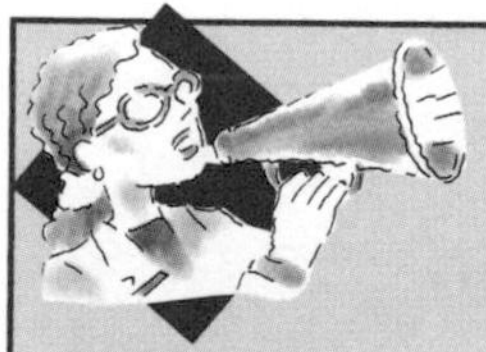

That's a wrap!

Male GU system review

Male GU structures

- Urinary structures: similar to those in the female GU system, including kidneys, ureters, bladder, and urethra; extra 6″ (15.2 cm) in male urethra to pass through the penis
- Penis: consists of the shaft, glans, urethral meatus, corona, and prepuce (foreskin); discharges urine as well as sperm
- Scrotum: loose, wrinkled sac that contains the testicles, epididymides, and portions of the spermatic cords
- Testicles: oval, rubbery structures that produce testosterone and sperm
- Epididymis: a reservoir for mature sperm located on the posterolateral surface of each testicle
- Vas deferens: storage site and pathway for sperm
- Seminal vesicles: saclike glands found on the lower posterior surface of the bladder whose secretions help form seminal fluid
- Prostate gland: produces a thin, milky fluid that mixes with seminal fluid to enhance sperm activity

The health history

- Determine the patient's chief complaint.
  - Common urinary problems include pain on urination and changes in voiding pattern or urine color or output.

(continued)

Male GU system review *(continued)*

– Common reproductive problems include penile discharge, erectile dysfunction, infertility, scrotal or inguinal masses, and pain or tenderness.

- Ask about past health and family health, especially about the presence or history of diabetes or hypertension.
- Ask about current health, such as circumcision status; penile sores, lumps, ulcers, or discharge; and scrotal swelling.
- Ask about sexual health and practices, including any history of sexually transmitted diseases and performance of testicular self-examination.

Assessment of the urinary system

- Performed similar to the female urinary assessment.
- Inspect the patient's skin and abdomen.
- Percuss and palpate the kidneys and bladder.
- Auscultate over the renal arteries to check for bruits.

Assessment of the reproductive system

- Inspect the penis for size, skin color, and abnormalities; compress the tip of the glans to inspect the urethral meatus.
- Inspect the scrotum, testicles, and pubic hair.
- Inspect the inguinal and femoral areas for bulges or hernias.
- Palpate the entire penile shaft.
- Gently palpate both testicles, assessing their size, shape, and response to pressure; transilluminate hard, irregular areas or lumps.
- Palpate the epididymides and both spermatic cords.
- Palpate for direct and indirect inguinal and femoral hernias.
- Palpate the prostate gland by performing a rectal examination.

Abnormal urinary findings

- Hematuria: presence of blood in urine
- Urinary frequency: abnormally frequent urination
- Urinary urgency: intense and immediate desire to urinate
- Urinary hesitancy: hesitancy in starting urine stream
- Nocturia: excessive urination at night

Abnormal reproductive system findings

- Paraphimosis: tight prepuce that, when retracted, gets caught behind the glans and can't be replaced
- Hypospadias: urethral meatus located on the underside of the penis
- Epispadias: urethral meatus located on top of the penis
- Hydrocele: collection of fluid in the testicle
- Hernia: protrusion of an organ through a muscle wall
- Erectile dysfunction: inability to achieve and maintain penile erection sufficient to complete satisfactory sexual intercourse
- Priapism: persistent, painful erection unrelated to sexual excitation

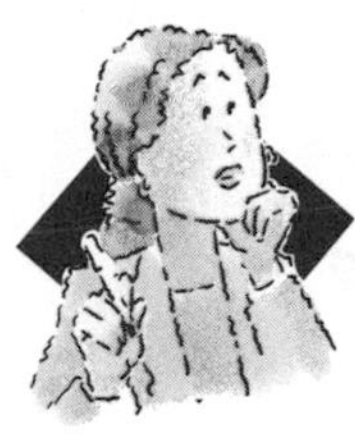

Quick quiz

1. Stress to the patient the importance of performing testicular self-examinations every:

- A. day.
- B. week.
- C. month.
- D. 6 months.

Answer: C. A monthly testicular self-examination can help detect testicular cancer early.

2. An inguinal hernia is best palpated with the patient:

- A. sitting.
- B. in a supine position.
- C. standing.
- D. lying on his right side.

Answer: C. To check for an inguinal hernia, have the patient stand and then hold his breath and bear down while you palpate the area.

3. Signs of benign prostatic hyperplasia include:

- A. an irregular, pea-shaped gland.
- B. an enlarged, hard gland with asymmetric swelling.
- C. smooth, firm symmetrical prostate enlargement.
- D. a firm, warm, tender prostate gland accompanied by a fever.

Answer: C. In men older than age 50, a smooth, firm, symmetrical enlargement of the prostate gland may be a normal finding.

4. Although the male and female urinary system functions in the same way, there's a difference in the length of the:

- A. bladder neck.
- B. ureter.
- C. epididymis.
- D. urethra.

Answer: D. Because a man's urethra passes through the erectile tissue of the penis, it's about 6″ (15 cm) longer than a woman's urethra.

Scoring

☆☆☆ If you answered all four questions correctly, incredible! You've shown that you're a hands-down master of the material in this chapter.

☆☆ If you answered three questions correctly, congratulations! You're making history as an awesome assessor.

☆ If you answered fewer than three questions correctly, hang in there! Why not take a break and then try the quiz again?

Musculoskeletal system

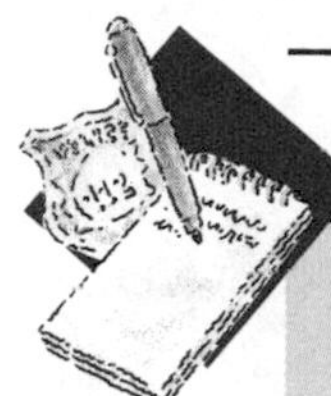

Just the facts

In this chapter, you'll learn:

- structures of the musculoskeletal system
- questions to ask during a health history
- techniques to assess the musculoskeletal system
- ways to identify abnormal findings and understand their significance.

A look at the musculoskeletal system

During a musculoskeletal assessment, you'll use sight, hearing, and touch to determine the health of the patient's muscles, bones, joints, tendons, and ligaments. These structures give the human body its shape and ability to move. Your sharp assessment skills will help uncover musculoskeletal abnormalities and evaluate the patient's ability to perform activities of daily living (ADLs).

The three main parts of the musculoskeletal system are the bones, joints, and muscles.

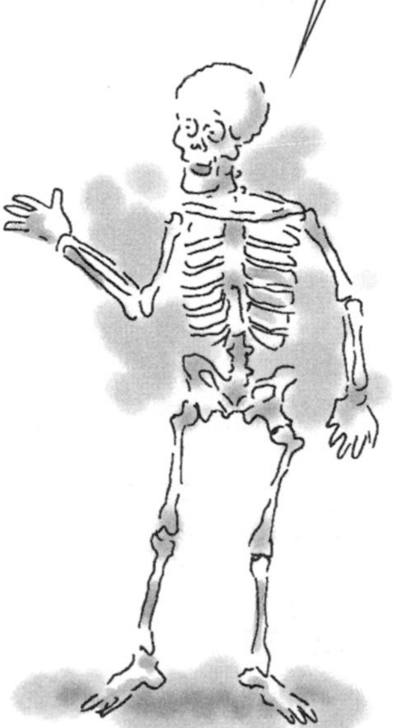

Bones

The 206 bones of the skeleton form the body's framework, supporting and protecting organs and tissues. The bones also serve as storage sites for minerals and contain bone marrow, the primary site for blood cell production. (See *A close look at the skeletal system*, page 298.)

A close look at the skeletal system

Of the 206 bones in the human skeletal system, 80 form the axial skeleton (skull, facial bones, vertebrae, ribs, sternum, and hyoid bone) and 126 form the appendicular skeleton (arms, legs, shoulders, and pelvis). Shown below are the body's major bones.

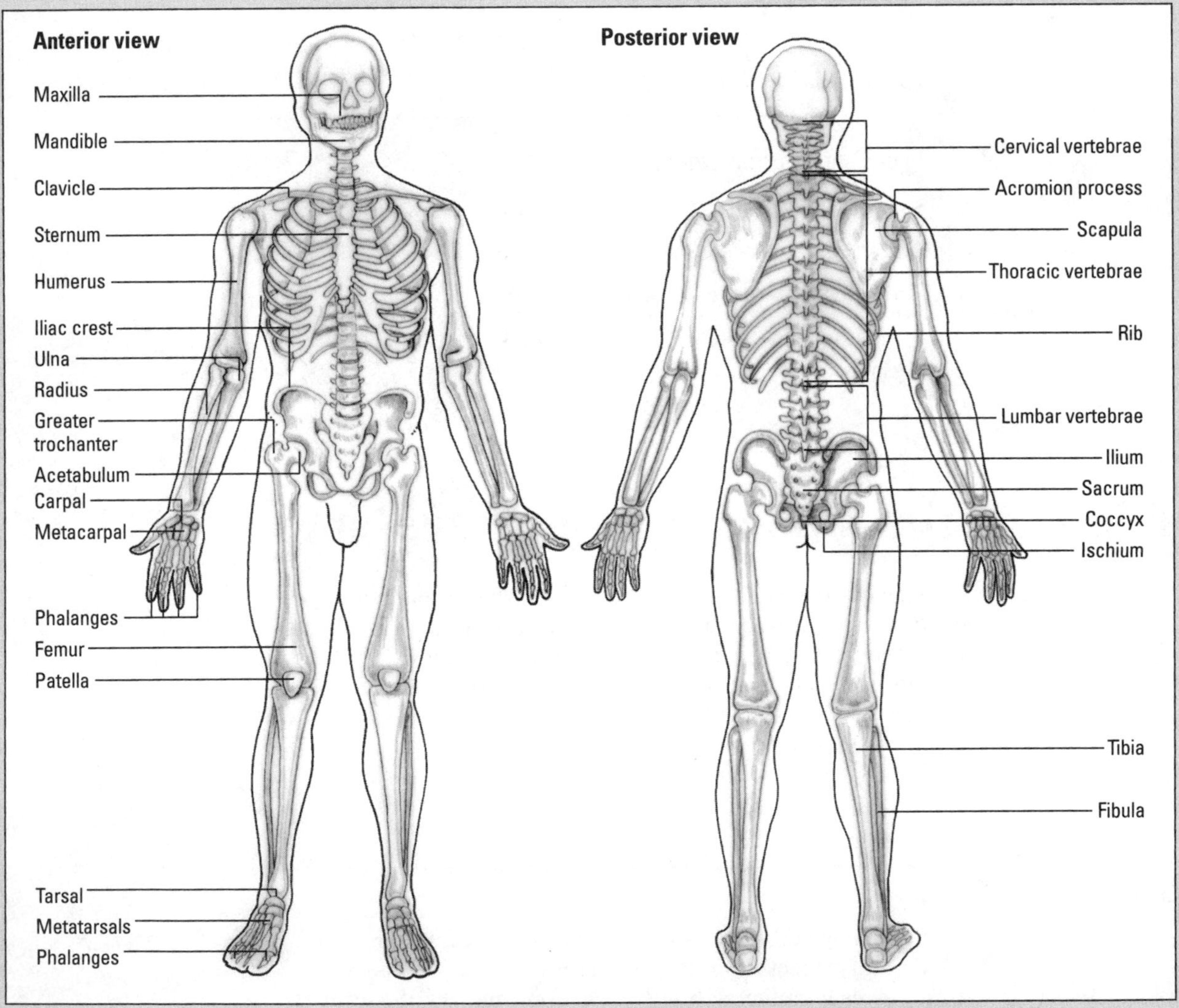

Anterior view

Maxilla
Mandible
Clavicle
Sternum
Humerus
Iliac crest
Ulna
Radius
Greater trochanter
Acetabulum
Carpal
Metacarpal
Phalanges
Femur
Patella
Tarsal
Metatarsals
Phalanges

Posterior view

Cervical vertebrae
Acromion process
Scapula
Thoracic vertebrae
Rib
Lumbar vertebrae
Ilium
Sacrum
Coccyx
Ischium
Tibia
Fibula

Joints

The junction of two or more bones is called a *joint.* Joints stabilize the bones and allow a specific type of movement. The two types of joints are nonsynovial and synovial.

Nonsynovial

In nonsynovial joints, the bones are connected by fibrous tissue, or cartilage. The bones may be immovable, like the sutures in the skull, or slightly movable, like the vertebrae.

Synovial

Synovial joints move freely; the bones are separate from each other and meet in a cavity filled with synovial fluid, a lubricant. (See *Synovial joint.*) In synovial joints, a layer of resilient cartilage covers the surfaces of opposing bones. This cartilage cushions the bones and allows full joint movement by making the surfaces of the bones smooth. (See *Types of joint motion*, page 300.) These joints are surrounded by a fibrous capsule that stabilizes the joint structures. The capsule also surrounds the joint's ligaments — the tough, fibrous bands that join one bone to another.

Synovial joint

Normally, bones fit together. Cartilage — a smooth, fibrous tissue — cushions the end of each bone, and synovial fluid fills the joint space. This fluid lubricates the joint and eases movement, much as the brake fluid functions in a car.

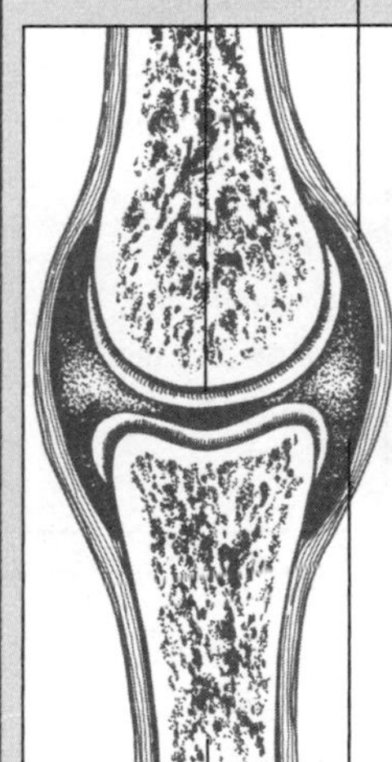

Popular joints

Synovial joints come in several types, including ball-and-socket joints and hinge joints. Ball-and-socket joints — the shoulders and hips being the only examples of this type — allow for flexion, extension, adduction, and abduction. These joints also rotate in their sockets and are assessed by their degree of internal and external rotation. Hinge joints, such as the knee and elbow, typically move in flexion and extension only.

Muscles

Muscles are groups of contractile cells or fibers that effect movement of an organ or a part of the body. Skeletal muscles, the focus of this chapter, contract and produce skeletal movement when they receive a stimulus from the central nervous system (CNS). The CNS is responsible for both involuntary and voluntary muscle function.

Tendons are tough fibrous portions of muscle that attach the muscles to bone. Bursae are sacs filled with friction-reducing synovial fluid; they're located in areas of high friction such as the knee. Bursae allow adjacent muscles or muscles and tendons to glide smoothly over each other during movement.

Obtaining a health history

The patient's reason for seeking care is important because it can determine the focus of your examination. Patients with joint injuries usually complain of pain, swelling, or stiffness, and they

Types of joint motion

The illustrations below show various areas of the body and what types of movements their joints allow.

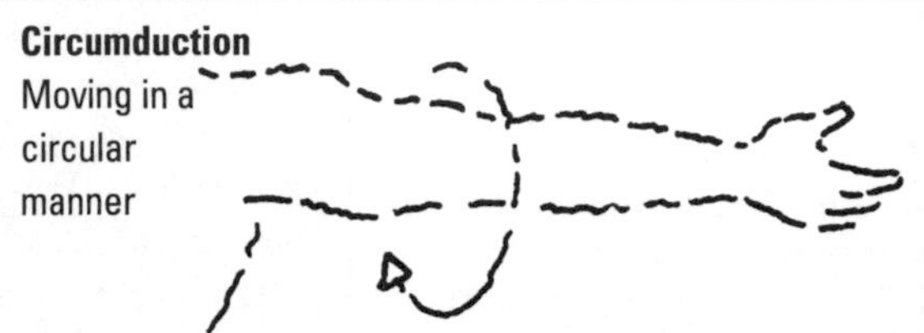

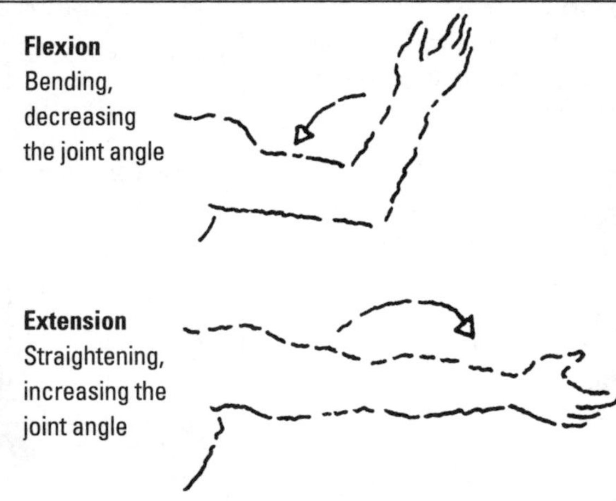

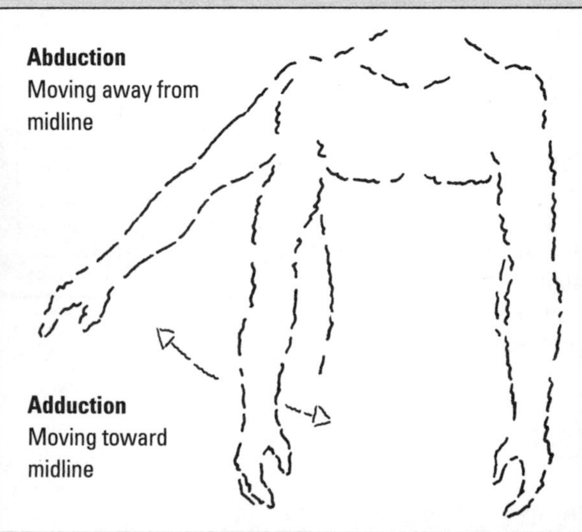

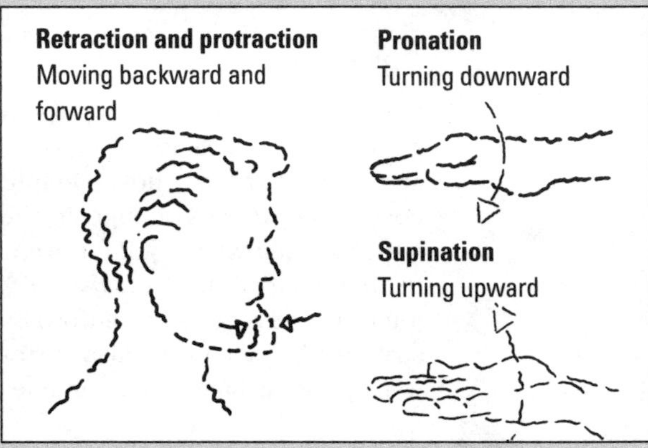

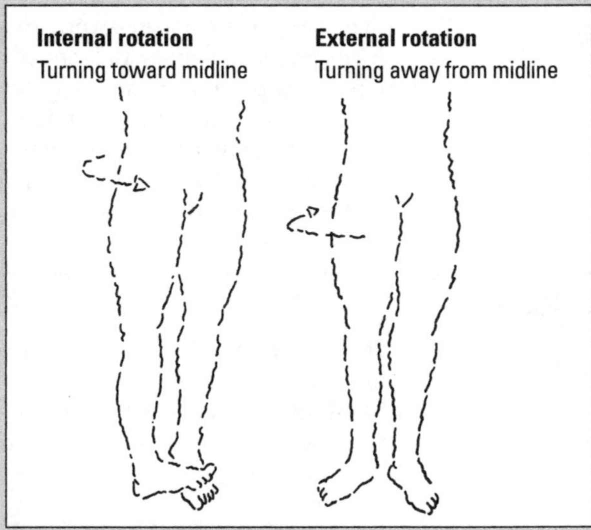

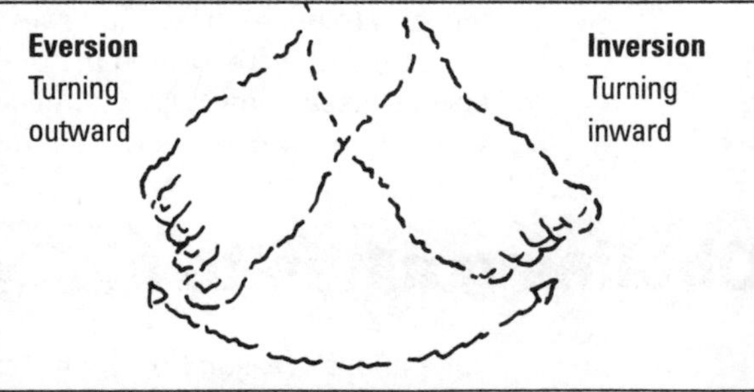

may have noticeable deformities. Deformity can also occur with a bone fracture, which causes sharp pain when the patient moves the affected area.

Muscular injury is commonly accompanied by pain, swelling, stiffness, and weakness. Because many musculoskeletal injuries are emergencies, you might not have time for a thorough assessment. In these cases, the PQRSTU device explained in chapter 1 can help you remember which key areas to focus on.

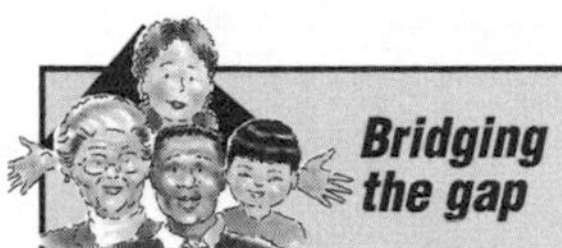

Biocultural variations in bone density

Studies of bone density have shown that black males have the densest bones. They also have a relatively low incidence of osteoporosis, a bone disorder characterized by a decrease in bone mass that leaves bones porous, brittle, and prone to being fractured. While the bone density of whites falls below that of blacks, whites tend to have higher bone densities than do Chinese, Japanese, and Inuit patients. Use this information to help you identify patients at risk for osteoporosis.

Asking about current and past health

Ask about the patient's past and current health status. Are the patient's ADLs affected by his condition? Ask whether he has noticed grating sounds when he moves certain parts of his body. Does he use ice, heat, or other remedies to treat the problem?

Ancient history

Inquire whether the patient has ever had gout, arthritis, tuberculosis, or cancer, which may cause bony metastases. Has the patient been diagnosed with osteoporosis? (See *Biocultural variations in bone density.*)

Ask whether he has had a recent blunt or penetrating trauma. If so, how did it happen? For example, did he suffer knee and hip injuries after being hit by a car, or did he fall from a ladder and land on his coccyx? This information can help guide your assessment and predict hidden trauma.

Also ask the patient whether he uses an assistive device, such as a cane, walker, or brace. If he does, watch him use the device to assess how he moves.

Asking about medications

Question the patient about the medications he takes regularly. Many drugs can affect the musculoskeletal system. Corticosteroids, for example, can cause muscle weakness, myopathy, osteoporosis, pathologic fractures, and avascular necrosis of the heads of the femur and humerus. Potassium-depleting diuretics can cause muscle cramping and weakness.

Asking about lifestyle

Ask the patient about his job, hobbies, and personal habits. Knitting, playing football or tennis, working at a computer, or doing construction work can all cause repetitive stress injuries or injure the musculoskeletal system in other ways. Even carrying a heavy knapsack or purse can cause injury or increase muscle size.

I'm really much larger when I have my muscles on.

Assessing the musculoskeletal system

Because the CNS and the musculoskeletal system are interrelated, you should assess them together. To assess the musculoskeletal system, use the techniques of inspection and palpation to test all the major bones, joints, and muscles. Perform a complete examination if the patient has generalized symptoms such as aching in several joints. Perform an abbreviated examination if he has pain in only one body area.

Go head to toe

Before starting your assessment, have the patient undress down to his underwear and have him put on a hospital gown. If possible, make sure the room is warm. Explain each procedure as you perform it. The only special equipment you'll need is a tape measure.

Begin your examination with a general observation of the patient. Then systematically assess the whole body, working from head to toe and from proximal to distal structures. Because muscles and joints are interdependent, interpret these findings together. As you work your way down the body, follow these general rules:

- Note the size and shape of joints, limbs, and body regions.
- Inspect and palpate the skin and tissues around the joint, limbs, and body regions.
- Have the patient perform active range-of-motion (ROM) exercises of a joint, if possible. Active ROM exercises are joint movements the patient can do without assistance.
- If he can't perform active ROM exercises, perform passive ROM exercises. Passive ROM exercises don't require the patient to exert any effort.
- During passive ROM exercises, support the joint firmly on either side and move it gently to avoid causing pain or spasm. Never force movement.

Walk the walk

Whenever possible, observe how the patient stands and moves. Watch him walk into the room or, if he's already in, ask him to walk to the door, turn around, and walk back toward you. His torso should sway only slightly, his arms should swing naturally at his sides, his gait should be even, and his posture should be erect.

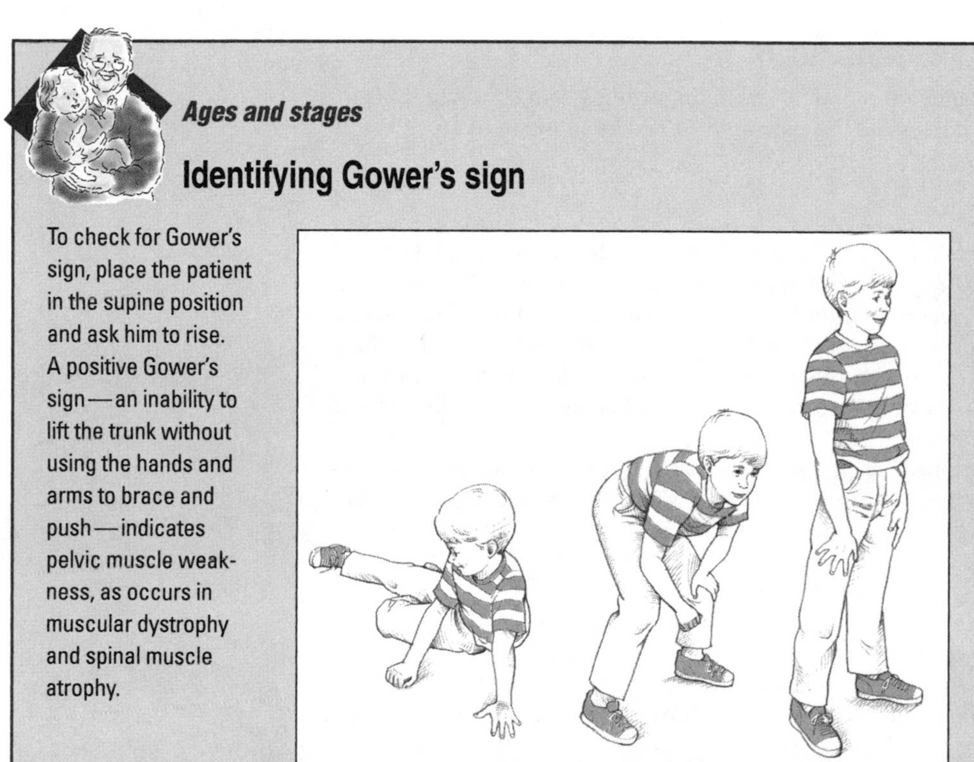

Ages and stages

Identifying Gower's sign

To check for Gower's sign, place the patient in the supine position and ask him to rise. A positive Gower's sign—an inability to lift the trunk without using the hands and arms to brace and push—indicates pelvic muscle weakness, as occurs in muscular dystrophy and spinal muscle atrophy.

As he walks, each foot should flatten and bear his weight completely, and his toes should flex as he pushes off with his foot. In midswing, his foot should clear the floor and pass the other leg. If you note a child with a waddling, ducklike gait (an important sign of muscular dystrophy), check for a positive Gower's sign, which indicates pelvic muscle weakness. (See *Identifying Gower's sign.*)

Assessing the bones and joints

Perform a head-to-toe evaluation of your patient's bones and joints using inspection and palpation. Then perform ROM exercises to help you determine whether the joints are healthy. Never force movement. Ask the patient to tell you when he experiences pain. Also, watch his facial expression for signs of pain or discomfort.

Head, jaw, and neck

First, inspect the patient's face for swelling, symmetry, and evidence of trauma. The mandible should be in the midline, not shifted to the right or left.

Is the TMJ A-OK?

Next, evaluate ROM in the temporomandibular joint (TMJ). Place the tips of your first two or three fingers in front of the middle of the ear. Ask the patient to open and close his mouth. Then place your fingers into the depressed area over the joint, and note the motion of the mandible. The patient should be able to open and close his jaw and protract and retract his mandible easily, without pain or tenderness.

If you hear or palpate a click as the patient's mouth opens, suspect an improperly aligned jaw. TMJ dysfunction may also lead to swelling of the area, crepitus, or pain.

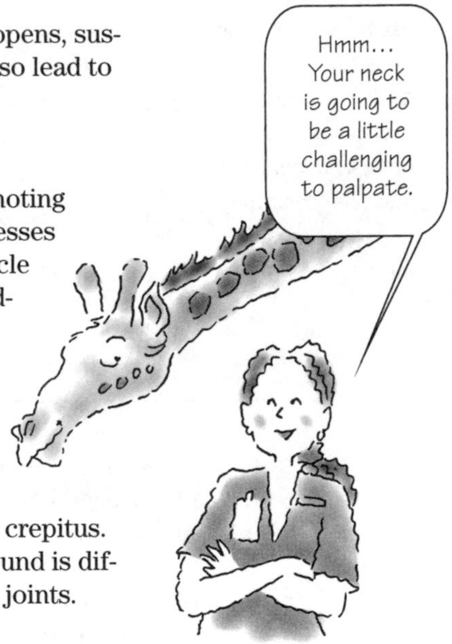

Check the neck

Inspect the front, back, and sides of the patient's neck, noting muscle asymmetry or masses. Palpate the spinous processes of the cervical vertebrae and the areas above each clavicle (supraclavicular fossae) for tenderness, swelling, or nodules.

To palpate the neck area, stand facing the patient with your hands placed lightly on the sides of the neck. Ask him to turn his head from side to side, flex his neck forward, and then extend it backward. Feel for any lumps or tender areas.

As the patient moves his neck, listen and palpate for crepitus. Crepitus is an abnormal grating sound. Note that this sound is different than the occasional crack that can be heard from joints.

Hmm... Your neck is going to be a little challenging to palpate.

Head circles and chin-ups

Now, check ROM in the neck. Ask the patient to try touching his right ear to his right shoulder and his left ear to his left shoulder. The usual ROM is 40 degrees on each side. Next, ask him to touch his chin to his chest and then to point his chin toward the ceiling. The neck should flex forward 45 degrees and extend backward 55 degrees.

To assess rotation, ask the patient to turn his head to each side without moving his trunk. His chin should be parallel to his shoulders. Finally, ask him to move his head in a circle — normal rotation is 70 degrees.

Spine

Ask the patient to remove his hospital gown so you can observe his spine. First check his spinal curvature as he stands in profile.

Kyphosis and lordosis

These illustrations show the difference between kyphosis and lordosis.

Kyphosis
If the patient has pronounced kyphosis, the thoracic curve is abnormally rounded, as shown below.

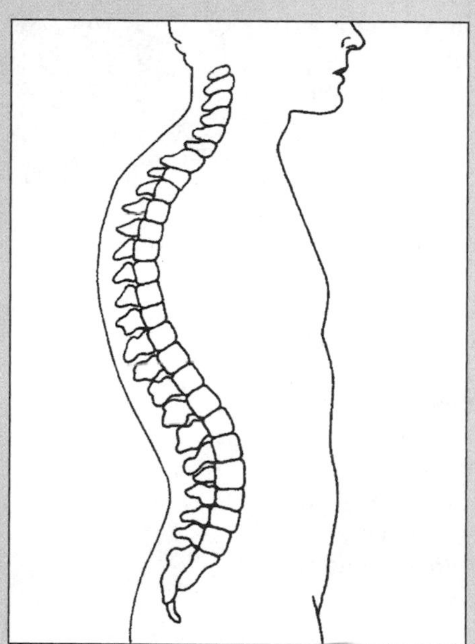

Lordosis
If the patient has pronounced lordosis, the lumbar spine is abnormally concave, as shown below. Lordosis (as well as a waddling gait) is normal in pregnant women and young children.

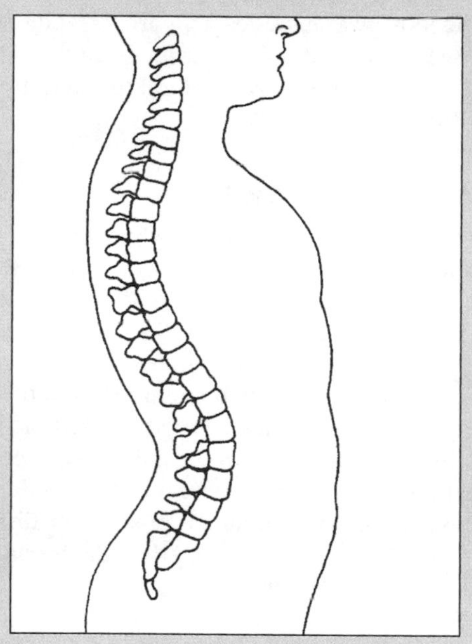

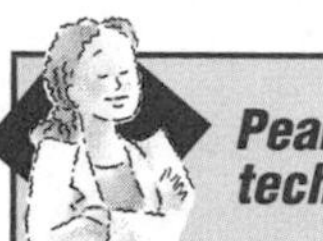

Peak technique

Testing for scoliosis

When testing for scoliosis, have the patient remove his shirt and stand as straight as possible with his back to you. Look for:

- uneven shoulder height and shoulder blade prominence
- unequal distance between the arms and the body
- asymmetrical waistline
- uneven hip height
- sideways lean.

Bent over
Then have the patient bend forward, keeping his head down and palms together. Look for:

- asymmetrical thoracic spine or prominent rib cage (rib hump) on either side
- asymmetrical waistline.

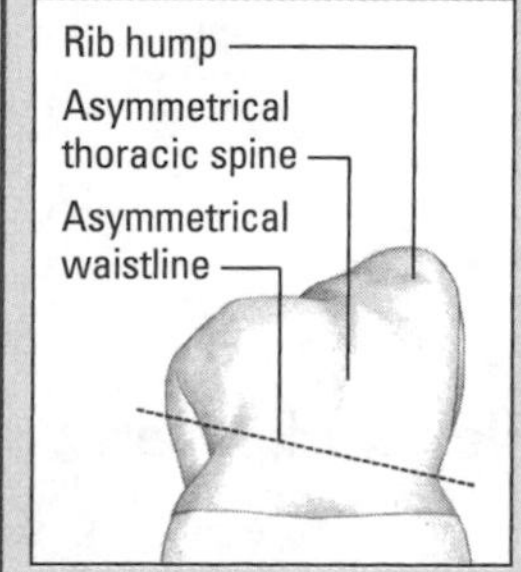

In this position, the spine has a reverse "S" shape. (See *Kyphosis and lordosis.*)

Next, observe the spine posteriorly. It should be in midline position, without deviation to either side. Lateral deviation suggests scoliosis. You may also notice that one shoulder is lower than the other. To assess for scoliosis, have the patient bend at the waist. This position makes deformities more apparent. Normally, the spine remains at midline. (See *Testing for scoliosis.*)

Spinal tape

Next, assess the range of spinal movement. Ask the patient to straighten up, and use a measuring tape to measure the distance from the nape of his neck to his waist. Then ask him to bend forward at the waist. Continue to hold the tape at his neck, letting it

How do I measure up? Nice spine, wouldn't you say?

slip through your fingers slightly to accommodate the increased distance as the spine flexes.

The length of the spine from neck to waist usually increases by at least 2″ (5 cm) when the patient bends forward. If it doesn't, the patient's mobility may be impaired, and you'll need to assess him further.

Spine-tingling procedure

Finally, palpate the spinal processes and the areas lateral to the spine. Have the patient bend at the waist and let his arms hang loosely at his sides. Palpate the spine with your fingertips. Then repeat the palpation using the side of your hand, lightly striking the areas lateral to the spine. Note tenderness, swelling, or spasm.

Shoulders and elbows

Start by observing the patient's shoulders, noting asymmetry, muscle atrophy, or deformity. Swelling or loss of the normal rounded shape could mean that one or more bones are dislocated or out of alignment. Remember, if the patient's reason for seeking care is shoulder pain, the problem may not have originated in the shoulder. Shoulder pain may be referred from other sources and may be due to a heart attack or ruptured ectopic pregnancy.

Palpate the shoulders with the palmar surfaces of your fingers to locate bony landmarks; note crepitus or tenderness. Using your entire hand, palpate the shoulder muscles for firmness and symmetry. Also palpate the elbow and the ulna for subcutaneous nodules that occur with rheumatoid arthritis.

Lift and rotate

If the patient's shoulders don't appear to be dislocated, assess rotation. Start with the patient's arm straight at his side — the neutral position. Ask him to lift his arm straight up from his side to shoulder level and then to bend his elbow horizontally until his forearm is at a 90-degree angle to his upper arm. His arm should be parallel to the floor, and his fingers should be extended with palms down.

To assess external rotation, have him bring his forearm up until his fingers point toward the ceiling. To assess internal rotation, have him lower his forearm until his fingers point toward the floor. Normal ROM is 90 degrees in each direction.

Flex and extend

To assess flexion and extension, start with the patient's arm in the neutral position (at his side). To assess flexion, ask him to move his arm anteriorly over his head, as if reaching for the sky. Full flexion is 180 degrees. To assess extension, have him move his arm from the neutral position posteriorly as far as possible. Normal extension ranges from 30 to 50 degrees.

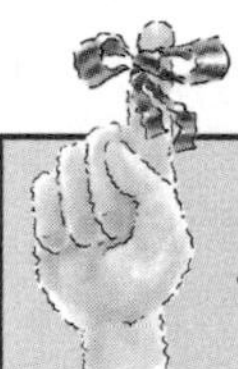

Memory jogger

Here's an easy way to keep adduction and abduction straight.

Adduction is moving a limb toward the body's midline; think of it as *adding* two things together.

Abduction is moving a limb away from the body's midline; think of it as taking something away, like *abducting*, or kidnapping.

Swing into position

To assess abduction, ask the patient to move his arm from the neutral position laterally as far as possible. Normal ROM is 180 degrees. To assess adduction, have the patient move his arm from the neutral position across the front of his body as far as possible. Normal ROM is 50 degrees.

He's up to his elbows

Next, assess the elbows for flexion and extension. Have the patient rest his arm at his side. Ask him to flex his elbow from this position and then extend it. Normal ROM is 90 degrees for both flexion and extension.

To assess supination and pronation of the elbow, have the patient place the side of his hand on a flat surface with the thumb on top. Ask him to rotate his palm down toward the table for pronation and upward for supination. The normal angle of elbow rotation is 90 degrees in each direction.

Wrists and hands

Inspect the wrists and hands for contour, and compare them for symmetry. Also check for nodules, redness, swelling, deformities, and webbing between fingers.

Use your thumb and index finger to palpate both wrists and each finger joint. Note any tenderness, nodules, or bogginess. To avoid causing pain, be especially gentle with elderly patients and those with arthritis.

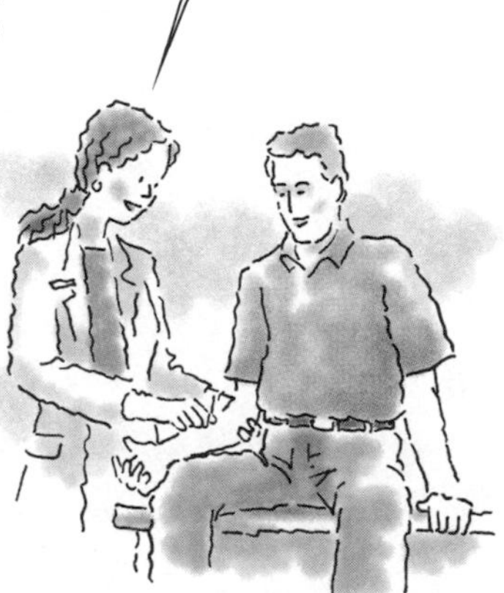

Wristy business

Assess ROM in the wrists. Ask the patient to rotate each wrist by moving his entire hand—first laterally then medially—as if he's waxing a car. Normal ROM is 55 degrees laterally and 20 degrees medially.

Observe the wrist while the patient extends his fingers up toward the ceiling and down toward the floor, as if he's flapping his hand. He should be able to extend his wrist 70 degrees and flex it 90 degrees. If these movements cause pain or numbness, he may have carpal tunnel syndrome. (See *Testing for carpal tunnel syndrome*, page 308.)

Lift a finger; make a fist

To assess extension and flexion of the metacarpophalangeal joints, ask the patient to keep his wrist still and move only

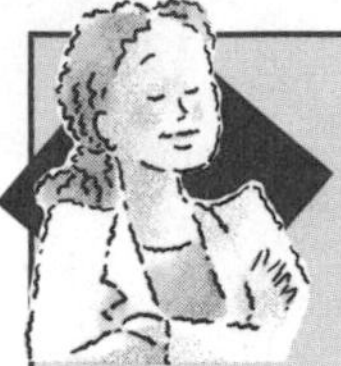

Peak technique

Testing for carpal tunnel syndrome

Two simple tests—Tinel's sign and Phalen's maneuver—can confirm carpal tunnel syndrome.

Tinel's sign

Lightly percuss the transverse carpal ligament over the median nerve where the patient's palm and wrist meet. If this action produces discomfort, such as numbness and tingling shooting into the palm and finger, the patient has Tinel's sign and may have carpal tunnel syndrome.

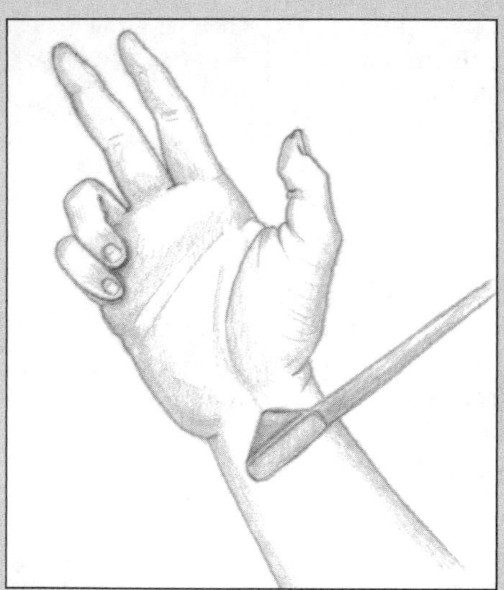

Phalen's maneuver

If flexing the patient's wrist for about 30 seconds causes pain or numbness in his hand or fingers, he has a positive Phalen's sign. The more severe the carpal tunnel syndrome, the more rapidly the symptoms develop.

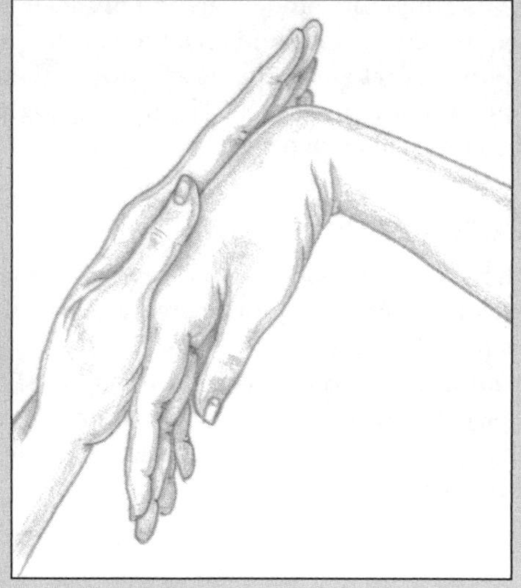

his fingers—first up toward the ceiling and then down toward the floor. Normal extension is 30 degrees; normal flexion, 90 degrees.

Next, ask the patient to touch his thumb to the little finger of the same hand. He should be able to fold or flex his thumb across the palm of his hand so that it touches or points toward the base of his little finger.

To assess flexion of all of the fingers, ask the patient to form a fist. Then have him spread his fingers apart to demonstrate abduction and draw them back together to demonstrate adduction.

At arm's length

If you suspect that one arm is longer than the other, take measurements. Put one end of the measuring tape at the acromial process of the shoulder and the other on the tip of the middle finger. Drape the tape over the outer elbow. The difference between the left and right extremities should be no more than ⅜″ (1 cm).

Hips and knees

Inspect the hip area for contour and symmetry. Inspect the position of the knees, noting whether the patient is bowlegged, with knees that point out, or knock-kneed, with knees that turn in. Then watch the patient walk.

Palpate each hip over the iliac crest and trochanteric area for tenderness or instability. Palpate both knees. They should feel smooth, and the tissues should feel solid. (See *Bulge sign*.)

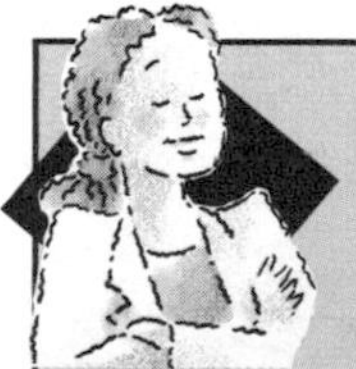

Peak technique

Bulge sign

The bulge sign indicates excess fluid in the joint. To assess the patient for this sign, ask him to lie down so that you can palpate his knee. Then give the medial side of his knee two to four firm strokes, as shown top right, to displace excess fluid.

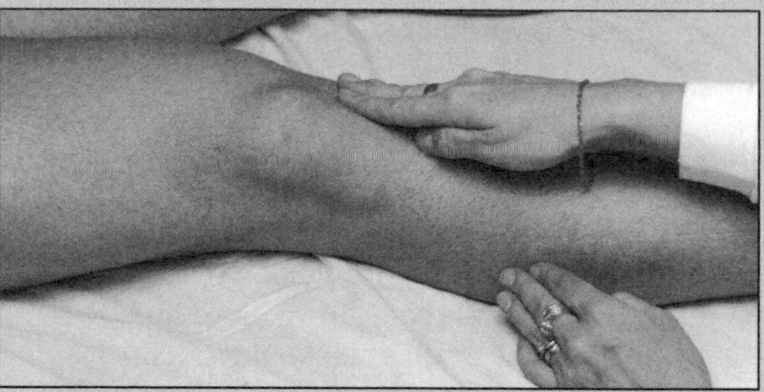

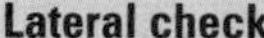

Lateral check

Next, tap the lateral aspect of the knee while checking for a fluid wave on the medial aspect, as shown bottom right.

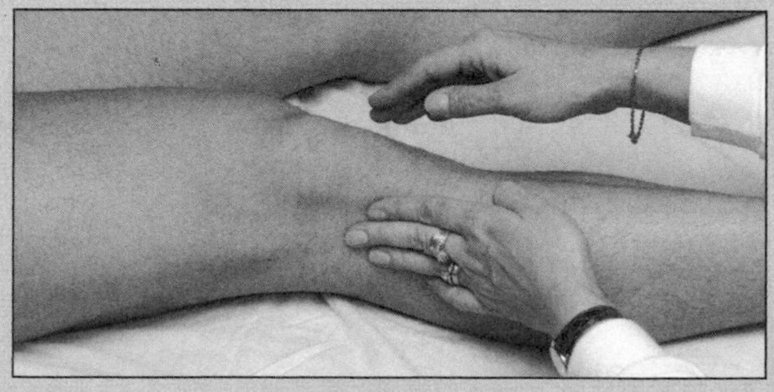

Hip, hip, hooray!

Assess ROM in the hip. These exercises are typically done with the patient in a supine position.

To assess hip flexion, place your hand under the patient's lower back and have the patient bend one knee and pull it toward his abdomen and chest as far as possible. You'll feel the patient's back touch your hand as the normal lumbar lordosis of the spine flattens. As the patient flexes his knee, the opposite hip and thigh should remain flat on the bed. Repeat on the opposite side.

To assess hip abduction, stand alongside the patient and press down on the superior iliac spine of the opposite hip with one hand to stabilize the pelvis. With your other hand, hold the patient's leg by the ankle and gently abduct the hip until you feel the iliac spine move. That movement indicates the limit of hip abduction. Then, while still stabilizing the pelvis, move the ankle medially across the patient's body to assess hip adduction. Repeat on the other side. Normal ROM is about 45 degrees for abduction and 30 degrees for adduction.

To assess hip extension, have the patient lie prone (facedown), and gently extend the thigh upward. Repeat on the other thigh.

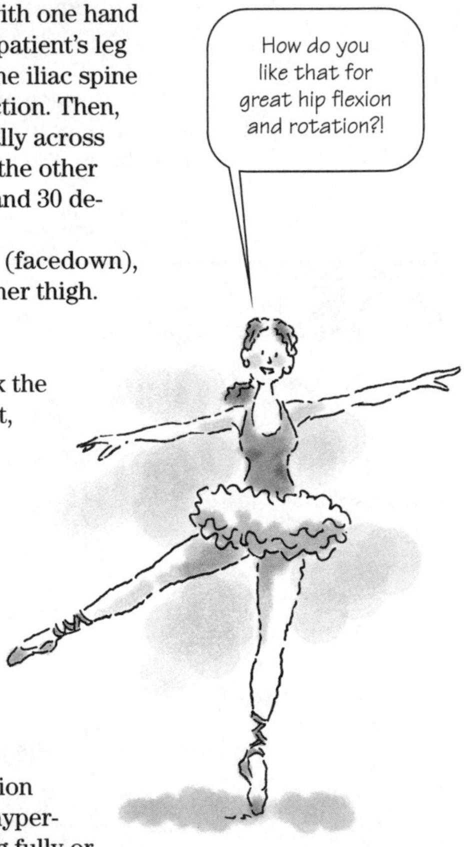

As the hip turns

To assess internal and external rotation of the hip, ask the patient to lift one leg up and, keeping his knee straight, turn his leg and foot medially and laterally. Normal ROM for internal rotation is 40 degrees; for external rotation, 45 degrees.

On bended knees

Assess ROM in the knee. If the patient is standing, ask him to bend his knee as if trying to touch his heel to his buttocks. Normal ROM for flexion is 120 to 130 degrees. If the patient is lying down, have him draw his knee up to his chest. His calf should touch his thigh.

Knee extension returns the knee to a neutral position of 0 degrees; however, some knees may normally be hyperextended 15 degrees. If the patient can't extend his leg fully or if his knee pops audibly and painfully, consider the response abnormal.

Other abnormalities include pronounced crepitus, which may signal a degenerative disease of the knee, and sudden buckling, which may indicate a ligament injury.

Ankles and feet

Inspect the ankles and feet for swelling, redness, nodules, and other deformities. Check the arch of the foot and look for toe deformities. Also note edema, calluses, bunions, corns, ingrown toenails, plantar warts, trophic ulcers, hair loss, or unusual pigmentation.

Use your fingertips to palpate the bony and muscular structures of the ankles and feet. Palpate each toe joint by compressing it with your thumb and fingers.

The ankle angle

To examine the ankle, have the patient sit in a chair or on the side of a bed. To test plantar flexion, ask him to point his toes toward the floor. Test dorsiflexion by asking him to point his toes toward the ceiling. Normal ROM for plantar flexion is about 45 degrees; for dorsiflexion, 20 degrees.

Next, assess ROM in the ankle. Ask the patient to demonstrate inversion by turning his feet inward, and eversion by turning his feet outward. Normal ROM for inversion is 45 degrees; for eversion, 30 degrees.

To assess the metatarsophalangeal joints, ask the patient to flex his toes and then straighten them.

The long and short of it

If you suspect that one leg is longer than the other, take measurements. Put one end of the tape at the medial malleolus at the ankle and the other end at the anterior iliac spine. Cross the tape over the medial side of the knee. A difference of more than ⅜″ (1 cm) is abnormal.

Assessing the muscles

Start assessing the muscles by inspecting all major muscle groups for tone, strength, and symmetry. If a muscle appears atrophied or hypertrophied, measure it by wrapping a tape measure around the largest circumference of the muscle on each side of the body and comparing the two numbers.

Other abnormalities of muscle appearance include contracture and abnormal movements, such as spasms, tics, tremors, and fasciculation.

This really isn't necessary to prove that you have good arm muscle tone.

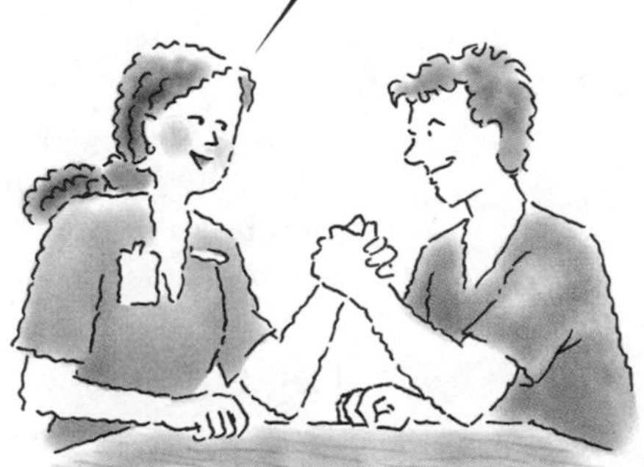

Tuning in to muscle tone

Muscle tone describes muscular resistance to passive stretching. To test the patient's arm muscle tone, move his shoulder through passive ROM exercises. You should feel a slight resistance. Then let his arm drop. It should fall easily to his side.

Test leg muscle tone by putting the patient's hip through passive ROM exercises and then letting the leg fall to the examination table or bed. Like the arm, the leg should fall easily.

Abnormal findings include muscle rigidity and flaccidity. Rigidity indicates increased muscle tone, possibly caused by an upper motor neuron lesion such as from a stroke. Flaccidity may result from a lower motor neuron lesion.

Wrestling with muscle strength

Observe the patient's gait and movements to form an idea of his general muscle strength. Grade muscle strength on a scale of 0 to 5, with 0 representing no strength and 5 representing maximum strength. Document the results as a fraction, with the score as the numerator and maximum strength as the denominator. (See *Grading muscle strength.*)

To test specific muscle groups, ask the patient to move the muscles while you apply resistance; then compare the contralateral muscle groups. (See *Testing muscle strength.*)

> **Grading muscle strength**
>
> Grade muscle strength on a scale of 0 to 5, as follows:
> - 5/5—Normal; Patient moves joint through full range of motion (ROM) and against gravity with full resistance.
> - 4/5—Good; Patient completes ROM against gravity with moderate resistance.
> - 3/5—Fair; Patient completes ROM against gravity only.
> - 2/5—Poor; Patient completes full ROM with gravity eliminated (passive motion).
> - 1/5—Trace; Patient's attempt at muscle contraction is palpable but without joint movement.
> - 0/5—Zero; No evidence of muscle contraction.

Shoulder, arm, wrist, and hand strength

Test the strength of the patient's shoulder girdle by asking him to extend his arms with the palms up and hold this position for 30 seconds. If he can't lift both arms equally and keep his palms up, or if one arm drifts down, he probably has shoulder girdle weakness on that side.

If he passes the first part of the test, gauge his strength by placing your hands on his arms and applying downward pressure as he resists you.

Testing the bi's and tri's

Next, have the patient hold his arm in front of him with the elbow bent. To test bicep strength, pull down on the flexor surface of his forearm as he resists. To test tricep strength, have him try to straighten his arm as you push upward against the extensor surface of his forearm.

Forcing his hand

Assess the strength of the patient's flexed wrist by pushing against it. Test the strength of the extended wrist by pushing down on it. Test the strength of finger abduction, thumb opposition, and handgrip the same way. (See *Testing handgrip strength.*)

Leg strength

Ask the patient to lie in a supine position on the examining table or bed and lift both legs at the same time. Note whether he lifts

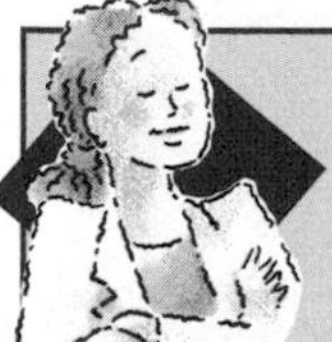

Peak technique

Testing muscle strength

To test the muscle strength of your patient's arm and ankle muscles, use the techniques shown here.

Biceps strength

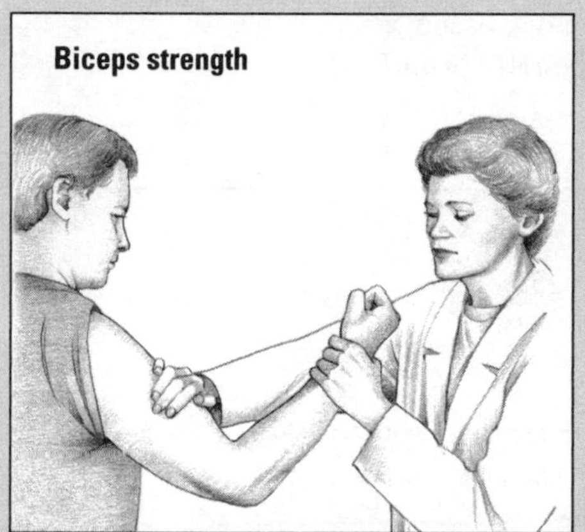

Ankle strength: Plantar flexion

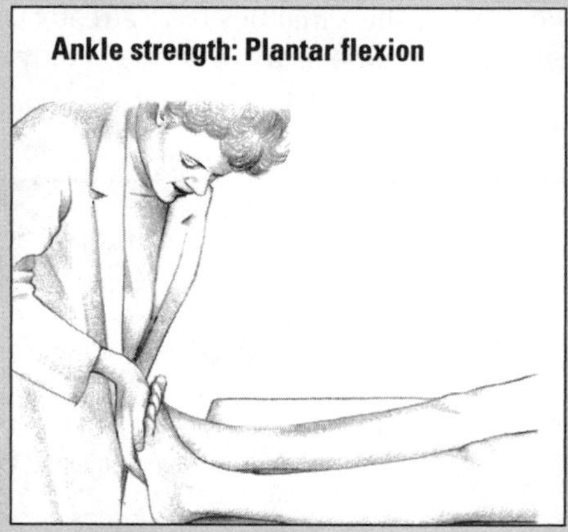

Triceps strength

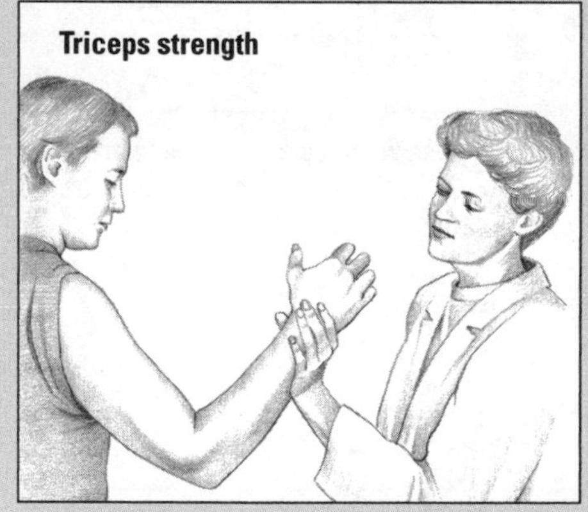

Ankle strength: Dorsiflexion

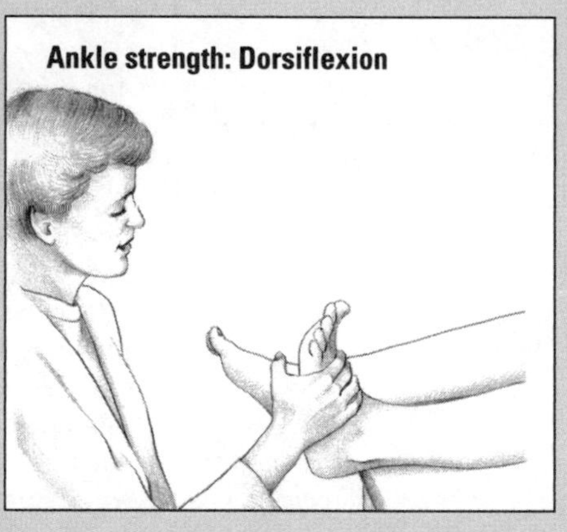

both legs at the same time and to the same distance. To test quadricep strength, have him lower his legs and raise them again while you press down on his anterior thighs.

Then ask the patient to flex his knees and put his feet flat on the bed. Assess lower-leg strength by pulling his lower leg forward as he resists and then by pushing it backward as he extends his knee.

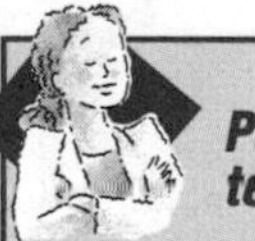

Peak technique

Testing handgrip strength

When testing handgrip strength, face the patient, extend the first and second fingers of each hand, and ask him to grasp your fingers and squeeze. Don't extend fingers with rings on them; a strong handgrip on those fingers can be painful.

Finally, assess ankle strength by having the patient push his foot down against your resistance and then pull his foot up as you try to hold it down.

Abnormal findings

Abnormalities in the musculoskeletal system occur for many reasons. Some general abnormalities have already been discussed; more specific abnormalities are described below. (See *Abnormal musculoskeletal findings.*)

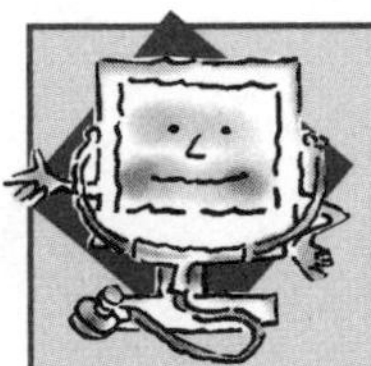

Interpretation station

Abnormal musculoskeletal findings

After you assess the patient, a group of findings may lead you to suspect a particular disorder. The chart below shows common groups of musculoskeletal system findings along with signs and symptoms and their probable causes.

Sign or symptom and findings	Probable cause
Arm pain	
• Pain radiating through the arm • Pain that worsens with movement • Crepitus, felt and heard • Deformity (if bones are misaligned) • Local ecchymosis and edema • Impaired distal circulation • Paresthesia	Fracture
• Left arm pain • Deep and crushing chest pain • Weakness • Pallor • Dyspnea • Diaphoresis • Apprehension	Myocardial infarction
***Arm pain** (continued)*	
• Severe arm pain with passive muscle stretching • Impaired distal circulation • Muscle weakness • Decreased reflex response • Paresthesia • Edema • Paralysis and absent pulse (ominous signs)	Compartment syndrome
Leg pain	
• Severe, acute leg pain, particularly with movement • Ecchymosis and edema • Leg unable to bear weight • Impaired neurovascular status distal to injury • Deformity, crepitus, and muscle spasms	Fracture

Abnormal musculoskeletal findings *(continued)*

Sign or symptom and findings	Probable cause
Leg pain *(continued)*	
• Shooting, aching, or tingling pain that radiates down the leg • Pain exacerbated by activity and relieved by rest • Limping • Difficulty moving from a sitting to a standing position	Sciatica
• Discomfort ranging from calf tenderness to severe pain • Edema and a feeling of heaviness in the affected leg • Warmth • Fever, chills, malaise, muscle cramps • Positive Homans' sign	Thrombophlebitis
Muscle spasm	
• Spasms and intermittent claudication • Loss of peripheral pulses • Pallor or cyanosis • Decreased sensation • Hair loss • Dry or scaling skin • Edema • Ulcerations	Arterial occlusive disease
• Localized spasms and pain • Swelling • Limited mobility • Bony crepitation	Fracture
Muscle spasm *(continued)*	
• Tetany (muscle cramps and twitching, carpopedal and facial muscle spasms, and seizures) • Positive Chvostek's and Trousseau's signs • Paresthesia of the lips, fingers, and toes • Choreiform movements • Hyperactive deep tendon reflexes • Fatigue • Palpitations • Cardiac arrhythmias	Hypocalcemia
Muscle weakness	
• Unilateral or bilateral weakness of the arms, legs, face, or tongue • Dysarthria • Aphasia • Paresthesia or sensory loss • Vision disturbances • Bowel and bladder dysfunction	Stroke
• Muscle weakness, disuse, and possible atrophy • Altered level of consciousness • Personality changes • Severe low back pain, possibly radiating to the buttocks, legs, and feet (usually unilateral) • Diminished reflexes • Sensory changes	Herniated disk
• Muscle weakness in one or more limbs, which may lead to atrophy, spasticity, and contractures • Diplopia, blurred vision, or vision loss • Hyperactive deep tendon reflexes • Paresthesia or sensory loss • Incoordination • Intention tremors	Multiple sclerosis

A call to arms

Arm pain (pain anywhere from the hand to the shoulder) usually results from musculoskeletal disorders, but it can also stem from neurovascular or cardiovascular disorders. In some cases, it may be referred pain from another area, such as the chest, neck, or abdomen.

Crunching crepitus

Crepitus is an abnormal crunching or grating you can hear and feel when a joint with roughened articular surfaces moves. It occurs in patients with rheumatoid arthritis or osteoarthritis or when broken pieces of bone rub together.

Unsure footing

Footdrop — plantar flexion of the foot with the toes bent toward the instep — results from weakness or paralysis of the dorsiflexor muscles of the foot and ankle. A characteristic and important sign of certain peripheral nerve or motor neuron disorders, footdrop may also stem from prolonged immobility when inadequate support, improper positioning, or infrequent passive exercise produces shortening of the Achilles tendon.

What kind of joint is this?

Heberden's and Bouchard's nodes are hard nodes that develop on the distal and proximal joints of the fingers in patients with osteoarthritis. (See *Heberden's and Bouchard's nodes.*) Patients with osteoarthritis may also experience joint swelling, pain, crepitus, limited movement, and contracture. Gait may be affected if knees and hips are involved.

Not a leg to stand on

Although leg pain commonly indicates a musculoskeletal disorder, it can also result from more serious vascular or neurologic disorders. The pain may occur suddenly or gradually and may be localized or affect the entire leg. Constant or intermittent, it may feel dull, burning, sharp, shooting, or tingling.

Wasting away

Muscle atrophy, or muscle wasting, results from denervation or prolonged muscle disuse. When deprived of regular exercise, muscle fibers lose both bulk and length, which produces a visible loss of muscle size and contour and apparent emaciation or deformity in the affected area. It usually results from neuromuscular disease or injury but may also stem from metabolic and endocrine disorders and prolonged immobility. Some muscle atrophy also occurs with aging.

Heberden's and Bouchard's nodes

Heberden's and Bouchard's nodes are typically seen in patients with osteoarthritis.

Heberden's nodes
Heberden's nodes appear on the distal interphalangeal joints. Usually hard and painless, these bony and cartilaginous enlargements typically occur in middle-aged and elderly patients with osteoarthritis.

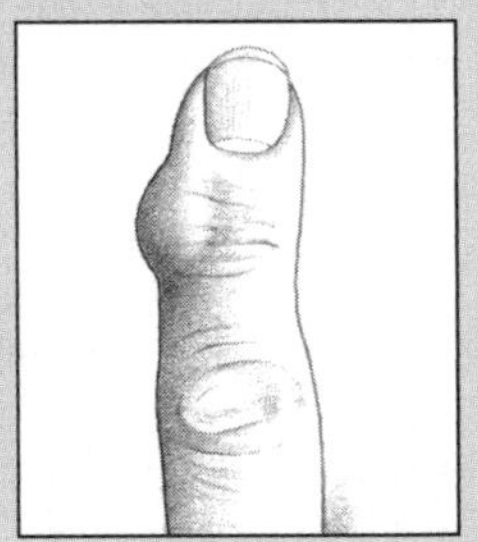

Bouchard's nodes
Bouchard's nodes are similar but less common and appear on the proximal interphalangeal joints.

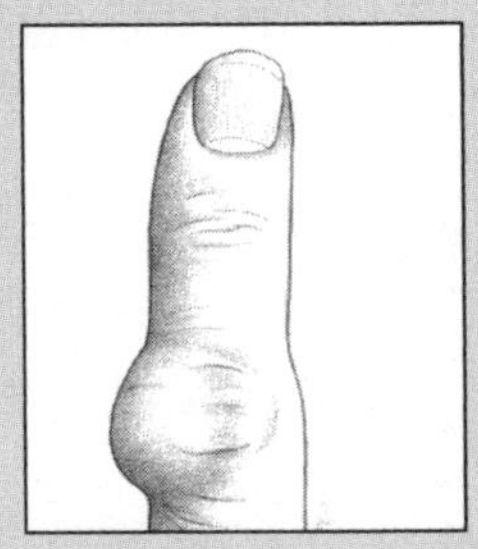

Spaz attack

Muscle spasms, or cramps, are strong, painful contractions. They can occur in virtually any muscle but are most common in the calf and foot. Muscle spasms typically occur from simple muscle fatigue, after exercise, and during pregnancy. However, they may also develop in electrolyte imbalances and neuromuscular disorders or as the result of certain drugs.

Feeble finding

Muscle weakness may be reported to you by the patient, or you may detect it by observing and measuring the strength of an individual muscle or muscle group. It can result from a malfunction in the cerebral hemispheres, brain stem, spinal cord, nerve roots, peripheral nerves, or myoneural junctions and within the muscle itself.

Feeling wounded

Most musculoskeletal emergencies result from trauma. Specific traumatic injuries include fractures, dislocations, amputations, crush injuries, and serious lacerations. The patient is usually alert and able to describe how the injury occurred.

If his level of consciousness deteriorates, suspect shock or drug or alcohol ingestion, and assess him further. Remember, even if the patient has ingested drugs or alcohol, he can still go into shock. (See *The 5 P's of musculoskeletal injury.*)

The 5 P's of musculoskeletal injury

To swiftly assess a musculoskeletal injury, remember the 5 P's: pain, paresthesia, paralysis, pallor, and pulse.

Pain
Ask the patient whether he feels pain. If he does, assess the location, severity, and quality of the pain.

Paresthesia
Assess the patient for loss of sensation by touching the injured area with the tip of an open safety pin. Abnormal sensation or loss of sensation indicates neurovascular involvement.

Paralysis
Assess whether the patient can move the affected area. If he can't, he might have nerve or tendon damage.

Pallor
Paleness, discoloration, and coolness on the injured side may indicate neurovascular compromise.

Pulse
Check all pulses distal to the injury site. If a pulse is decreased or absent, blood supply to the area is reduced.

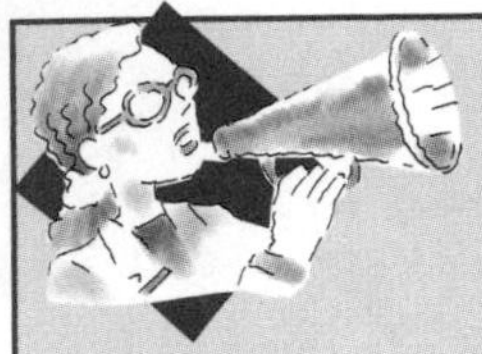

That's a wrap!

Musculoskeletal system review

Structures

Bones

- Support and protect organs and tissues
- Serve as storage sites for minerals
- Produce blood cells in bone marrow

Joints

- Defined as the junction of two or more bones
- Consist of two types
  - Nonsynovial: immovable or slightly movable bones connected by fibrous tissue or cartilage (such as the skull and vertebrae)
  - Synovial: freely movable bones that meet in a cavity filled with synovial fluid (a lubricant); include ball-and-socket and hinge joints
- Perform different types of motion:
  - Circumduction: moving in a circular manner
  - Flexion: bending, decreasing the joint angle
  - Extension: straightening, increasing the joint angle
  - Abduction: moving away from midline
  - Adduction: moving toward midline
  - Retraction and protraction: moving backward and forward
  - Pronation: turning downward
  - Supination: turning upward
  - Internal rotation: turning toward midline
  - External rotation: turning away from midline
  - Eversion: turning outward
  - Inversion: turning inward

Muscles

- Consist of groups of contractile cells or fibers
- Attach to bone by tendons (tough fibrous portions of muscle)

The health history

- Determine the patient's reason for seeking care, such as pain, swelling, stiffness, and obvious deformities.
- Ask about current health, such as effects on ADLs and the use of ice, heat, or other remedies to treat the problem.
- Ask about past health, including arthritis, cancer, osteoporosis, and trauma, and inquire about the patient's use of assistive devices, such as a walker or cane.
- Ask about medications, especially those that may affect the musculoskeletal system (such as corticosteroids and potassium-depleting diuretics).
- Ask about lifestyle, including the patient's job, hobbies, and personal habits.

Assessing the musculoskeletal system

- Work from head to toe and from proximal to distal.
- Note the size and shape of joints, limbs, and body regions.
- Inspect and palpate around joints, limbs, and body regions.
- Have the patient perform active ROM exercises; if he can't, perform passive ROM exercises. Never force any movement!
- Observe the patient's posture and gait whenever possible.

Assessing bones and joints

Head, jaw, and neck

- Inspect the patient's face.
- Evaluate ROM in the TMJ.
- Inspect the front, back, and sides of the patient's neck.
- Palpate the cervical vertebrae and the neck area. Listen for crepitus as the patient moves his neck.
- Assess ROM in the neck.

Spine

- Inspect the patient's spine posteriorly and as he stands in profile.
- Assess for scoliosis by having the patient bend at the waist.
- Assess the range of spinal movement.
- Palpate the spinal processes and areas lateral to the spine as the patient bends at the waist.

Shoulders and elbows

- Inspect and palpate the shoulders.
- Assess internal and external rotation, flexion and extension, and abduction and adduction of the shoulders.
- Assess flexion and extension and supination and pronation of the elbows.

Musculoskeletal system review *(continued)*

Wrists and hands

- Inspect and palpate the wrists and hands. Also palpate each finger joint.
- Assess ROM in the wrist: rotation, flexion, and extension. Assess for carpal tunnel syndrome if these movements cause pain or numbness.
- Assess extension and flexion of the metacarpophalangeal joints.
- Assess flexion, extension, abduction, and adduction of all the fingers.
- Measure both arms if you suspect one is longer than the other.

Hips and knees

- Inspect the hip area and knees.
- Palpate the hips and knees.
- Perform the bulge sign to assess for excess fluid in the knee joint.
- Assess hip flexion, extension, abduction, and adduction as well as internal and external hip rotation.
- Assess flexion and extension in the knee.

Ankles and feet

- Inspect and palpate the ankles and feet.
- Assess dorsiflexion, plantar flexion, inversion, and eversion of the ankles.
- Assess the metatarsophalangeal joints by having the patient flex and extend his toes.
- Measure both legs if you suspect one is longer than the other.

Assessment of the muscles

- Assess muscle tone as you move each limb through passive ROM exercises.
- Assess shoulder, arm, wrist, and hand strength.
- Assess leg strength.

Abnormal musculoskeletal findings

- Crepitus: abnormal crunching or grating that may be heard or felt when a joint with roughened articular surfaces moves
- Footdrop: plantar flexion of the foot with the toes bent toward the instep
- Heberden's nodes: hard nodes on the distal interphalangeal joints in patients with osteoarthritis
- Bouchard's nodes: hard nodes on the proximal interphalangeal joints in patients with osteoarthritis
- Muscle atrophy: muscle wasting
- Muscle spasms: muscle cramps; strong, painful muscle contractions

The 5 P's of musculoskeletal injury

- Pain
- Paresthesia
- Paralysis
- Pallor
- Pulse

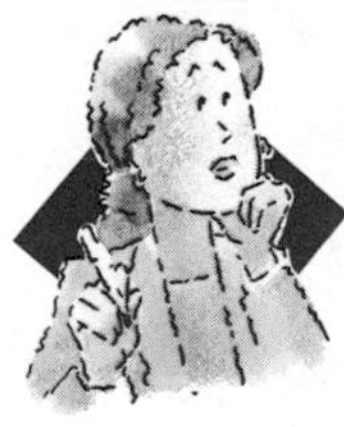

Quick quiz

1. If you hear crepitus while moving a patient's joint, the joint must be:

A. synovial.
B. nonsynovial.
C. fixed.
D. slightly movable.

Answer: A. Crepitus occurs when roughened articular surfaces of bone or bone fragments rub together. Thus it can only occur in joints that are freely movable such as the synovial joints.

2. If your patient's arm drifts down after he extends it for 10 seconds, he probably has:

A. carpal tunnel syndrome.
B. broken metatarsal bones.
C. shoulder-girdle weakness.
D. a fractured rib.

Answer: C. Inability to lift and extend an arm for 30 seconds indicates weakness of the shoulder girdle muscles on that side.

3. A patient with kyphosis has an:

A. exaggerated lateral spinal curvature.
B. unusually rounded thoracic curve.
C. abnormally concave lumbar spine.
D. inability to bend forward at the waist.

Answer: B. Kyphosis causes a rounded back in the thoracic region.

4. Your patient can't move his right arm away from his side, so you document this as impaired:

A. supination.
B. abduction.
C. adduction
D. eversion.

Answer: B. Abduction is the ability to move a limb away from the midline. In adduction, the limb is moved toward the midline.

5. To assess a swollen knee, perform the:

A. bulge sign test.
B. straight-leg-raising test.
C. Ortolani's sign test.
D. Phalen's maneuver test.

Answer: A. A swollen knee suggests excess fluid in the joint. The bulge sign occurs when you apply pressure to the knee and a bulge of fluid appears on the opposite side.

Scoring

☆☆☆ If you answered all five questions correctly, hooray! No bones about it, you're a master of musculoskeletal assessments.

☆☆ If you answered four questions correctly, yeah! You're really beginning to flex your assessment muscles.

☆ If you answered fewer than four questions correctly, that's okay! Building knowledge, just like building muscles, takes persistence.

Neurologic system

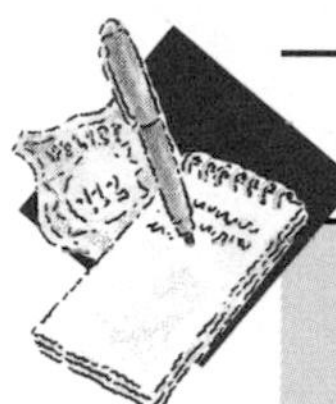

Just the facts

In this chapter, you'll learn:

- characteristics of the organs and structures of the neurologic system
- methods to obtain a patient history of neurologic function
- techniques to conduct a physical assessment of the neurologic system
- ways to recognize neurologic abnormalities.

A look at the neurologic system

The neurologic system controls body function and is related to every other body system. Consequently, patients who suffer from diseases of other body systems can develop neurologic impairments related to the disease. For example, a patient who has heart surgery may then suffer a stroke.

Because the neurologic system is so complex, evaluating it can seem overwhelming at first. Although tests for neurologic status are extensive, they're also basic and straightforward. In fact, your daily nursing care may routinely include some of these tests.

Just talking with a patient helps you assess his orientation, level of consciousness (LOC), and ability to formulate and produce speech. Having him perform a simple task such as walking allows you to evaluate motor ability. Your knowledge of neurologic assessment techniques will enhance your patient care and may save some patients from irreversible neurologic damage.

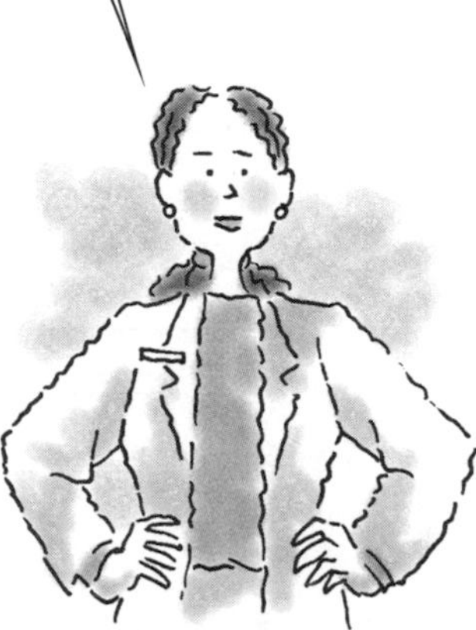

Divvy it up

The neurologic system is divided into the central nervous system (CNS), the peripheral nervous system, and the autonomic nervous system. Through complex and coordinated interactions, these three parts integrate all physical, intellectual, and emotional activities. Understanding how each part works is essential to conducting an accurate neurologic assessment.

Central nervous system

The CNS includes the brain and spinal cord. These two structures collect and interpret voluntary and involuntary motor and sensory stimuli. (See *A close look at the CNS.*)

Brain

The brain consists of the cerebrum (or *cerebral cortex*), the brain stem, and the cerebellum. It collects, integrates, and interprets all stimuli and initiates and monitors voluntary and involuntary motor activity.

The reasons for your cerebrum

The cerebrum gives us the ability to think and reason. It's encased by the skull and enclosed by three membrane layers (the dura

A close look at the CNS

This illustration shows a cross section of the brain and spinal cord, which together make up the central nervous system (CNS). The brain joins the spinal cord at the base of the skull and ends near the second lumbar vertebrae. Note the H-shaped mass of gray matter in the spinal cord.

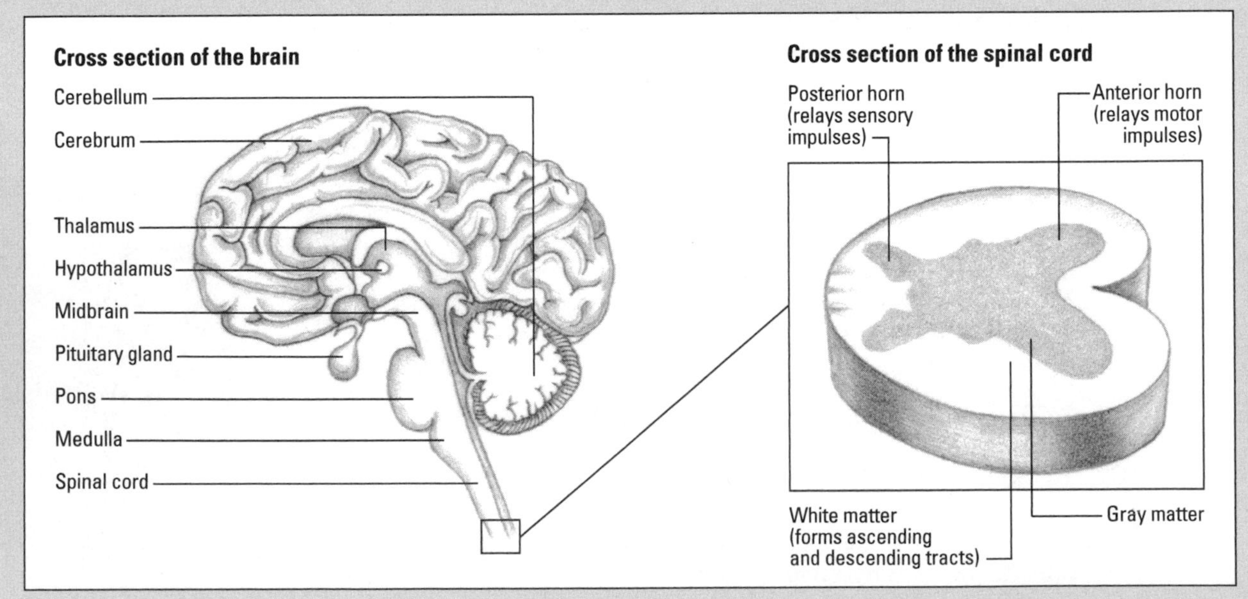

A close look at the cerebrum and its functions

The cerebrum is divided into four lobes, based on anatomic landmarks and functional differences. The lobes—parietal, occipital, temporal, and frontal—are named for the cranial bones that lie over them.

This illustration shows the locations of the cerebral lobes and explains their functions. It also shows the location of the cerebellum.

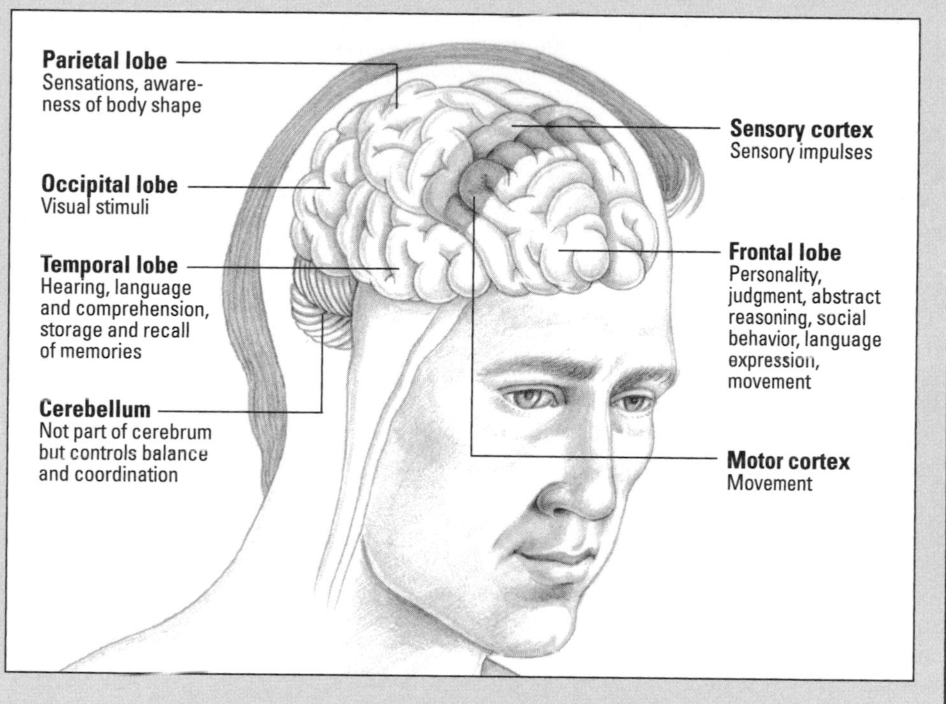

mater, arachnoid mater, and pia mater) called *meninges*. The space under the arachnoid layer (called the *subarachnoid space*) contains cerebrospinal fluid (CSF). If blood or fluid accumulates between these layers, pressure builds inside the skull and compromises brain function.

The cerebrum is divided into four lobes and two hemispheres. The right hemisphere controls the left side of the body, and the left hemisphere controls the right side of the body. Each lobe controls different functions. Cranial nerves I and II originate in the cerebrum. (See *A close look at the cerebrum and its functions.*)

Meet the muses, Thala and Hypothala

The diencephalon, a division of the cerebrum, contains the thalamus and hypothalamus. The thalamus is a relay station for sensory impulses. The hypothalamus has many regulatory functions, including temperature control, pituitary hormone production, and water balance.

Quite the sy-stem!

The brain stem lies below the diencephalon and is divided into three parts: the midbrain, pons, and medulla. The brain stem contains cranial nerves III through XII, also known as the *nuclei*, and is a major sensory and motor pathway for impulses running to and from the cerebral cortex. It also regulates automatic body functions, such as heart rate, breathing, swallowing, and coughing.

Go to the back of the brain

The cerebellum, the most posterior part of the brain, contains the major motor and sensory pathways. It facilitates smooth, coordinated muscle movement and helps maintain equilibrium.

Spinal cord

The spinal cord is the primary pathway for messages traveling between the peripheral areas of the body and the brain. It also mediates the sensory-to-motor transmission path known as the *reflex arc*. Because the reflex arc enters and exits the spinal cord at the same level, reflex pathways don't need to travel up and down the way other stimuli do. (See *Reflex arc*.)

The spinal cord extends from the upper border of the first cervical vertebrae to the lower border of the first lumbar vertebrae. It's encased by a continuation of the meninges and CSF that surround and protect the brain and is also protected by the bony vertebrae of the spine.

The dorsal white matter contains the ascending tracts that carry impulses up the spinal cord to higher sensory centers. The ventral white matter contains the descending motor tracts that transmit motor impulses down from the higher motor centers to the spinal cord.

Mapping out the body

For the purpose of documenting sensory function, the body is divided into dermatomes. Each dermatome represents an area supplied with afferent, or sensory, nerve fibers from an individual spinal root—either cervical, thoracic, lumbar, or sacral. This body map is used when testing sensation and trying to identify the source of a lesion.

Reflex arc

Spinal nerves, which have sensory and motor portions, control deep tendon and superficial reflexes. A simple reflex arc requires a sensory (or afferent) neuron and a motor (or efferent) neuron. The knee-jerk, or *patellar,* reflex illustrates the sequence of events in a normal reflex arc.

First, a sensory receptor detects the mechanical stimulus produced by the reflex hammer striking the patellar tendon. Then the sensory neuron carries the impulse along its axon by way of the spinal nerve to the dorsal root, where it enters the spinal column.

Patellar reflex arc

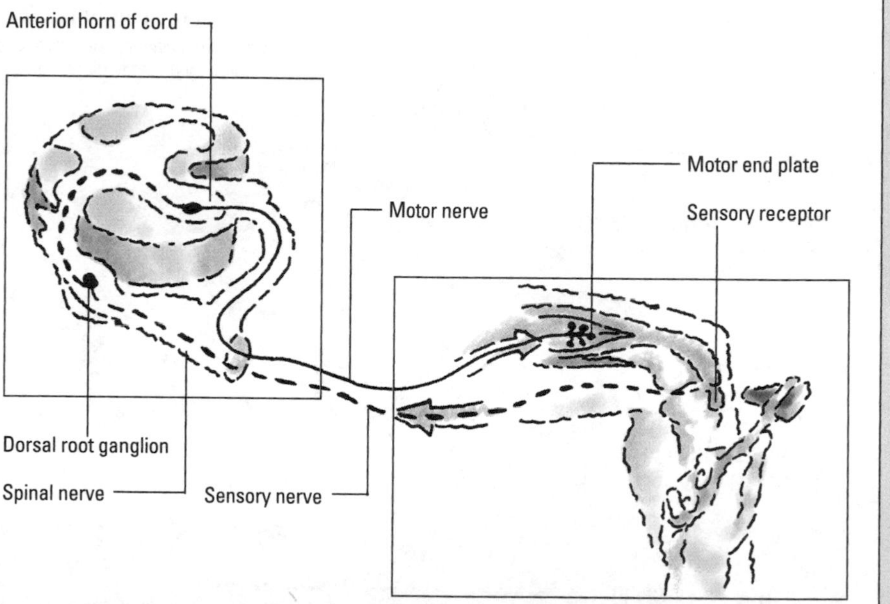

Next, in the anterior horn of the spinal cord, the sensory neuron joins with a motor neuron, which carries the impulse along its axon by way of a spinal nerve to the muscle. The motor neuron transmits the impulse to the muscle fibers through stimulation of the motor end plate. This impulse triggers the muscle to contract and the leg to extend. *Don't stand directly in front of a patient when testing this reflex!*

Peripheral nervous system

The peripheral nervous system includes the peripheral and cranial nerves. Peripheral sensory nerves transmit stimuli to the posterior horn of the spinal cord from sensory receptors located in the skin, muscles, sensory organs, and viscera. The upper motor neurons of the brain and the lower motor neurons of the cell bodies in the anterior horn of the spinal cord carry impulses that affect movement.

The 12 pairs of cranial nerves are the primary motor and sensory pathways between the brain, head, and neck. (See *Identifying cranial nerves,* page 326.)

Identifying cranial nerves

The cranial nerves have sensory function, motor function, or both. They're assigned Roman numerals and are written this way: *CN I, CN II, CN III,* and so forth. This illustration lists the function of each cranial nerve.

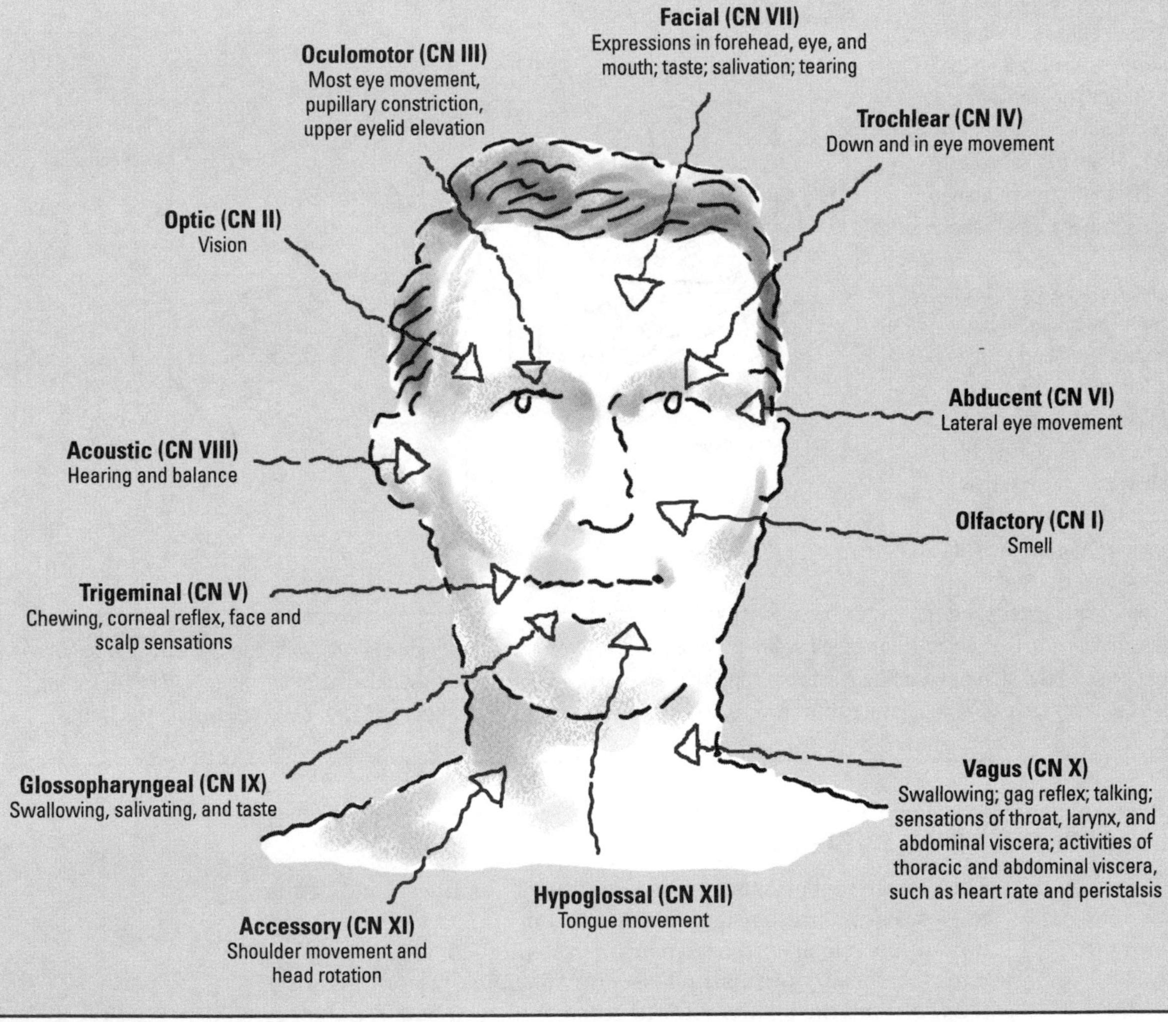

Facial (CN VII)
Expressions in forehead, eye, and mouth; taste; salivation; tearing

Oculomotor (CN III)
Most eye movement, pupillary constriction, upper eyelid elevation

Trochlear (CN IV)
Down and in eye movement

Optic (CN II)
Vision

Abducent (CN VI)
Lateral eye movement

Acoustic (CN VIII)
Hearing and balance

Olfactory (CN I)
Smell

Trigeminal (CN V)
Chewing, corneal reflex, face and scalp sensations

Glossopharyngeal (CN IX)
Swallowing, salivating, and taste

Vagus (CN X)
Swallowing; gag reflex; talking; sensations of throat, larynx, and abdominal viscera; activities of thoracic and abdominal viscera, such as heart rate and peristalsis

Hypoglossal (CN XII)
Tongue movement

Accessory (CN XI)
Shoulder movement and head rotation

Autonomic nervous system

The autonomic nervous system contains motor neurons that regulate the activities of the visceral organs and affect the smooth and cardiac muscles and the glands. It consists of two parts:

 sympathetic division, which controls fight-or-flight reactions

parasympathetic division, which maintains baseline body functions.

Obtaining a health history

The most common complaints about the neurologic system include headache, dizziness, faintness, confusion, impaired mental status, disturbances in balance or gait, and changes in LOC. When documenting the reason for seeking care, record the information in the patient's own words.

So, fill me in on the details

When you learn the patient's reason for seeking care, ask about the onset and frequency of the problem, what precipitates or exacerbates it, and what alleviates it. Ask whether other symptoms accompany the patient's problem and whether he has had adverse effects from treatments.

Also ask about other aspects of his current health and about his past health and family history. Help him describe problems by asking pertinent questions such as those mentioned here.

Asking about current health

Ask the patient whether he has headaches. If so, how often and what seems to bring them on? Does light bother his eyes during a headache? What other symptoms occur with the headache?

Does the patient have dizziness, numbness, tingling, seizures, tremors, weakness, or paralysis? Does he have problems with any of his senses or walking, keeping his balance, swallowing, or urinating?

How does he rate his memory and ability to concentrate? Does he ever have trouble speaking or understanding people? Does he have trouble reading or writing? If he has these problems, how much do they interfere with his daily activities?

Keep in mind that some neurologic changes, such as decreased reflexes, hearing, and vision, are a normal part of aging. (See *Aging and the neurologic system.*)

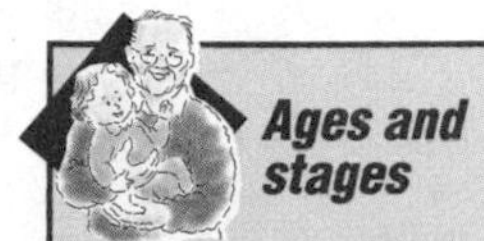

Ages and stages

Aging and the neurologic system

Because neurons undergo various degenerative changes, aging can lead to:

- diminished reflexes
- decreased hearing, vision, taste, and smell
- slowed reaction time
- decreased agility
- decreased vibratory sense in the ankles
- development of muscles tremors, such as in the head and hands.

Look beyond age

Remember, not all neurologic changes in elderly patients are caused by aging. Some drugs can cause them as well. See whether the changes are asymmetric, indicating a pathologic condition, or whether other abnormalities need further investigation.

Asking about past health

Because many chronic diseases can affect the neurologic system, ask the patient about his past health. Inquire about major illnesses, recurrent minor illnesses, accidents or injuries, surgical procedures, and allergies. Don't forget to ask what medications he's taking, because many medications can affect the neurologic system.

Asking about family history

Finally, ask about his family history. Some genetic diseases are degenerative; others cause muscle weakness. For example, the incidence of seizures is higher in patients whose family history shows idiopathic epilepsy, and more than half of patients with migraine headaches have a family history of the disorder.

Assessing the neurologic system

A complete neurologic examination is so long and detailed that you probably won't ever perform one in its entirety. However, if your initial screening examination suggests a neurologic problem, you may want to perform a detailed assessment.

Always examine the patient's neurologic system in an orderly fashion. Begin with the highest levels of neurologic function and work down to the lowest, covering these five areas:

- mental status and speech
- cranial nerve function
- sensory function
- motor function
- reflexes.

Assessing mental status and speech

Your mental status assessment actually begins when you talk to the patient during the health history. How he responds to your questions gives clues to his orientation and memory and guides you during your physical assessment.

Be sure to ask questions that require more than yes or no answers. Otherwise, confusion or disorientation may not be immediately apparent. If you have doubts about a patient's mental status, perform a screening examination. (See *A quick check of mental status.*)

When assessing mental status, be sure to ask more than just yes-or-no questions.

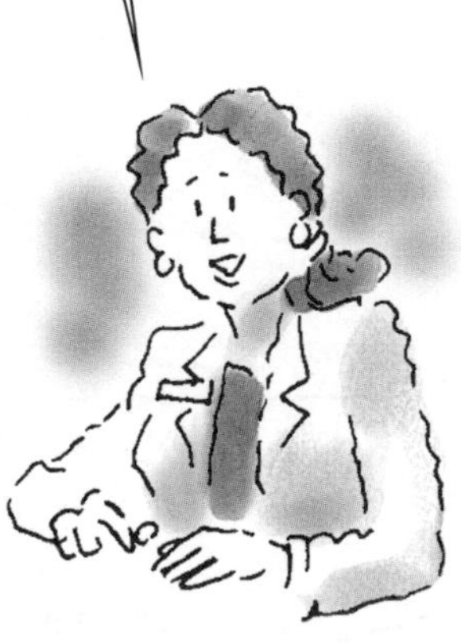

Another guide during the physical assessment is the patient's reason for seeking care. For example, if he complains about confusion or memory problems, you'll want to concentrate on the mental status part of the examination, which consists of checking:

- LOC
- appearance and behavior
- speech

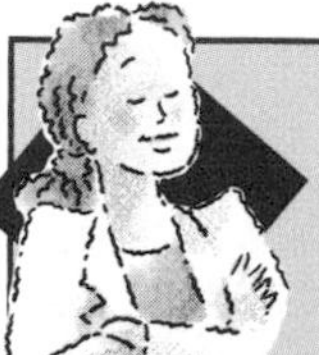

Peak technique

A quick check of mental status

To quickly screen patients for disordered thought processes, ask the questions below. An incorrect answer to any question may indicate the need for a complete mental status examination. Make sure you know the correct answers before asking the questions.

Question	Function screened
What's your name?	Orientation to person
What's your mother's name?	Orientation to other people
What year is it?	Orientation to time
Where are you now?	Orientation to place
How old are you?	Memory
Where were you born?	Remote memory
What did you have for breakfast?	Recent memory
Who's currently the U.S. president?	General knowledge
Can you count backward from 20 to 1?	Attention span and calculation skills

- cognitive function
- constructional ability.

Level of consciousness

A change in the patient's LOC is the earliest and most sensitive indicator that his neurologic status has changed. Many terms are used to describe LOC, but their definitions may differ slightly among practitioners. To avoid confusion, clearly describe the patient's response to various stimuli using these guidelines:

- alert — follows commands and responds completely and appropriately to stimuli
- lethargic — is drowsy; has delayed responses to verbal stimuli; may drift off to sleep during examination
- stuporous — requires vigorous stimulation for a response

- comatose — doesn't respond appropriately to verbal or painful stimuli; can't follow commands or communicate verbally.

Perky or drowsy?

During your assessment, observe the patient's LOC. Is he alert, or is he falling asleep? Can he focus his attention and maintain it, or is he easily distracted? If you need to use a stronger stimulus than your voice, record what it is and how strong it needs to be to get a response from the patient. The Glasgow Coma Scale offers a more objective way to assess the patient's LOC. (See *Glasgow Coma Scale.*)

Appearance and behavior

Also note how the patient behaves, dresses, and grooms himself. Are his appearance and behavior inappropriate? Is his personal hygiene poor? If so, discuss your findings with the family to determine whether this is a change. Even subtle changes in a patient's behavior can signal a new onset of a chronic disease or a more acute change that involves the frontal lobe.

Speech

Next, listen to how well the patient can express himself. Is his speech fluent or fragmented? Note the pace, volume, clarity, and spontaneity of his speech. To assess for dysarthria (difficulty forming words), ask him to repeat the phrase "No ifs, ands, or buts." Assess comprehension by determining his ability to follow instructions and cooperate with your examination.

Cognitive function

Assessing cognitive function involves testing the patient's memory, orientation, attention span, calculation ability, thought content, abstract thinking, judgment, insight, and emotional status.

Telltale testing

To quickly test your patient's orientation, memory, and attention span, use the mental status screening questions previously discussed. Orientation to time is usually disrupted first; orientation to person, last.

Always consider the patient's environment and physical condition when assessing orientation. For example, an elderly patient admitted to the hospital for several days may not be oriented to time, especially if he has been bedridden. Also, when the person is intubated and can't speak, ask questions that require only a nod, such as "Do you know you're in the hospital?" and "Are we in Pennsylvania?"

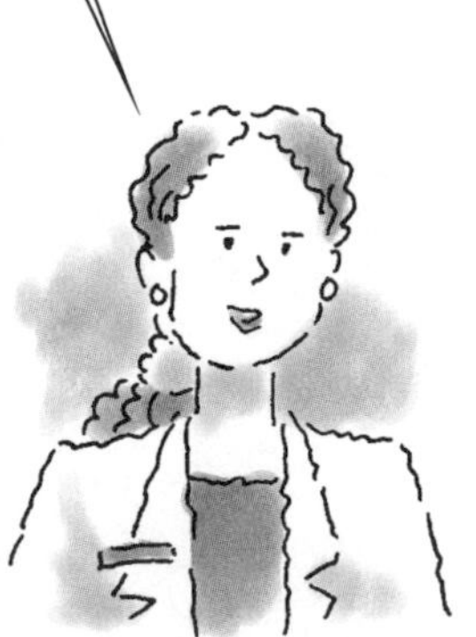

Glasgow Coma Scale

The Glasgow Coma Scale provides an easy way to describe the patient's baseline mental status and to help detect and interpret changes from baseline findings. To use the Glasgow Coma Scale, test the patient's ability to respond to verbal, motor, and sensory stimulation, and grade your findings according to the scale. If a patient is alert, can follow simple commands, and is oriented to person, place, and time, his score will total 15 points. A decreased score in one or more categories may signal an impending neurologic crisis. A total score of 7 or less indicates severe neurologic damage.

Test	Score	Patient's response
Eye-opening response		
Spontaneously	4	Opens eyes spontaneously
To speech	3	Opens eyes when told to
To pain	2	Opens eyes only on painful stimulus
None	1	Doesn't open eyes in response to stimulus
Motor response		
Obeys	6	Shows two fingers when asked
Localizes	5	Reaches toward painful stimulus and tries to remove it
Withdraws	4	Moves away from painful stimulus
Abnormal flexion	3	Assumes a decorticate posture (shown below)
Abnormal extension	2	Assumes a decerebrate posture (shown below)
None	1	No response; just lies flaccid — an ominous sign
Verbal response		
Oriented	5	Tells current date
Confused	4	Tells incorrect year
Inappropriate words	3	Replies randomly with incorrect word
Incomprehensible	2	Moans or screams
None	1	No response
Total score		

The patient with an intact short-term memory can generally repeat five to seven nonconsecutive numbers right away and again 10 minutes later. Remember that short-term memory is commonly affected first in patients with neurologic disease.

When testing attention span and calculation skills, keep in mind that lack of mathematical ability and anxiety can affect the patient's performance. If he has difficulty with numerical computation, ask him to spell the word "world" backward. While he's performing these functions, note his ability to pay attention.

Clear and cogent?

Assess thought content by evaluating the clarity and cohesiveness of the patient's ideas. Is his conversation smooth, with logical transitions between ideas? Does he have hallucinations (sensory perceptions that lack appropriate stimuli) or delusions (beliefs not supported by reality)? Disordered thought patterns may indicate delirium or psychosis.

Extract the abstract

Test the patient's ability to think abstractly by asking him to interpret a common proverb such as "A stitch in time saves nine." A patient with dementia may interpret this proverb literally. If the patient's primary language isn't English, he'll probably have difficulty interpreting the proverb. Engage the assistance of family members when English isn't the patient's primary language. Have them ask the patient to explain a saying in his native language.

What if...?

Test the patient's judgment by asking him how he would respond to a hypothetical situation. For example, what would he do if he were in a public building and the fire alarm sounded? Evaluate the appropriateness of his answer.

Feelings, nothing more than feelings

Throughout the interview, assess the patient's emotional status. Note his mood, his emotional lability or stability, and the appropriateness of his emotional responses. Also, assess his mood by asking how he feels about himself and his future. Keep in mind that symptoms of depression in elderly patients may be atypical—for example, decreased function or increased agitation rather than the usual sad affect.

Constructional ability

Constructional disorders affect the patient's ability to perform simple tasks and use various objects.

Assessing cranial nerve function

There are 12 pairs of cranial nerves. These nerves transmit motor or sensory messages, or both, primarily between the brain and brain stem and the head and neck.

Something smells!

Assess cranial nerve I, the olfactory nerve, first. Make sure the patient's nostrils are patent. Have him identify at least two common substances, such as coffee and cinnamon or cloves. Avoid stringent odors, such as ammonia or peppermint, which stimulate the trigeminal nerve.

Seeing eye to eye

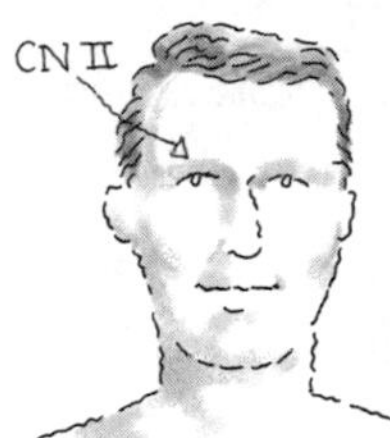

Next, assess cranial nerve II, the optic nerve. To test visual acuity quickly and informally, have the patient read a newspaper, starting with large headlines and moving to small print.

Test visual fields with a technique called *confrontation*. To do this, stand 2′ (0.6 m) in front of the patient, and have him cover one eye. Then close your eye on the side directly facing the patient's closed eye and bring your moving fingers into the patient's visual field from the periphery. Ask him to tell you when he sees the object. Test each quadrant of the patient's visual field, and compare his results with your own. Chart any defects you find. (See *Visual field defects*, page 334.)

Finally, examine the fundus of the optic nerve, as described in chapter 6. Blurring of the optic disc may indicate increased intracranial pressure (ICP).

Three real lookers

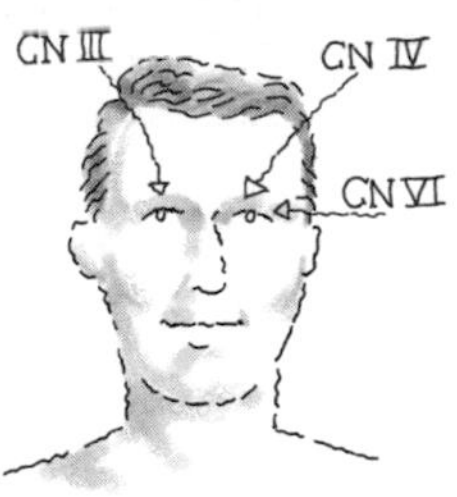

The oculomotor nerve (cranial nerve III), the trochlear nerve (cranial nerve IV), and the abducent nerve (cranial nerve VI) all control eye movement. So assess these nerves together.

The oculomotor nerve controls most extraocular movement; it's also responsible for elevation of the eyelid and pupillary constriction. Abnormalities include ptosis, or drooping of the upper lid, and pupil inequality. Make sure that the patient's pupils constrict when exposed to light and that his eyes accommodate for seeing objects at various distances.

To assess the oculomotor nerve, trochlear nerve (responsible for down and in eye movement), and abducent nerve (responsible for lateral eye movement), ask the patient to follow your finger through the six cardinal positions of gaze: left superior, left lateral, left inferior, right superior, right lateral, and right inferior. Pause slightly before moving from one position to the next; this helps to assess the patient for involuntary eye movement (or nystagmus) and the ability to hold the gaze in that particular position.

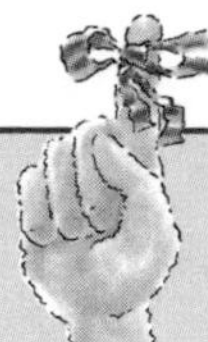

Memory jogger

Cranial nerves I, II, and VIII have sensory functions. Cranial nerves III, IV, VI, XI, and XII have motor functions. Cranial nerves V, VII, IX, and X have sensory and motor functions. How will you ever remember which does what?

Use the following mnemonic to help you remember which cranial nerves have sensory functions (S), motor functions (M), or both (B). The mnemonic begins with cranial nerve I and ends with cranial nerve XII.

I: Some
II: Say
III: Marry
IV: Money
V: But
VI: My
VII: Brother
VIII: Says
IX: Bad
X: Business
XI: Marries
XII: Money

"Tri" chewing without this nerve

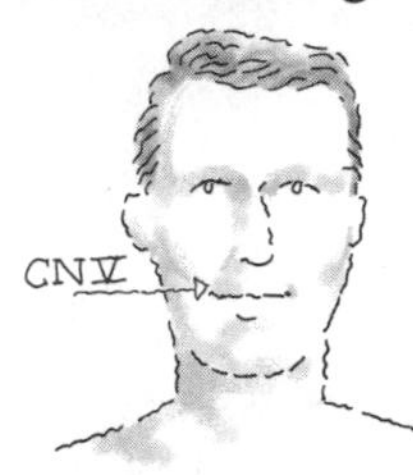

The trigeminal nerve (cranial nerve V) is both a sensory and a motor nerve. It supplies sensation to the corneas, nasal and oral mucosa, and facial skin and also supplies motor function for the jaw and all chewing muscles.

To assess the sensory component, check the patient's ability to feel light touch on his face. Ask him to close his eyes; then touch him with a wisp of cotton on his forehead, cheek, and jaw on each side. Next, test pain perception by touching the tip of a safety pin to the same three areas. Ask the patient to describe and compare both sensations.

Alternate the touches between sharp and dull to test the patient's reliability in comparing sensations. Proper assessment of the nerve requires that the patient identify sharp stimuli. To test the motor component of cranial nerve V, ask the patient to clench his teeth while you palpate the temporal and masseter muscles.

Taking a taste test

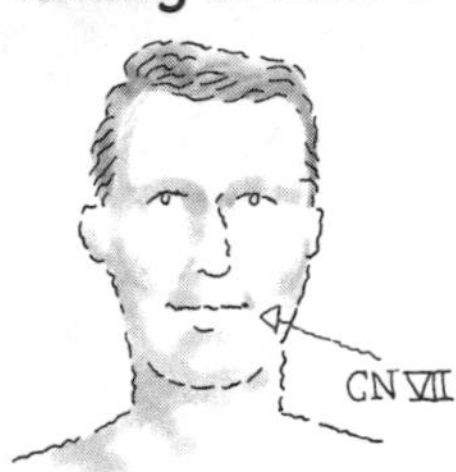

The facial nerve (cranial nerve VII) also has a sensory and motor component. The sensory component controls taste perception on the anterior part of the tongue. You can assess taste by placing items with various tastes on the anterior portion of the patient's tongue—for example, sugar (sweet), salt, lemon juice (sour), and quinine (bitter). Simply have the patient wash away each taste with a sip of water.

The motor component is responsible for the facial muscles. Assess it by observing the patient's face for symmetry at rest and while he smiles, frowns, and raises his eyebrows.

If a weakness caused by a stroke or other condition damages the cortex, the patient will be able to raise his eyebrows and wrinkle his forehead. If the weakness is due to an interruption of the facial nerve or other peripheral nerve involvement, the entire side of the face will be immobile.

Let's hear it for the acoustic nerve!

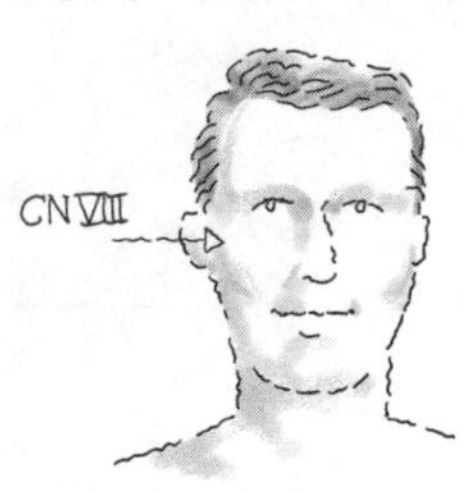

The acoustic nerve (cranial nerve VIII) is responsible for hearing and equilibrium. The cochlear division controls hearing, and the vestibular division controls balance.

To test hearing, ask the patient to cover one ear, and then stand on his opposite side and whisper a few words. See whether he can repeat what you said. Test the other ear the same way.

To test the vestibular portion of this nerve, observe the patient for nystagmus and disturbed balance, and note reports of dizziness or the room spinning.

Visual field defects

Here are some examples of visual field defects. The black areas represent visual loss.

Left	Right
A: Blindness of right eye	
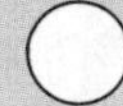	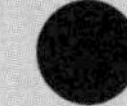
B: Bitemporal hemianopsia, or loss of half the visual field	
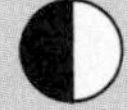	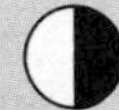
C: Left homonymous hemianopsia	
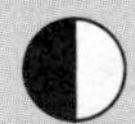	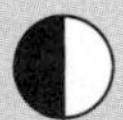
D: Left homonymous hemianopsia, superior quadrant	
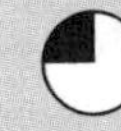	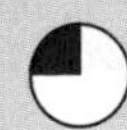

Not so hard to swallow

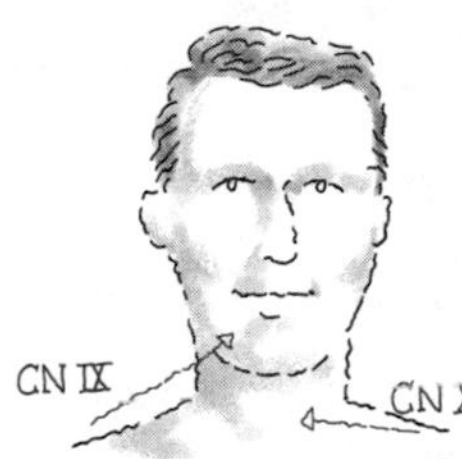

The glossopharyngeal nerve (cranial nerve IX) and the vagus nerve (cranial nerve X) are tested together because their innervation overlaps in the pharynx. The glossopharyngeal nerve is responsible for swallowing, salivation, and taste perception on the posterior one-third of the tongue. The vagus nerve controls swallowing and is also responsible for voice quality.

Start your assessment by listening to the patient's voice. Then check his gag reflex by touching the tip of a tongue blade against his posterior pharynx and asking him to open wide and say "ah." Watch for the symmetrical upward movement of the soft palate and uvula and for the midline position of the uvula.

A very important accessory

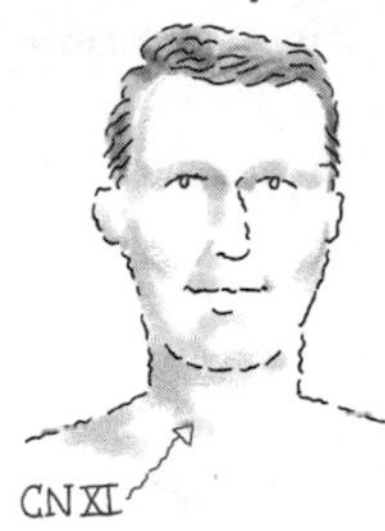

The spinal accessory nerve (cranial nerve XI) is a motor nerve that controls the sternocleidomastoid muscles and the upper portion of the trapezius muscle. To assess this nerve, test the strength of both muscles. First, place your palm against the patient's cheek; then ask him to turn his head against your resistance.

Test the trapezius muscle by placing your hands on the patient's shoulder and asking him to shrug his shoulders against your resistance. Repeat each test on the other side, comparing muscle strength.

Speaking about the tongue

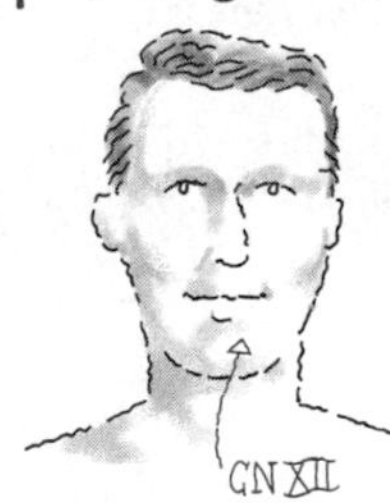

The hypoglossal nerve (cranial nerve XII) controls tongue movement involved in swallowing and speech. The tongue should be midline, without tremors or fasciculations. Test tongue strength by asking the patient to push his tongue against his cheek as you apply resistance. Observe his tongue for symmetry.

Assessing sensory function

Sensory system evaluation involves checking five areas of sensation:

- pain
- light touch
- vibration
- position
- discrimination.

This may hurt a bit

To test the patient for pain sensation, have him close his eyes; then touch all the major dermatomes, first with the sharp end of a safety pin and then with the dull end. Proceed in this order: fingers, shoulders, toes, thighs, and trunk. Ask him to identify when he feels the sharp stimulus.

If the patient has major deficits, start in the area with the least sensation, and move toward the area with the most sensation to help you determine the level of deficit.

Getting in touch

To test for the sense of light touch, follow the same routine as above but use a wisp of cotton. Lightly touch the patient's skin—don't swab or sweep the cotton, because you might miss an area of loss. A patient with a peripheral neuropathy might retain his sensation for light touch after he has lost pain sensation.

Good vibrations

To test vibratory sense, apply a tuning fork over certain bony prominences while the patient keeps his eyes closed. Start at the distal interphalangeal joint of the index finger and move proximally. Test only until the patient feels the vibration, because everything above that level will be intact. (See *Evaluating vibratory sense.*) If vibratory sense is intact, you won't have to check position sense because the same pathway carries both.

Fingers and toes on the move

To assess position sense, have the patient close his eyes. Then grasp the sides of his big toe, move the toe up and down, and ask him what position it's in. To be tested for position sense, the patient needs intact vestibular and cerebellar function. To perform the same test on the patient's upper extremities, grasp the sides of his index finger and move it back and forth.

Rate ability to discriminate

Discrimination testing assesses the ability of the cerebral cortex to interpret and integrate information. *Stereognosis* is the ability to discriminate the shape, size, weight, texture, and form of an object by touching and manipulating it. To test this, ask the patient to close his eyes and open his hand. Then place a common object, such as a key, in his hand and ask him to identify it.

If he can't identify the object, test graphesthesia next. Have the patient keep his eyes closed and hold out his hand while you draw a large number on the palm. Ask him to identify the number. Both of these tests assess the ability of the cortex to integrate sensory input.

To test point localization, have the patient close his eyes; then touch one of his limbs, and ask him where you touched him. Test two-point discrimination by touching the patient simultaneously in two contralateral areas. He should be able to identify both

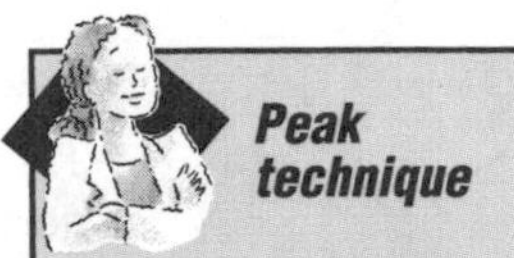

Evaluating vibratory sense

To evaluate vibratory sense, apply the base of a vibrating tuning fork to the interphalangeal joint of the patient's great toe, as shown below.

Ask him what he feels. If he feels the sensation, he'll typically report a feeling of buzzing or vibration. If he doesn't feel the sensation at the toe, try the medial malleolus. Then continue moving proximally until he feels the sensation. Note where he feels it, and then repeat the process on the other leg.

touches. Failure to perceive touch on one side is called *extinction.*

Assessing motor function

Assessing the motor system includes inspecting the muscles and testing muscle tone and muscle strength. Cerebellar testing is also done because the cerebellum plays a role in smooth-muscle movements, such as tics, tremors, or fasciculation.

Muscle tone

Muscle tone represents muscular resistance to passive stretching. To test arm muscle tone, move the patient's shoulder through passive range-of-motion (ROM) exercises. You should feel a slight resistance. Then let the arm drop to the patient's side. It should fall easily.

To test leg muscle tone, guide the hip through passive ROM exercises; then let the leg fall to the bed. The leg shouldn't fall into an externally rotated position; this is an abnormal finding.

Muscle strength

To perform a general examination of muscle strength, observe the patient's gait and motor activities. To evaluate muscle strength, ask the patient to move major muscles and muscle groups against resistance. For instance, to test shoulder girdle strength, have him extend his arms with his palms up and maintain this position for 30 seconds.

If he can't maintain this position, test further by pushing down on his outstretched arms. If he does lift both arms equally, look for pronation of the hand and downward drift of the arm on the weaker side.

Cerebellum

Cerebellar testing looks at the patient's coordination and general balance. Can he sit and stand without support? If so, observe him as he walks across the room, turns, and walks back. Note imbalances or abnormalities.

With cerebellar dysfunction, the patient will have a wide-based, unsteady gait. Deviation to one side may indicate a cerebellar lesion on that side. Ask the patient to walk heel to toe, and observe his balance. Then perform Romberg's test. (See *Romberg's test.*)

Romberg's test

Observe the patient's balance as he stands with his eyes open, feet together, and arms at his sides. Then ask him to close his eyes. Hold your arms out on either side of him to protect him if he sways. If he falls to one side, the result of Romberg's test is positive.

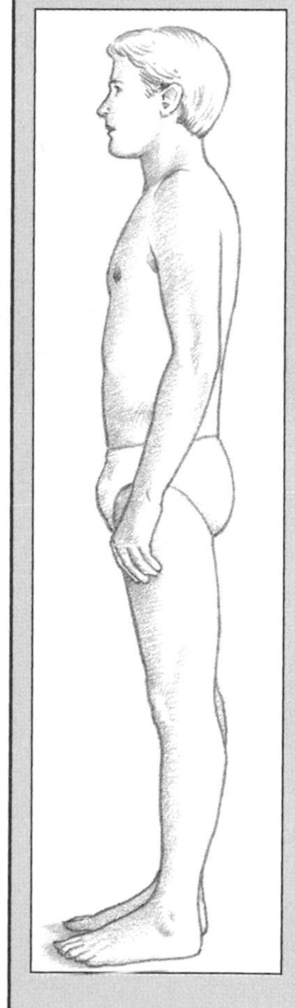

Nose-to-finger test

Test extremity coordination by asking the patient to touch his nose and then touch your outstretched finger as you move it. Have him do this faster and faster. His movements should be accurate and smooth.

Quick, do these tests!

Other tests of cerebellar function assess rapid alternating movements. In these tests, the patient's movements should be accurate and smooth.

First, ask the patient to touch the thumb of his right hand to his right index finger and then to each of his remaining fingers. Observe the movements for accuracy and smoothness. Next, ask him to sit with his palms on his thighs. Tell him to turn his palms up and down, gradually increasing his speed.

Sole tapping

Finally, have the patient lie in a supine position. Then stand at the foot of the table or bed and hold your palms near the soles of his feet. Ask him to alternately tap the sole of his right foot and the sole of his left foot against your palms. He should increase his speed as you observe his coordination.

Assessing reflexes

Evaluating reflexes involves testing deep tendon and superficial reflexes and observing for primitive reflexes.

Deep tendon reflexes

The key to testing deep tendon reflexes is to make sure the patient is relaxed and the joint is flexed appropriately. First, distract the patient by asking him to focus on a point across the room. Always test deep tendon reflexes by moving from head to toe and comparing side to side. (See *Assessing deep tendon reflexes*.)

Grade deep tendon reflexes using the following scale:

- 0 — absent impulses
- +1 — diminished impulses
- +2 — normal impulses
- +3 — increased impulses (may be normal)
- +4 — hyperactive impulses.

I'm supposed to assess your deep tendon reflexes.
You may find this hard to believe, but I used to have great tendons.

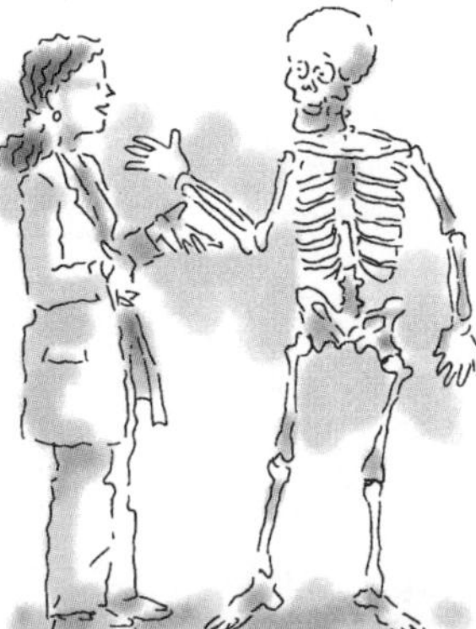

Superficial reflexes

Stimulating the skin or mucous membranes is a method of testing superficial reflexes. Because these are cutaneous reflexes, the

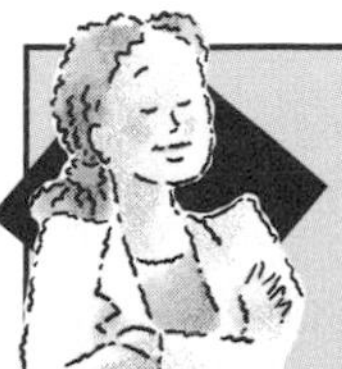

Peak technique

Assessing deep tendon reflexes

During a neurologic examination, you'll assess the patient's deep tendon reflexes. Test the biceps, triceps, brachioradialis, patellar or quadriceps, and Achilles reflexes.

Biceps reflex

Position the patient's arm so his elbow is flexed at a 45-degree angle and his arm is relaxed. Place your thumb or index finger over the biceps tendon and your remaining fingers loosely over the triceps muscle. Strike your finger with the pointed end of the reflex hammer, and watch and feel for the contraction of the biceps muscle and flexion of the forearm.

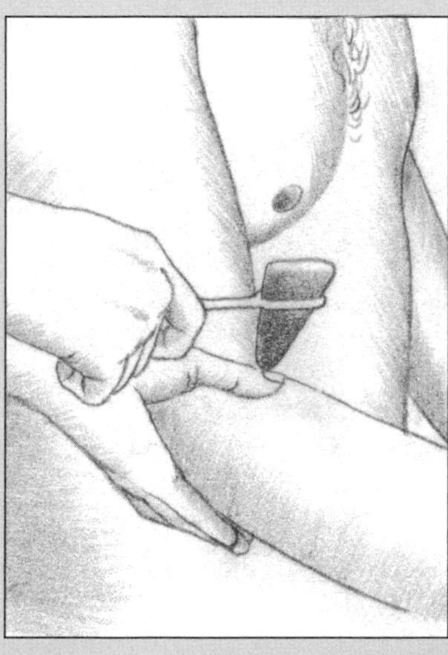

Triceps reflex

Have the patient adduct his arm and place his forearm across his chest. Strike the triceps tendon about 2" (5 cm) above the olecranon process on the extensor surface of the upper arm. Watch for contraction of the triceps muscle and extension of the forearm.

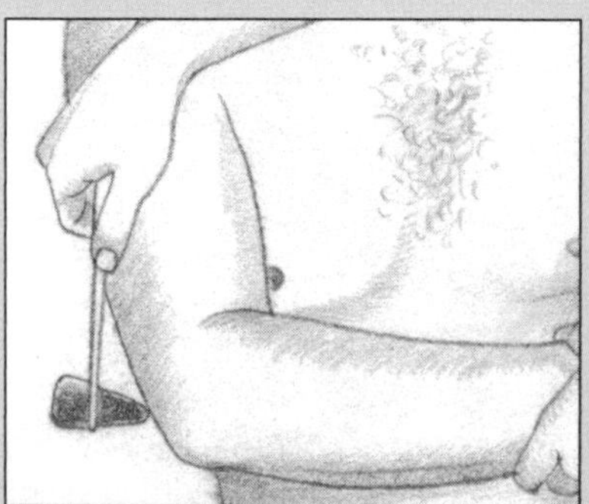

Brachioradialis reflex

Ask the patient to rest the ulnar surface of his hand on his abdomen or lap with the elbow partially flexed. Strike the radius, and watch for supination of the hand and flexion of the forearm at the elbow.

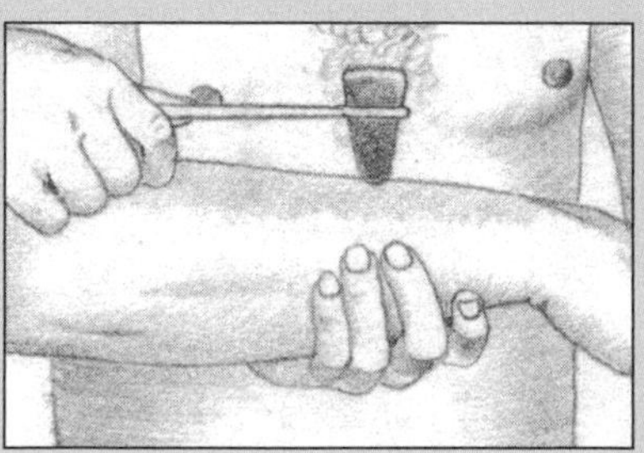

Patellar reflex

Have the patient sit with his legs dangling freely. If he can't sit up, flex his knee at a 45-degree angle and place your nondominant hand behind it for support. Strike the patellar tendon just below the patella, and look for contraction of the quadriceps muscle in the thigh with extension of the leg.

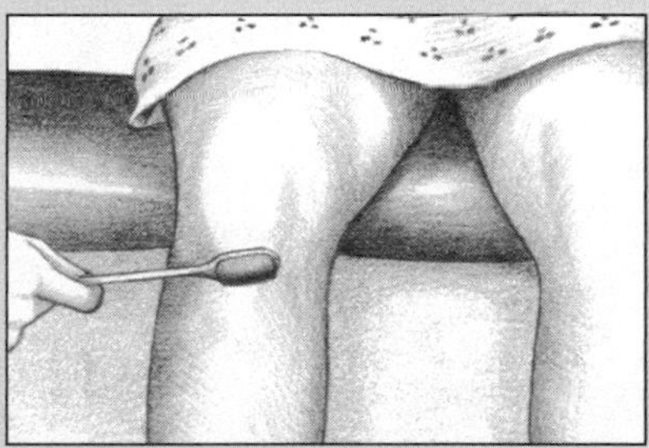

Achilles reflex

Have the patient flex his foot. Then support the plantar surface. Strike the Achilles tendon, and watch for plantar flexion of the foot at the ankle.

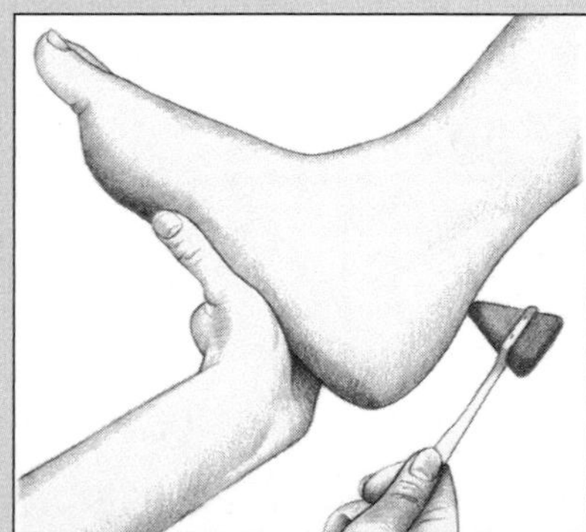

more you try to elicit them in succession, the less of a response you'll get. So observe carefully the first time you stimulate.

Tickling the feet

Using an applicator stick, tongue blade, or key, slowly stroke the lateral side of the patient's sole from the heel to the great toe. The normal response in an adult is plantar flexion of the toes. Upward movement of the great toe and fanning of the little toes — called *Babinski's reflex* — is abnormal. (See *Babinski's reflex in infants*.)

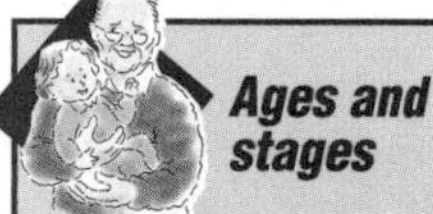

Babinski's reflex in infants

The Babinski reflex can be elicited in some normal infants — sometimes until age 2 years. However, plantar flexion of the toes is seen in more than 90% of normal infants.

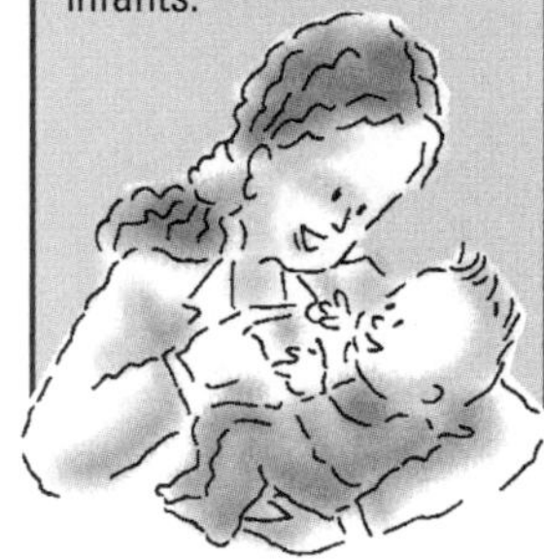

For men only

The cremasteric reflex is tested in men by using an applicator stick to stimulate the inner thigh. Normal reaction is contraction of the cremaster muscle and elevation of the testicle on the side of the stimulus.

Tickling the tummy

Test the abdominal reflexes with the patient in the supine position with his arms at his sides and his knees slightly flexed. Briskly stroke both sides of the abdomen above and below the umbilicus, moving from the periphery toward the midline. Movement of the umbilicus toward the stimulus is normal.

Primitive reflexes

Primitive reflexes are abnormal in an adult but normal in an infant, whose CNS is immature. As the neurologic system matures, these reflexes disappear. The primitive reflexes you'll assess for are the grasp, snout, sucking, and glabella reflexes.

Just gotta grasp

Assess the grasp reflex by applying gentle pressure to the patient's palm with your fingers. If he grasps your fingers between his index finger and thumb, suspect cortical or premotor cortex damage.

Read my lip

The snout reflex is assessed by lightly tapping on the patient's upper lip. Pursing of the lip is a positive snout reflex that indicates frontal lobe damage.

The urge to suck

Observe the patient while you're feeding him or if he has an oral airway or endotracheal tube in place. If you see a sucking motion, this indicates cortical damage. This reflex is commonly seen in patients with advanced dementia.

Tap, tap, blink, blink

The glabella response is elicited by repeatedly tapping the bridge of the patient's nose. The abnormal response is persistent blinking, which indicates diffuse cortical dysfunction.

Abnormal findings

During your assessment, you may detect abnormalities caused by neurologic dysfunction. The most common categories of abnormalities include altered LOC, cranial nerve impairment, abnormal muscle movements, and abnormal gaits. (See *Abnormal neurologic findings*.)

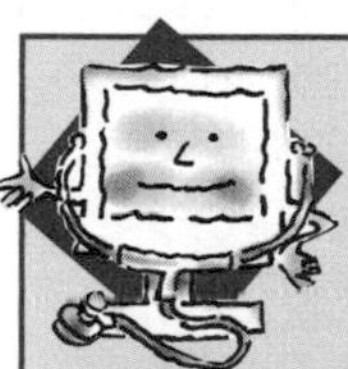

Interpretation station

Abnormal neurologic findings

Your assessment will reveal a group of findings that may lead you to suspect a particular disorder. The chart below shows common groups of findings for the neurologic system along with signs and symptoms and their probable causes.

Sign or symptom and findings	Probable cause
Aphasia	
• Wernicke's, Broca's, or global aphasia • Decreased level of consciousness (LOC) • Right-sided hemiparesis • Homonymous hemianopsia • Paresthesia and loss of sensation	Stroke
• Any type of aphasia occurring suddenly (may be transient or permanent) • Blurred or double vision • Headache • Cerebrospinal otorrhea and rhinorrhea • Disorientation • Behavioral changes • Signs of increased intracranial pressure	Head trauma
Aphasia *(continued)*	
• Any type of aphasia occurring suddenly and resolving within 24 hours • Transient hemiparesis • Hemianopsia • Paresthesia • Dizziness and confusion	Transient ischemic attack
Decreased LOC	
• Slowly decreasing LOC, from lethargy to coma • Apathy, behavior changes • Memory loss • Decreased attention span • Morning headache • Sensorimotor disturbances	Brain tumor

(continued)

Abnormal neurologic findings *(continued)*

Sign or symptom and findings	Probable cause
Decreased LOC *(continued)*	
• Slowly decreasing LOC, from lethargy to possible coma • Malaise • Tachycardia • Tachypnea • Orthostatic hypotension • Hot, flushed, and diaphoretic skin	Heatstroke
• Lethargy progressing to coma • Confusion, anxiety, and restlessness • Hypotension • Tachycardia • Weak pulse with narrowing pulse pressure • Dyspnea • Oliguria • Cool, clammy skin	Shock
Tremors	
• Tremors in fingers, progressing to feet, eyelids, jaws, lips, and tongue • Characteristic pill-rolling tremor • Lead-pipe rigidity • Bradykinesia • Propulsive gait with forward-leaning posture • Masklike face • Drooling	Parkinson's disease
• Intention tremor that waxes and wanes • Visual and sensory impairments • Muscle weakness, paralysis, or spasticity • Hyperreflexia • Ataxic gait • Dysphagia • Dysarthria	Multiple sclerosis

Sign or symptom and findings	Probable cause
Tremors *(continued)*	
• Intention tremor • Ataxia • Nystagmus • Muscle weakness and atrophy • Hypoactive or absent deep tendon reflexes	Cerebellar tumor
Apraxia	
• Gradual and irreversible apraxia • Amnesia • Anomia • Decreased attention span • Apathy • Aphasia	Alzheimer's disease
• Progressive apraxia • Decreased mental activity • Headache • Dizziness • Seizures • Pupillary changes	Brain tumor
• Sudden onset of apraxia • Headache • Confusion • Aphasia • Agnosia • Stupor or coma • Hemiplegia • Visual field defects	Stroke

Altered level of consciousness

Consciousness may be impaired by any one of several disorders that can affect the cerebral hemisphere of the brain stem. Consciousness is the most sensitive indicator of neurologic dysfunction and may be a valuable adjunct to other findings. When assessing LOC, make sure that you provide a stimulus that's strong enough to get a true picture of the patient's baseline. (See *Detecting increased ICP.*)

Consciousness-altering disorders

Disorders that affect LOC include toxic encephalopathy, hemorrhage, and extensive, generalized cortical atrophy. Compression of brain-stem structures by tumor or hemorrhage can also affect consciousness by depressing the reticular activating system that

Detecting increased ICP

The earlier you can recognize the signs of increased intracranial pressure (ICP), the more quickly you can intervene and better the patient's chance of recovery. By the time late signs appear, interventions may be useless.

	Early signs	Late signs
Level of consciousness	• Requires increased stimulation • Subtle orientation loss • Restlessness and anxiety • Sudden quietness	Unarousable
Pupils	• Pupil changes on side of lesion • One pupil constricts but then dilates (unilateral hippus) • Sluggish reaction of both pupils • Unequal pupils	Pupils fixed and dilated or "blown"
Motor response	• Sudden weakness • Motor changes on side opposite the lesion • Positive pronator drift; with palms up, one hand pronates	Profound weakness
Vital signs	• Intermittent increases in blood pressure	Increased systolic pressure, profound bradycardia, abnormal respirations (Cushing's syndrome)

maintains wakefulness. In addition, sedatives and opioids can depress LOC.

Compression of brain-stem structures can affect consciousness. Oof. That doesn't sound good.

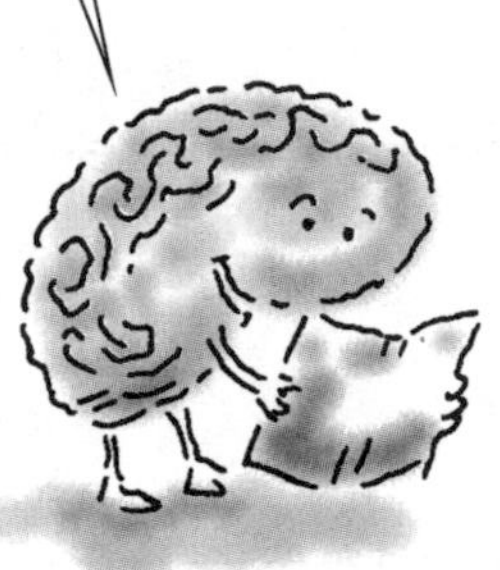

Cranial nerve impairment

Damage to the cranial nerves causes many abnormalities, including olfactory, visual, auditory, and muscle problems. Vertigo and dysphagia can also indicate cranial nerve damage.

Olfactory impairment

If the patient can't detect odors with both nostrils, he may have a dysfunction in cranial nerve I. This dysfunction can result from any disease that affects the olfactory tract, such as a tumor, hemorrhage or, more commonly, a facial bone fracture that crosses the cribriform plate (portion of the ethmoid bone that separates the roof of the nose from the cranial cavity).

Visual impairment

Visual problems include visual field defects, pupillary changes, eye muscle impairment, and facial nerve impairment.

Far afield

Visual fields are affected by tumors or infarcts of the optic nerve head, optic chiasm, or optic tracts.

Peer at the pupils

If the patient's pupillary response to light is affected, he may have damage to the optic nerve and oculomotor nerve. Pupils are also sensitive indicators of neurologic dysfunction. Increased ICP causes dilation of the pupil ipsilateral to the mass lesion; without treatment, both pupils become fixed and dilated. (See *Understanding pupillary changes*.) Unequal pupils, or *anisocoria*, is normal in about 20% of people. In normal anisocoria, pupil size doesn't change with the amount of illumination.

Don't move a muscle!

Weakness or paralysis of the eye muscles can result from cranial nerve damage. Increased ICP and intracranial lesions can affect the motor nuclei of the oculomotor, trochlear, and abducent nerves.

The drifters

Damage to the peripheral labyrinth, brain stem, or cerebellum can cause nystagmus. The eyes drift slowly in one direction and then jerk back to the other.

Understanding pupillary changes

Use this chart as a guide to pupillary changes.

Pupillary change	Possible causes
Unilateral, dilated (4 mm), fixed, and nonreactive 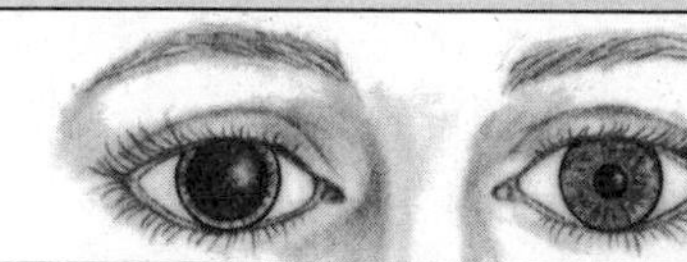	• Uncal herniation with oculomotor nerve damage • Brain stem compression • Increased intracranial pressure • Tentorial herniation • Head trauma with subdural or epidural hematoma • Normal in some people
Bilateral, dilated (4 mm), fixed, and nonreactive 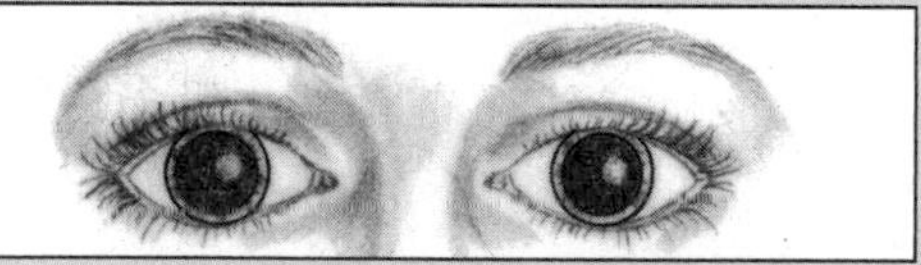	• Severe midbrain damage • Cardiopulmonary arrest (hypoxia) • Anticholinergic poisoning
Bilateral, midsize (2 mm), fixed, and nonreactive 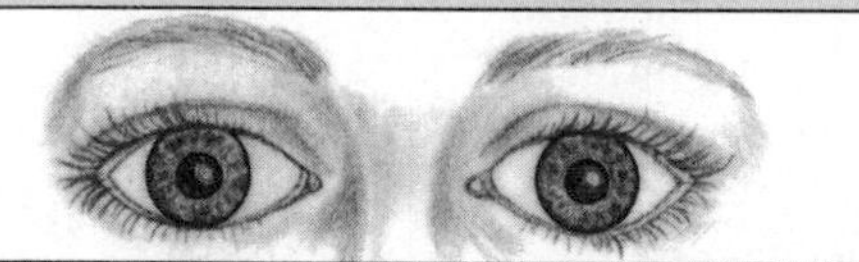	• Midbrain involvement caused by edema, hemorrhage, infarctions, lacerations, contusions
Bilateral, pinpoint (<1 mm), and usually nonreactive 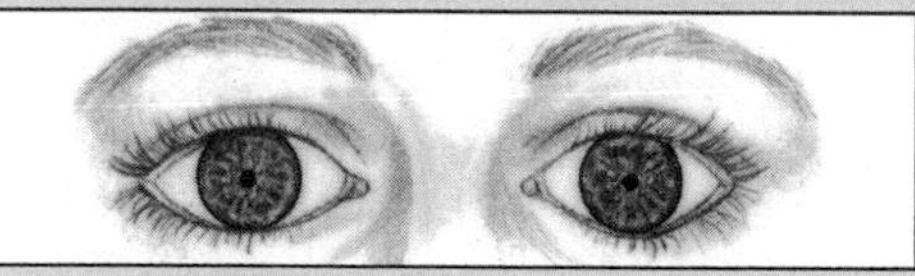	• Lesions of pons, usually after hemorrhage
Unilateral, small (1.5 mm), and nonreactive 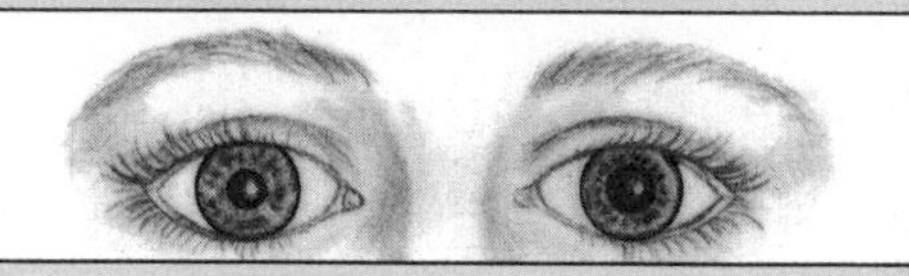	• Disruption of sympathetic nerve supply to the head caused by spinal cord lesion above the first thoracic vertebrae

Feeling droopy

Drooping of the eyelid, or *ptosis*, can result from a defect in the oculomotor nerve. To assess ptosis more accurately, have the patient sit upright.

Facing the pain

If the patient responds inadequately to sensory stimulation of the skin or eye, the trigeminal nerve may be affected. Trigeminal neuralgia causes severe piercing or stabbing pain over one or more of the facial dermatomes.

Auditory impairment

Sensorial hearing loss can result from lesions of the cochlear branch of the acoustic nerve or from lesions in any part of the nerve's pathway to the brain stem. A patient with this type of hearing loss may have trouble hearing high-pitched sounds, or he may have a total loss of hearing in the affected ear.

Which end is up?

Vertigo is the illusion of movement and can result from a disturbance of the vestibular centers. If it's caused by a peripheral lesion, vertigo and nystagmus will occur 10 to 20 seconds after the patient changes position, and symptoms will gradually lessen with the repetition of the position change. If the vertigo is of central origin, there's no latent period, and the symptoms won't diminish with repetition.

Dysphagia (difficulty swallowing) commonly occurs after stroke but can also result from a mass lesion affecting cranial nerves IX and X.

Speech impairment

Aphasia is a speech disorder caused by injury to the cerebral cortex. Several types of aphasia exist, including:

- *expressive or Broca's aphasia* — impaired fluency and difficulty finding words; impairment located in the frontal lobe, the anterior speech area
- *receptive or Wernicke's aphasia* — inability to understand written words or speech and the use of made-up words; impairment located in the posterior speech cortex, which involves the temporal and parietal lobes
- *global aphasia* — lack of both expressive and receptive language; impairment of both speech areas.

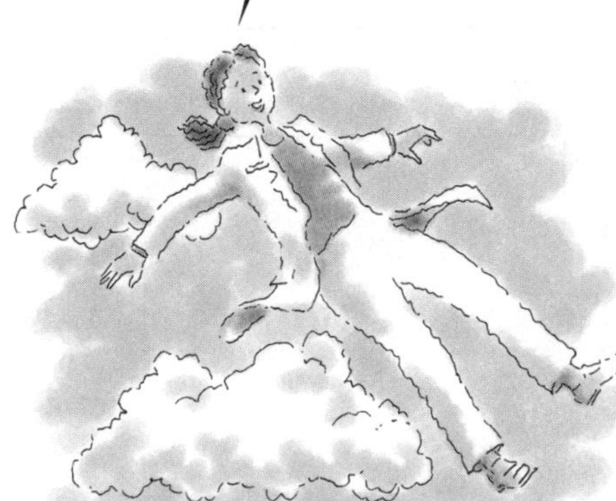

Constructional impairment

Apraxia and agnosia are two types of constructional disorders.

What's the purpose of this?

Apraxia is the inability to perform purposeful movements and make proper use of objects. It's commonly associated with parietal lobe dysfunction and can appear in four types:
- *ideomotor apraxia* — inability to understand the effect of motor activity; ability to perform simple activities but without awareness of performing them; inability to perform actions on command
- *ideational apraxia* — awareness of actions that should be done but inability to perform them
- *constructional apraxia* — inability to copy a design such as the face of a clock
- *dressing apraxia* — inability to understand the meaning of various articles of clothing or the sequence of actions required to get dressed.

What did you say this was?

Agnosia is the inability to identify common objects. It may indicate a lesion in the sensory cortex. Types of agnosia include:
- *visual* — inability to identify common objects without touching
- *auditory* — inability to identify common sounds
- *body image* — inability to identify body parts by sight or touch; inability to localize a stimulus; denial of existence of half the body.

Abnormal muscle movements

Neurologic disorders can cause a wide range of abnormal muscle movements from facial tics to motor restlessness. Findings may or may not indicate serious neurologic disease.

It's a tic...

Sudden, uncontrolled movements of the face, shoulders, and extremities, called *tics*, are caused by abnormal neural stimuli. Tics are normal movements that appear repetitively and inappropriately. They include blinking, shoulder shrugging, and facial twitching.

...no, a tremor...

Like tics, tremors are involuntary, repetitive movements usually seen in the fingers, wrist, eyelids, tongue, and legs. They can occur when the affected body part is at rest or with voluntary movement. For example, the patient with Parkinson's disease has a characteristic pill-rolling resting tremor, and the patient with cerebellar disease has an intention tremor as he reaches for an object.

...no, a fasciculation!

Fasciculations, which are fine twitchings in small muscle groups, are most commonly associated with lower motor neuron dysfunction.

Abnormal gaits

During your assessment, you may identify gait abnormalities. These abnormalities may result from disorders of the cerebellum, posterior columns, corticospinal tract, basal ganglia, and lower motor neurons. (See *Identifying gait abnormalities.*)

Spastic gait

Spastic gait — sometimes referred to as *paretic* or *weak gait*—is a stiff, foot-dragging walk caused by unilateral leg muscle hypertonicity. The leg doesn't swing normally at the hip or knee, so the

Identifying gait abnormalities

The illustrations below identify five gait abnormalities.

Spastic gait

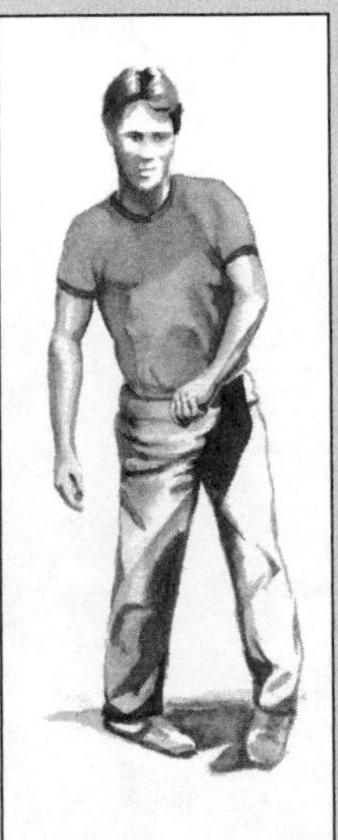

Scissors gait

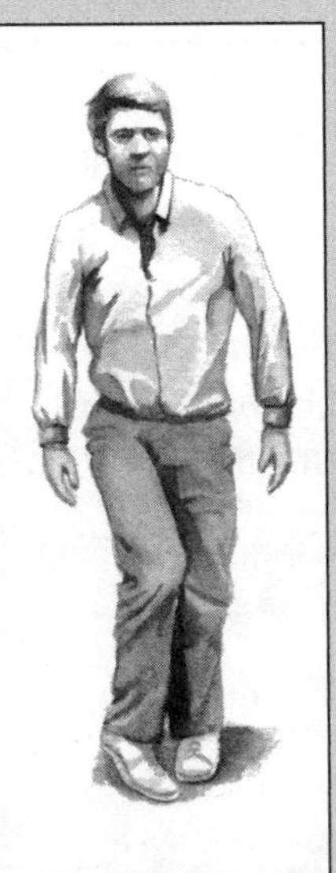

Propulsive gait

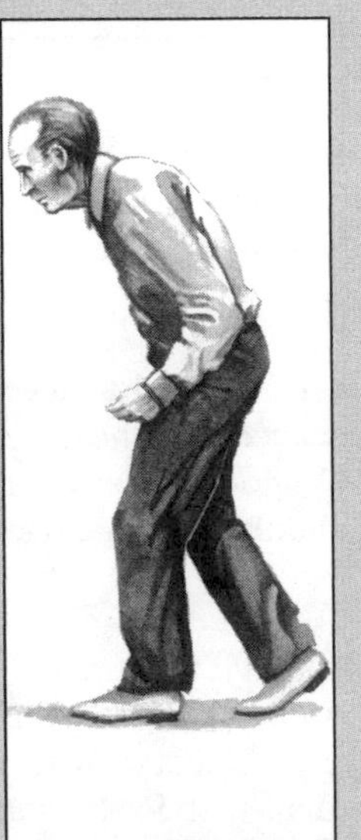

Steppage gait

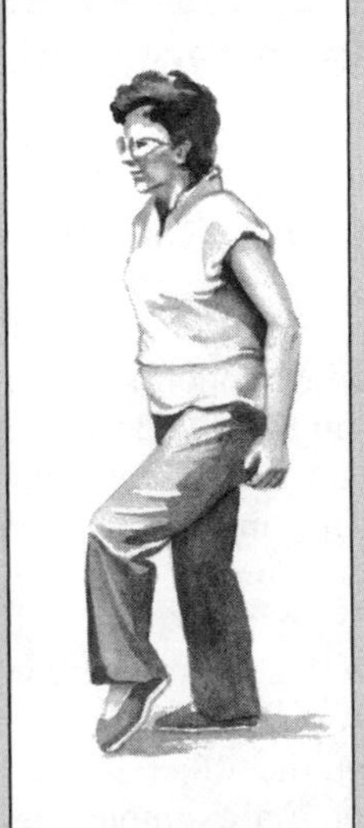

Waddling gait

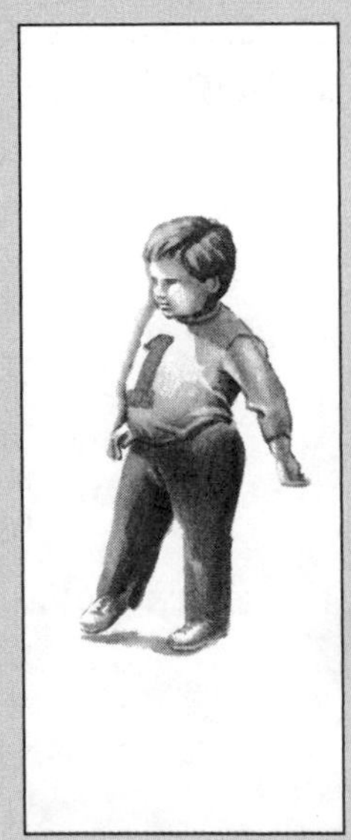

patient's foot tends to drag or shuffle, scraping his toes on the ground. This gait indicates focal damage to the corticospinal tract and is usually permanent once it develops.

Scissors gait

Resulting from bilateral spastic paresis, scissors gait affects both legs but has little or no effect on the arms. The patient's legs flex slightly at the hips and knees, so he looks as if he's crouching. With each step, his thighs adduct and his knees hit or cross in a scissorslike movement.

Propulsive gait

Propulsive gait is characterized by a stooped, rigid posture — the patient's head and neck are bent forward; his flexed, stiffened arms are held away from the body; his fingers are extended; and his knees and hips are stiffly bent. Propulsive gait is a cardinal sign of advanced Parkinson's disease.

Steppage gait

Steppage gait typically results from footdrop caused by weakness or paralysis of pretibial and peroneal muscles, usually from lower motor neuron lesions. Footdrop causes the foot to hang with the toes pointing down, causing the toes to scrape the ground during ambulation. To compensate, the hip rotates outward and the hip and knee flex in an exaggerated fashion to lift the advancing leg off the ground. The foot is thrown forward and the toes hit the ground first, producing an audible slap.

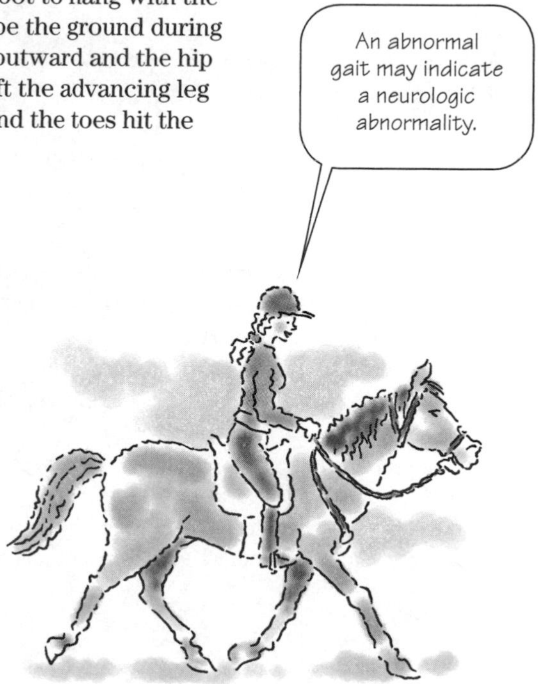

An abnormal gait may indicate a neurologic abnormality.

Waddling gait

Waddling gait, a distinctive ducklike walk, is an important sign of muscular dystrophy, spinal muscle atrophy or, rarely, developmental dysplasia of the hip. It may be present when the child begins to walk or may appear only later in life. The gait results from deterioration of the pelvic girdle muscles.

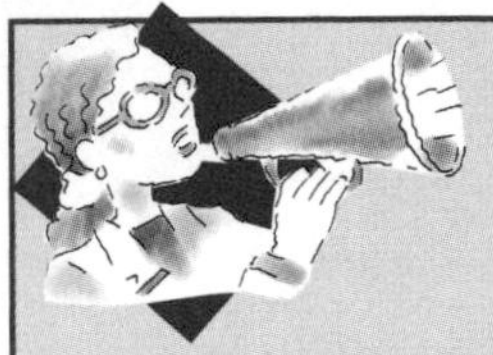

That's a wrap!

Neurologic system review

Central nervous system

Brain

- Cerebrum (cerebral cortex): enables thinking and reasoning
- Brainstem: acts as a major sensory and motor pathway for impulses to and from the cerebral cortex; regulates automatic body functions, such as heart rate and breathing
- Cerebellum: facilitates coordinated muscle movement and maintains equilibrium

Spinal cord

- Acts as the primary pathway for messages traveling between the peripheral areas of the body and the brain
- Mediates the reflex arc

Peripheral nervous system

- Peripheral nerves: serve the skin, muscles, sensory organs, and viscera
- Cranial nerves: serve the brain, head, and neck

Autonomic nervous system

- Regulates the activities of the visceral organs
- Affects smooth and cardiac muscles and glands
- Consists of the sympathetic division (controls fight-or-flight reactions) and parasympathetic division (maintains baseline body functions)

The health history

- Determine the patient's reason for seeking care, which may include headache, dizziness, faintness, confusion, impaired mental status, or balance or gait disturbances.
- Ask the patient about his current health, including his memory and ability to concentrate as well as his current medications.
- Ask him about his past health, including illnesses, accidents or injuries, surgeries, and allergies.
- Inquire about a family history of neurologic disorders that may have a genetic component, such as seizures and migraine headaches.

Assessment of mental status and speech

- Observe for any changes in LOC.
- Note the patient's appearance and behavior.
- Listen to how well the patient speaks and expresses himself.
- Assess cognitive function by testing memory, orientation, attention span, calculation ability, thought content, abstract thinking, judgment, insight, and emotional status.
- Observe the patient's constructional ability (ability to perform simple tasks and use various objects).

Assessment of cranial nerves

- *Cranial nerve I (olfactory nerve):* Have the patient identify at least two smells.
- *Cranial nerve II (optic nerve):* Test visual acuity and visual fields with confrontation; examine the fundus of the optic nerve.
- *Cranial nerves III (oculomotor nerve), IV (trochlear nerve), and VI (abducent nerve):* Test extraocular movement using the six cardinal positions of gaze.
- *Cranial nerve V (trigeminal nerve):* Check the patient's ability to feel light touch and pain perception over his face; have him clench his teeth to assess temporal and masseter muscles.
- *Cranial nerve VII (facial nerve):* Test taste perception; observe the patient's face for symmetry at rest and when smiling, frowning, and raising eyebrows.
- *Cranial nerve VIII (acoustic nerve):* Test hearing and check balance.
- *Cranial nerves IX (glosssopharyngeal nerve) and X (vagus nerve):* Check the gag reflex.
- *Cranial nerve XI (spinal accessory nerve):* Check the strength of the sternocleidomastoid and trapezius muscles.
- *Cranial nerve XII (hypoglossal nerve):* Assess tongue position, movement, and strength; observe for tongue symmetry.

Assessment of sensory function

- Test pain perception in all dermatomes with the sharp and dull ends of a safety pin.
- Test light touch sensation in all dermatomes using a wisp of cotton.

Neurologic system review *(continued)*

- Test vibratory sense with a tuning fork over bony prominences.
- Assess position sense by having the patient identify whether his toe or finger is positioned up or down as you move it.
- Assess discrimination by testing stereognosis, graphesthesia, and point localization.

Assessment of motor function

- Assess muscle tone by guiding the shoulders and hips through passive ROM exercises.
- Assess muscle strength by having the patient move major muscles and muscle groups against resistance.
- Assess cerebellar function by observing the patient's coordination and general balance, testing extremity coordination, and having the patient perform rapid alternating movements.

Assessment of reflexes

- Test deep tendon reflexes:
  - –biceps reflex
  - –triceps reflex
  - –brachioradialis reflex
  - –patellar reflex
  - –Achilles reflex.
- Test superficial reflexes:
  - –Babinski's reflex (normally absent)
  - –cremasteric reflex (in males)
  - –abdominal reflexes.
- Check for primitive reflexes (shouldn't be present in an adult but are normal in infants):
  - –grasp reflex
  - –snout reflex
  - –suck reflex
  - –glabella response.

Abnormal cranial nerve findings

- Olfactory impairment: inability to detect odors
- Visual impairment: visual field defects, pupillary changes, eye muscle impairment, and facial nerve impairment
- Auditory problems: difficulty hearing high-pitched sounds or total hearing loss
- Vertigo: illusion of movement resulting from a disturbance of vestibular centers
- Dysphagia: difficulty swallowing, typically occurring after a stroke
- Speech disorders: impaired fluency or expression
- Constructional problems: apraxia (inability to perform purposeful movement) and agnosia (inability to identify common objects)

Abnormal muscle movements

- Tics: sudden uncontrolled movements of the face, shoulders, and extremities
- Tremors: involuntary, repetitive movements in the fingers, wrists, eyelids, tongue, and legs
- Fasciculations: fine twitchings in small muscle groups
- Abnormal gaits: spastic, scissoring, propulsive, steppage, waddling

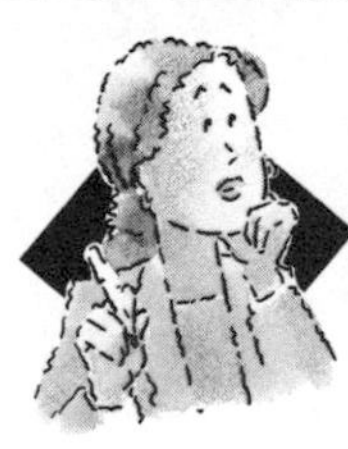

Quick quiz

1. If a patient can't recognize the sound of a ringing phone, he probably has:

A. agnosia.
B. apraxia.
C. aphasia.
D. ataxia.

Answer: A. Agnosia, or the inability to identify common objects, occurs in three forms: visual, auditory, or body image.

2. The most sensitive indicator of a change in a patient's neurologic status is his:

A. gross motor movement.
B. LOC.
C. speech patterns.
D. vision.

Answer: B. While gross motor movement, speech patterns, and vision may change with an alteration in neurologic status, LOC is the most sensitive and earliest indicator of a change in neurologic status.

3. Normal findings in the assessment of gross motor function include:

A. downward drift of the arm when it's outstretched.
B. positive Romberg's test result.
C. ability to distinguish odors.
D. smooth, coordinated gait.

Answer: D. A smooth, coordinated gait is a normal gross motor finding as is a negative Romberg's test result.

4. One of the primitive reflexes is the:

A. patellar reflex.
B. grasping reflex.
C. brachial reflex.
D. triceps reflex.

Answer: B. The grasping, snout, sucking, and glabella reflexes occur normally in infants, whose neurologic systems are immature. These reflexes are abnormal in adults.

5. To test sensation, you'll need a:

A. key and tongue blade.
B. pencil and paper.
C. safety pin and cotton wisp.
D. measuring tape and reflex hammer.

Answer: C. A safety pin and a cotton wisp are used to assess pain and light touch.

Scoring

☆☆☆ If you answered all five questions correctly, wow! There's obviously nothing wrong with your cerebral cortex.

☆☆ If you answered four questions correctly, fantastic! Your alert attention to the details in this chapter really paid off.

☆ If you answered fewer than four questions correctly, don't let it get on your nerves! Try reading the chapter one more time.

Appendices and index

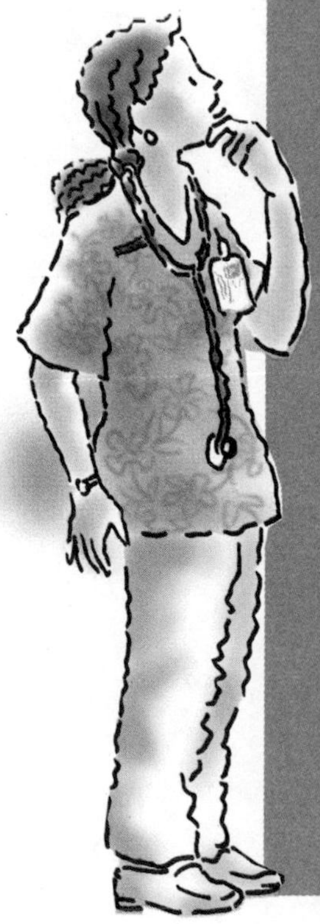

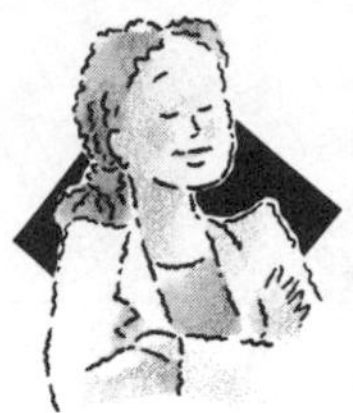

Practice makes perfect

1. An 82-year-old patient is admitted with pneumonia. What's your first priority as you perform his admission assessment?

A. Having the patient sign the admission forms
B. Establishing rapport with the patient
C. Obtaining the necessary equipment
D. Taking the patient's vital signs

2. An 86-year-old patient is admitted to your floor with a diagnosis of syncope. He tells you, "When I get up in the morning, I feel dizzy." You reply, "You feel dizzy when you get out of bed in the morning?" What communication strategy are you using?

A. Reflection
B. Facilitation
C. Confirmation
D. Summarization

3. As an occupational health nurse, you must perform a physical assessment on a prospective company employee. Which of the following areas should be assessed first?

A. Vital signs
B. Presence of skin lesions
C. Anthropometric measurements
D. Appearance

4. A 52-year-old patient is admitted to your facility with unstable angina. When you assess his pulse, you note an irregular rhythm. To further assess the irregular pulse, you determine the patient's pulse deficit. Which pulses help identify the pulse deficit?

A. Carotid and apical
B. Apical and radial
C. Radial and brachial
D. Carotid and radial

5. You're assessing the blood pressure of a patient with diabetic ketoacidosis. How high should you inflate the blood pressure cuff before releasing the valve and listening for the blood pressure?

A. Inflate the cuff until the radial pulse disappears, and then inflate it an additional 30 mm Hg.
B. Inflate the cuff to 200 mm Hg; if you hear the sound immediately, inflate to 220 mm Hg.
C. Inflate the cuff until the needle on the manometer stops bouncing.
D. Inflate the cuff until the patient reports feeling a tingling sensation in his hand.

6. A 52-year-old patient who underwent a right-sided thoracotomy 2 days ago complains of nausea. You perform an abdominal assessment. Which sound should you hear when percussing over dense tissue?

A. Tympany
B. Dullness
C. Flatness
D. Resonance

7. A 73-year-old female patient with Alzheimer's disease is admitted to the hospital with dehydration. Her daughter, who has been caring for the patient at home, verbalizes frustration that the patient refuses to eat or drink because she thinks her family is trying to poison her. You perform anthropometric arm measurements on the patient, and the result is 85% of the standard. What does this result suggest?

A. Caloric deprivation
B. Normalcy
C. Protein malnutrition
D. Caloric excess

8. Your 76-year-old patient is diagnosed with iron deficiency anemia. What would you expect to find when assessing her nails?

A. Dark, yellowish nails
B. Transverse bands of white covering the nails
C. White patches on the nails
D. Spoon-shaped nails

9. A 23-year-old patient is admitted to the inpatient psychiatric unit with severe depression. In developing rapport with her, you initiate a contract. What should the contract include?

A. Expectations and responsibilities for you and the patient
B. A description of the therapies the patient will undergo
C. A prediction of the length of the hospitalization
D. The patient's insurance and financial information

10. You assess a child's visual acuity using the Snellen chart. The result is 20/50 in both eyes. Which explanation should you give to her parent?

A. "What normal eyes see at a distance of 50 feet, your child's eyes see at a distance of 20 feet."
B. "What normal eyes see at a distance of 20 feet, your child's eyes see at a distance of 50 feet."
C. "To see what the normal eye sees at a distance of 20 feet, your child's eyes need a 50% magnification increase."
D. "Your child's eyes see 20% of what children with normal vision see at 50 feet."

11. During an assessment, an 18-year-old states that she uses an addictive substance. What's the most appropriate nursing response?

- A. "How do you obtain the substance?"
- B. "What substance do you use?"
- C. "Does your employer know about this?"
- D. "You really shouldn't do that."

12. During an interview, your patient has episodes in which she jumps abruptly from topic to topic. Which term identifies this type of speech?

- A. Neologisms
- B. Echolalia
- C. Pressured speech
- D. Flight of ideas

13. After making violent threats against her husband, a patient who has just gone through a painful divorce is brought to the inpatient psychiatric unit by the police. Her threats of violence toward her ex-husband are most consistent with which diagnosis?

- A. Schizophrenia
- B. Personality disorder
- C. Anxiety disorder
- D. Obsessive-compulsive disorder

14. A patient is admitted with vomiting after eating at a buffet. You need to assess his skin turgor for signs of dehydration. How should you proceed?

- A. Squeeze the skin on his forearm or sternum.
- B. Palpate the skin on the dorsum of his hand.
- C. Press on his nail beds to cause blanching.
- D. Transilluminate the skin over the forearm.

15. As you assess your patient's skin, you notice a number of small, firm, round, raised lesions on the patient's body. You would chart these findings as:

- A. macules.
- B. pustules.
- C. papules.
- D. plaques.

16. A 49-year-old patient with a history of alcohol abuse is admitted with bleeding esophageal varices. When you assess him you note several small, weblike, vascular lesions on the his cheeks. You would chart these findings as:

- A. purpura.
- B. telangiectases.
- C. angiomas.
- D. petechiae.

17. A 65-year-old patient comes to the plastic surgeon's office for a follow-up appointment after having a basal cell lesion removed from his face. You need to teach him to inspect his skin for signs of melanoma. What should you tell him to look for?

A. Pale patches on the skin
B. Skin flaking that won't go away
C. Black or purple irregularly shaped nodules
D. Flat areas of discoloration.

18. You're working as a school nurse in a local elementary school. A child tells you that his eye itches and tears much more than usual. When you examine his eye, his sclera is reddened. Which eye abnormality do these signs and symptoms most suggest?

A. Cataracts
B. Ptosis
C. Glaucoma
D. Conjunctivitis

19. You're inspecting a child's pupils as part of a routine examination. You shine indirect light into his right eye. What's the normal response?

A. Both eyes dilate.
B. Both eyes constrict.
C. The right eye constricts, and the left eye dilates.
D. There should be no response.

20. You need to perform a mental health assessment of a patient who comes to the clinic seeking help to control her overwhelming anxiety. During the mental health assessment, what should be your focus?

A. To state goals for care of the patient
B. To determine outcomes for the patient
C. To distinguish medical problems from mental health problems
D. To gather information from the patient

21. You're filling in as a substitute school nurse. When an 11-year-old child with an earache and a sore throat reports to the school nurse's office, you inspect the tympanic membrane using an otoscope. Which color suggests a normal eardrum?

A. Pink
B. White
C. Gray
D. Red

22. You're performing an otoscopic examination on a child who has an earache and a fever. In which direction should you pull his auricle to straighten the ear canal?

A. Down and forward
B. Up and forward
C. Up and back
D. Down and back

23. A mother states that her daughter has been complaining for 3 days of a sore throat, which has increased in severity. You palpate the girl's neck and identify a swollen lymph node directly under the chin. Which lymph node is this?
A. Preauricular
B. Submandibular
C. Submental
D. Supraclavicular

24. A 19-year-old college student is brought to the emergency department with dyspnea and asymmetrical breathing patterns after falling down a flight of steps at a party. His admission chest X-ray shows right-sided pneumothorax. During inspection, what other characteristic of pneumothorax might you observe?
A. Funnel chest
B. Barrel chest
C. Intercostal bulging
D. Tracheal deviation

25. After a fall from a scaffold, a 32-year-old construction worker complains of shortness of breath and has labored breathing. His admission chest X-ray reveals right-sided pneumothorax. What sound should you expect when you percuss over the right lung?
A. Tympany
B. Dullness
C. Hyperresonance
D. Flatness

26. You're performing the admission assessment of a 63-year-old patient with pneumonia. While auscultating his lungs, you ask him to repeatedly say "ninety-nine." What are you checking for?
A. Bronchophony
B. Egophony
C. Pectoriloquy
D. Crepitus

27. Your patient develops pneumothorax after an attempted central line insertion. What breath sounds should you expect to hear over the affected lung?
A. Crackles
B. Rhonchi
C. Diminished sounds
D. Wheezes

28. You're evaluating a 46-year-old patient with left lower lobe pneumonia who reports shortness of breath. Identify the area where you may hear fine crackles associated with this condition.

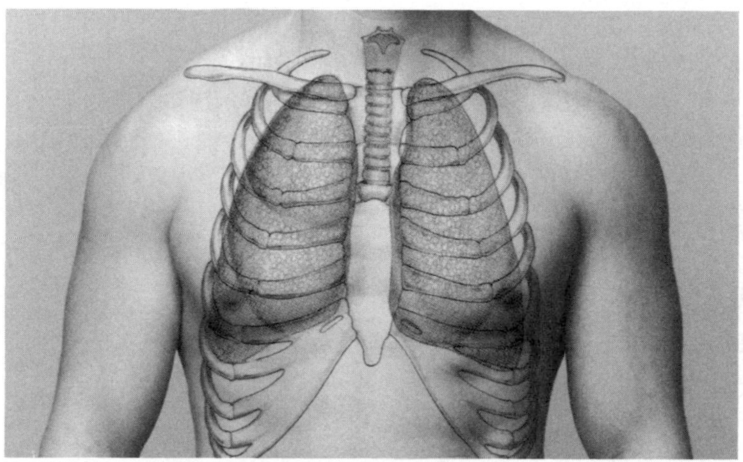

29. A 63-year-old man is hospitalized in the coronary care unit after experiencing an anterior myocardial infarction. As you perform your initial assessment, you palpate the pulses on top of his feet. What are these pulses?

A. Popliteal pulses
B. Dorsalis pedis pulses
C. Posterior tibial pulses
D. Anterior tibial pulses

30. A 57-year-old obese man comes to the emergency department complaining of chest pain that developed while he was eating. You ask the patient to describe his chest pain. Which type of chest pain is most commonly associated with a myocardial infarction (MI)?

A. Sore and aching
B. Dull and stabbing
C. Sharp and burning
D. Tightness and pressure

31. A 19-year-old patient is admitted to the coronary care unit after experiencing a syncopal episode while playing basketball. When auscultating his heart sounds, you hear a "lub-dub" sound. What mechanical event in the heart is associated with the "lub" sound?

A. Closure of the mitral and aortic valves
B. Closure of the tricuspid and aortic valves
C. Closure of the aortic and pulmonic valves
D. Closure of the mitral and tricuspid valves

32. You're inspecting a 58-year-old patient's chest wall to locate the apical impulse. Where should you look?

A. At the fifth intercostal space medial to the left midclavicular line

B. Over the base of the heart

C. Over the aortic area

D. At the third intercostal space to the left of the sternum

33. Which of the following findings is a normal change associated with menopause?

A. Breast enlargement

B. Flattened nipples

C. Asymmetrical areolae

D. Inverted nipples

34. Identify on the illustration below where you should place the diaphragm of your stethoscope to auscultate the pulmonic valve.

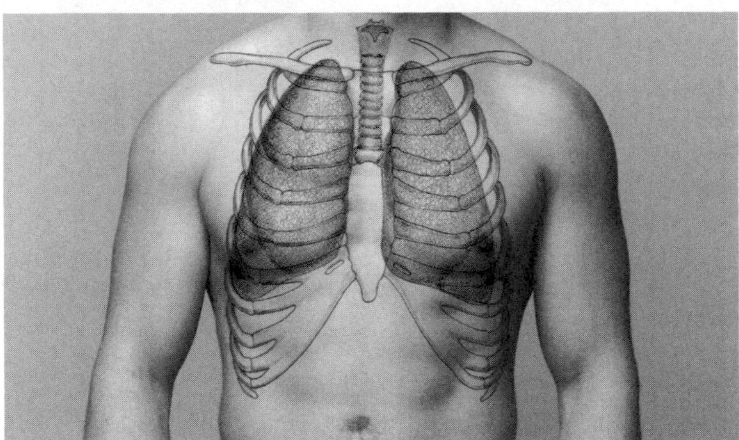

35. During your examination of a 36-year-old woman's right breast, you palpate a lump. Which characteristic most suggests that the lump may be malignant?

A. Softness

B. Mobility

C. Irregular shape

D. Nontender

36. A 28-year-old patient asks, "When should I perform breast self-examination (BSE)?" Which response is best?

A. "On the first day of your menstrual cycle each month."

B. "On the last day of your menstrual cycle each month."

C. "On the first day of every month."

D. "7 to 10 days after your menstrual cycle begins each month."

37. When palpating a patient's breast, it's preferable to use:
- A. the whole palm of the palpating hand.
- B. one index finger.
- C. three middle finger pads.
- D. the pad of the thumb.

38. Burning abdominal pain is most commonly associated with:
- A. cholecystitis.
- B. appendicitis.
- C. peptic ulcer disease.
- D. pancreatitis.

39. A patient comes to the emergency department complaining of right lower quadrant pain and nausea. His temperature is 100.7° F (38.2° C). How should you proceed with his abdominal assessment?
- A. Palpation, percussion, inspection, auscultation
- B. Inspection, auscultation, percussion, palpation
- C. Auscultation, inspection, palpation, percussion
- D. Auscultation, palpation, percussion, inspection

40. The doctor orders daily measurement of abdominal girth for a 35-year-old patient with upper-GI bleeding. At which point on the abdomen should you take your measurement?
- A. Just below the rib cage
- B. Just above the pelvis
- C. Across the umbilicus
- D. At the fullest point

41. Deep palpation of the abdomen shouldn't be performed if the patient:
- A. has ascites.
- B. reports constipation.
- C. is ticklish.
- D. has abdominal rigidity.

42. You're assisting a doctor with a routine pelvic examination. What should you use to lubricate the speculum?
- A. Water-soluble jelly
- B. Petroleum jelly
- C. Warm water
- D. Mineral oil

43. You're teaching a group of fifth-grade girls about menstruation. You tell them that menses occurs every 21 to 38 days and that the duration is normally:
- A. 2 to 4 days.
- B. 2 to 8 days.
- C. 3 to 5 days.
- D. 4 to 7 days.

44. A patient with a urinary tract infection reports pain when you percuss her back at the costovertebral angle. This suggests:

A. a ureteral stone.
B. an ovarian cyst.
C. kidney inflammation.
D. bladder cancer.

45. To assess for scoliosis, you should:

A. palpate for crepitus.
B. measure the length of the spine from neck to waist.
C. ask the patient to bend forward at the waist.
D. palpate the spinous processes.

46. A 28-year-old man tells you that he noticed a lump in his scrotum. Before palpating his testicles, you should know that a normal testicle is:

A. irregularly shaped.
B. round.
C. rubbery.
D. nodular.

47. You're assessing a patient with an abdominal aortic aneurysm. Identify in the illustration below the area of the abdomen where you would auscultate for a bruit over the aorta.

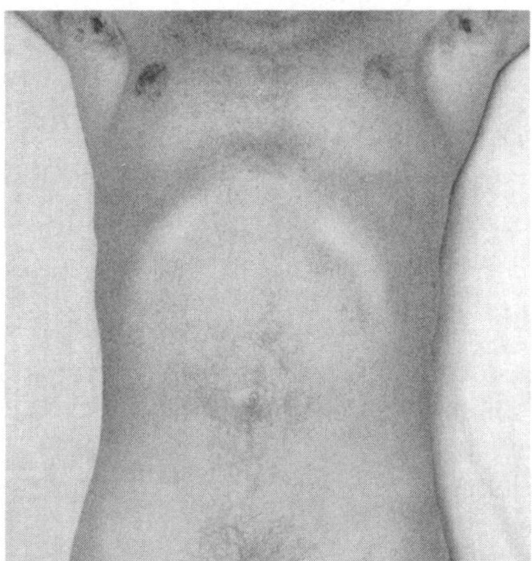

48. A 46-year-old construction worker comes to the clinic for his annual physical examination. During the assessment, you palpate his inguinal area. Why?

A. To check for herniation
B. To locate a pulse
C. To check for a nondescended testicle
D. To assess the prostate gland

49. A 62-year-old comes to the clinic complaining of urinary hesitancy. During the assessment, you palpate his prostate gland. You should know that a normal prostate gland is about the size of a:

A. marble.
B. grape.
C. walnut.
D. peach.

50. After slipping in her bathroom, an 80-year-old patient is brought to the emergency department with a deformed right hip and hip pain that she rates as an 8 on a scale of 1 to 10. When you examine her, you notice gross internal rotation of the right hip. Which of the following signs alerts you to this?

A. A misshapen pelvis
B. Inward pointing of the foot
C. Outward pointing of the foot
D. Unequal leg lengths

51. A 34-year-old patient is complaining of pain and tingling in her right wrist. During your examination, the patient reports pain when the wrist is flexed for 30 seconds. This finding indicates:

A. a fractured wrist.
B. carpal tunnel syndrome.
C. a stroke.
D. paralysis.

52. A 58-year-old man comes to the clinic for his annual physical examination. You collect a urine specimen from him and notice that his urine has a brown appearance. What does this finding suggest?

A. Hypervolemia
B. Benign prostatic hyperplasia
C. Biliary obstruction
D. Hematuria

53. You are assessing the leg of a patient who has come to the emergency department with a suspected fractured femur. To perform a quick and accurate assessment, you should evaluate the affected leg for which of the following signs and symptoms?

Select all that apply.

A. Pain
B. Pliability
C. Paresthesia
D. Paralysis
E. Pallor
F. Pulses

54. A 30-year-old is brought to the emergency department with head injuries from a motorcycle accident. During your neurologic assessment, the patient displays Babinski's reflex. This finding is:
- A. an abnormal response.
- B. a normal response.
- C. a hyperactive response.
- D. a diminished response.

55. During a routine physical examination, a 68-year-old patient can't identify a pencil or a cotton ball when manipulating the objects with his hands, keeping his eyes closed. This abnormal finding indicates impaired:
- A. apraxia.
- B. aphasia.
- C. graphesthesia.
- D. stereognosis.

56. You're assessing the cranial nerves of a 62-year-old patient who had a stroke. How should you assess the function of the facial nerve (cranial nerve VII)?
- A. Test the patient's hearing and ask him if he ever experiences dizziness or vertigo.
- B. Test the patient's ability to feel light touch on his face as well as his ability to differentiate sharp and dull sensations on his face.
- C. Test the patient's ability to identify tastes, and observe his face for symmetry at rest and while making facial expressions, such as smiling or frowning.
- D. Test the patient's gag reflex and his ability to swallow.

57. A patient's muscle tone is assessed by performing:
- A. deep tendon reflex testing.
- B. passive range-of-motion (ROM) exercises.
- C. Romberg's test.
- D. point localization testing.

Answers

1. B. The first priority of a successful physical assessment is establishing rapport with the patient.

2. A. Reflection is repeating something a patient has just said. This technique can help you obtain more-specific information.

3. D. After assembling the necessary equipment, you should perform the first part of your assessment—forming your initial impression of the patient by observing his appearance.

4. B. When determining a pulse deficit, you should palpate the radial pulse while auscultating the apical pulse. The apical pulse rate minus the radial pulse rate equals the pulse deficit.

5. A. You should neither underinflate nor overinflate the cuff. The ideal method is to palpate the radial pulse while inflating the cuff. When the radial pulse disappears, inflate the cuff an additional 30 mm Hg and then close the valve.

6. C. When percussing over dense tissue, such as muscle, you should expect to hear flatness.

7. A. Anthropometric arm measurements help assess nutritional status. Less than 90% of the standard indicates caloric deprivation.

8. D. Patients with iron deficiency anemia typically have spoon-shaped nails.

9. A. A contract with a psychiatric patient should include your expectations and responsibilities as well as the patient's.

10. A. The Snellen chart measures visual acuity and provides readings such as 20/50. A person with 20/50 vision can view from 20′ that which a person with normal vision can view from 50′.

11. B. When a patient identifies a history of substance abuse, it's important for you to assess the risk of withdrawal, which includes determining the substance being used.

12. D. A continuous flow of speech in which the patient jumps abruptly from topic to topic is called *flight of ideas.*

13. B. Pervasive maladaptive patterns of behavior suggest a personality disorder.

14. A. To evaluate skin turgor, gently squeeze the skin on the forearm or sternum. If the skin quickly returns to its original shape, the patient's skin turgor is normal. If it returns to its original shape slowly over 30 seconds or maintains a tented position, the skin has poor turgor, which is a sign of dehydration.

15. C. Papules are small, raised, circumscribed, solid lesions.

16. B. Telangiectases are small, dilated vessels that form a web-like pattern. They're commonly seen on the face, especially in patients with a history of alcohol abuse.

17. C. Typically, melanomas are black or purple nodules that are irregularly shaped.

18. D. Conjunctivitis causes redness of the eye as well as itching and increased tearing.

19. B. Shining a light in the right eye should cause right eye constriction (direct) and left eye constriction (consensual).

20. D. The focus of the mental health assessment should be to gather information from the patient so you can develop a plan of care.

21. C. The normal eardrum (tympanic membrane) is gray.

22. C. To perform an otoscopic examination on a patient age 3 or older, pull the auricle up and back to straighten the ear canal.

23. C. The submental lymph node is located directly under the chin.

24. D. With any type of pneumothorax, you may observe intercostal retractions; with right-sided pneumothorax, tracheal deviation to the left may also be present.

25. C. For a patient with pneumothorax, the pleural space on the affected side is increased, which produces a hyperresonant sound on percussion.

26. A. When testing for bronchophony, the patient must say "ninety-nine" or "blue moon" while you auscultate his lungs. Over normal tissue, the words sound muffled; over consolidated areas, such as those that occur with pneumothorax, the words sound unusually loud.

27. C. With pneumothorax, air movement is diminished or absent in the affected lung, so breath sounds are diminished in that area.

28. To auscultate the left lower lobe from the anterior chest, use the landmarks of the left anterior axillary line, between the fifth and sixth intercostal spaces.

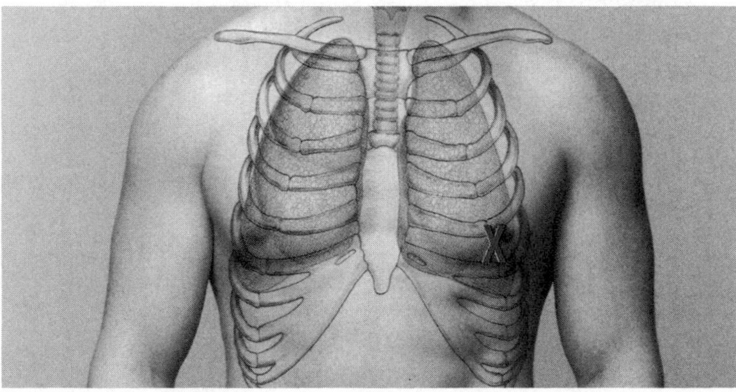

29. B. The pulses on the tops of the feet are the dorsalis pedis pulses.

30. D. The pain typically associated with an MI is characterized by tightness and pressure.

31. D. The first heart sound, S_1, which produces the "lub" sound, is associated with closure of the mitral and tricuspid valves.

32. A. The apical impulse, also usually the point of maximum impulse, can be found at the fifth intercostal space medial to the left midclavicular line.

33. B. After menopause, glandular tissues atrophy and are replaced with fatty deposits. The breasts become flabbier and smaller, and the nipples flatten and become less erectile.

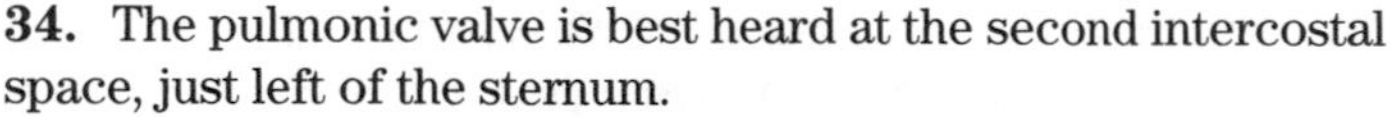

34. The pulmonic valve is best heard at the second intercostal space, just left of the sternum.

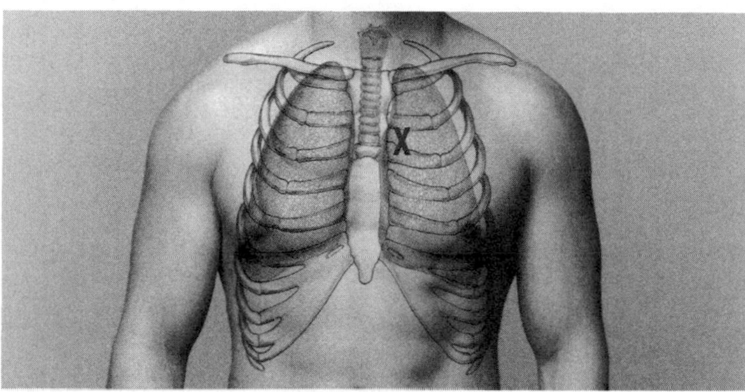

35. C. An irregularly shaped lump in the breast suggests malignancy.

36. D. Because certain changes take place in the breasts during the menstrual cycle, it's best for a menstruating woman to perform BSE 7 to 10 days after the beginning of her cycle.

37. C. When palpating a patient's breast, it's preferable to use three middle finger pads and to gently rotate them around the breast, moving in concentric circles.

38. C. Burning abdominal pain is most commonly associated with peptic ulcer disease.

39. B. The proper order for abdominal assessment is inspection, auscultation, percussion, and palpation.

40. D. When measuring abdominal girth, you should measure the abdomen at its fullest point.

41. D. Because abdominal rigidity may indicate peritoneal inflammation, palpation should be avoided because it may lead to pain or organ rupture.

42. C. Water should be used to lubricate the speculum before an internal vaginal examination. Other lubricants are discouraged because they can alter the results of a Papanicolaou test.

43. B. The duration of menses in a normal menstrual cycle is 2 to 8 days.

44. C. Pain during percussion over the costovertebral angle suggests kidney inflammation.

45. C. To assess for scoliosis, inspect the spine for abnormalities while the patient is bending forward at the waist. This position can make spinal deformities more apparent.

46. C. A normal testicle is oval and rubbery.

47. An aortic bruit is best heard with the stethoscope bell placed at the midline of the abdomen, slightly below the xiphoid process.

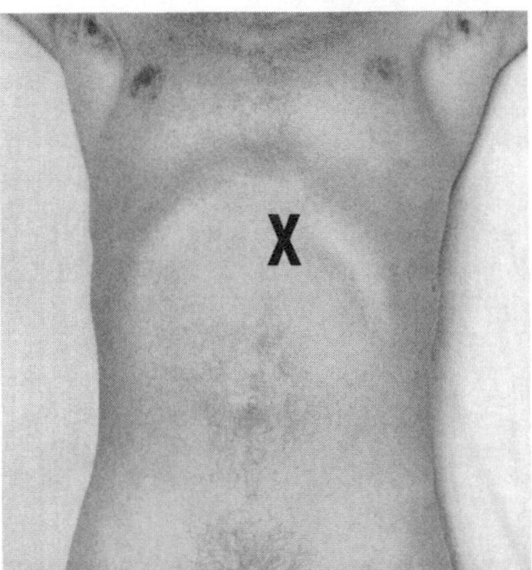

48. A. The purpose of palpating a patient's inguinal area during assessment is to check for herniation.

49. C. A normal prostate gland is about the size of a walnut.

50. B. With internal rotation of the hip, inward turning and pointing of the foot to a pigeon-toed position occurs.

51. B. Pain or numbness in the hand or fingers that occurs when the patient's wrist is flexed is called *Phalen's sign.* This finding is indicative of carpal tunnel syndrome.

52. D. A patient with hematuria may have brown or bright red urine.

53. A, C, D, E, F. To perform a swift assessment of a musculoskeletal injury, remember the 5 P's: pain, paresthesia, paralysis, pallor, and pulses.

54. A. Although Babinski's reflex is a normal finding in infants and children younger than age 2, it's always an abnormal finding in adults.

55. D. The ability to identify a common object by touching and manipulating it is called *stereognosis.* If the patient has impaired stereognosis, test graphesthesia next.

56. C. The facial nerve has sensory and motor components. Assess the sensory component by testing the patient's taste perception, and test the motor component by observing the function of the facial muscles.

57. B. Muscle tone, which represents muscular resistance to passive stretching, is assessed by performing passive ROM exercises.

Glossary

accommodation: a change in the shape of the lens that allows the eye to focus on a nearby object; accompanied by constriction of the pupils and convergence of the eyes

adnexa: appendages of the uterus, including the ovaries, fallopian tubes, and supporting tissues

alert: term used to describe a patient who can follow commands, comprehend verbal and written language, and express ideas freely and is oriented to time, place, and person

alopecia: hair loss

amplitude: strength of a pulse or other force; recorded as bounding, normal, weak, or absent

anisocoria: unequal pupils

ankylosis: fixation of a joint due to fibrous or bony union; results from a disease process

anorexia: loss of appetite

anthropometric measurements: measurements of the human body taken as part of a comprehensive nutritional assessment; include midarm circumference, skin-fold thickness, and midarm muscle circumference

aphasia: language disorder characterized by difficulty expressing or comprehending speech

apraxia: inability to perform coordinated movements, even though no motor deficit is present

ascites: accumulation of fluid in the abdominal cavity

ataxia: uncoordinated actions when voluntary muscle movements are attempted

auscultation: physical assessment technique by which the examiner listens (usually with a stethoscope) for sounds coming from the heart, lungs, abdomen, or other organs

bimanual palpation: method of palpation involving the use of two hands to locate body structures and assess their texture, size, consistency, mobility, and tenderness

borborygmus: loud, gurgling, splashing sounds caused by gas passing through the intestine; normally heard over the large intestine

bruit: abnormal sound heard over peripheral vessels that indicates turbulent blood flow

cardiac cycle: the period from the beginning of one heartbeat to the beginning of the next; includes two phases, systole and diastole

cataract: opacity of the lens of the eye

cerumen: waxlike secretion in the external ear

closed questions: questions that elicit yes-or-no answers

coma: unconscious state in which the patient appears to be asleep, doesn't speak, and responds to neither body nor environmental stimuli

consensual light reflex: reflex constriction of the pupil of one eye when the other eye is illuminated

crackles: intermittent, nonmusical, crackling breath sounds that are caused by collapsed or fluid-filled alveoli popping open

cremasteric reflex: superficial reflex in men; elicited by stroking the upper inner thigh, which causes brisk retraction of the testis on the side of the stimulus

crepitus: noise or vibration produced by rubbing together irregular cartilage surfaces or broken ends of a bone; also the sound heard when air in subcutaneous tissue is palpated

dimpling: puckering or depression of the skin of the breast possibly caused by underlying growth; also called *retraction*

diplopia: double vision

dorsal lithotomy position: position commonly used for female pelvic examinations in which the patient lies on her back with her hips and knees flexed and her thighs abducted and rotated externally

dysarthria: speech defect commonly related to a motor deficit of the tongue or speech muscles

dysphagia: difficulty swallowing

Erb's point: auscultatory point on the precordium at the third intercostal space to the left of the sternum

exophthalmos: abnormal protrusion of the eyeball

expressive aphasia: inability to express words or thoughts

flaccidity: decreased muscle tone, which causes muscle to become weak or flabby

fluid wave: rippling across the abdomen during percussion; indicative of the presence of ascites

fremitus: palpable vibration that results from air passing through the bronchopulmonary system and transmitting vibrations to the chest wall

gynecomastia: enlargement of breast tissue in a male

hematuria: presence of blood in the urine

hernia: abnormal protrusion of a structure through an opening; for example, the protrusion of a loop of bowel through a muscle wall

hirsutism: excessive hair growth; may be hereditary, a sign of an endocrine disorder, or an effect of certain drugs

hordeolum: inflammation of the sebaceous gland of the eyelid; also called *stye*

hydrocele: accumulation of serous fluid in a saclike structure such as the testis

hyperopia: defect in vision that allows a person to see objects clearly at a distance but not at close range; also called *farsightedness*

hyperresonance: increased resonance produced by percussion

inspection: critical observation of the patient during which the examiner may use sight, hearing, or smell to make informed observations

intensity: degree of strength; for example, the loudness of a heart murmur recorded as soft, medium, or loud

introitus: entrance to a canal or cavity, such as the vagina

jaundice: yellowish discoloration of the skin caused by the accumulation of bilirubin

kwashiorkor: protein-deficiency malnutrition that occurs in young children and involves a loss of visceral protein

lethargy: slowed responses, sluggish speech, and slowed mental and motor processes in a person oriented to time, place, and person

lichenification: thickening of the skin related to eczema that occurs especially in the antecubital and popliteal fossae

mammogram: X-ray of the breast used to detect tumors and other abnormalities

marasmus: protein and calorie malnutrition that primarily affects children ages 6 to 18 months; results from a chronic lack of nutrients

meatus: opening or passageway in the body

menarche: first menstrual period

menopause: cessation of the menstrual period

murmur: abnormal sound heard on auscultation of the heart; caused by abnormal blood flow through a valve

mydriasis: dilation of the pupil due to paralysis of the oculomotor muscles or the effects of drugs

myopia: defect in vision that allows a person to see objects clearly at close range but not at a distance; also called *nearsightedness*

nipple inversion: inward turning or depression of the central portion of the nipple

nystagmus: involuntary, rhythmic movement of the eye

objective data: information verifiable through direct observation, laboratory tests, screening procedures, or physical examination

occult blood: blood hidden in stool or urine that can be detected with a guaiac test

open-ended question: question that requires an answer in a sentence form rather than a yes-or-no form

palpation: physical assessment technique by which the examiner uses the sense of touch to feel pulsations and vibrations or to locate body structures and assess their texture, size, consistency, mobility, and tenderness

peau d'orange: orange-peel appearance of breast skin caused by edema; associated with breast cancer

percussion: physical assessment technique by which the examiner taps on the skin surface with his fingers to assess the size, border, and consistency of internal organs and to detect and evaluate fluid in a body cavity

peristalsis: sequence of muscle contractions that propels food through the GI tract

pitch: frequency of a sound, measured in the number of sound waves generated per second

point of maximum impulse (PMI): point at which the upward thrust of the heart against the chest wall is greatest, usually over the apex of the heart

precordium: area of the chest over the heart

protein-calorie malnutrition (PCM): spectrum of disorders resulting from either prolonged or chronic inadequate protein or calorie intake or from high metabolic requirements for protein and energy

pruritus: severe itching

ptosis: drooping of the eyelid

rebound tenderness: sharp, stabbing pain that occurs when the abdomen is pushed in deeply and then suddenly released; usually associated with peritoneal inflammation

receptive aphasia: inability to understand spoken word

resonance: clear, hollow, low-pitched sound produced by percussion; typically heard over normal lungs

rhonchi: low-pitched, snoring, rattling breath sounds that may be heard on inhalation or exhalation

strabismus: lack of coordination of eye muscles

striae: stripes or lines of tissue differing in color and texture from the surrounding tissue

stridor: loud, high-pitched crowing sound usually heard during inspiration without the need for a stethoscope

stupor: state in which a patient lies quietly with minimal spontaneous movement and is unresponsive except to vigorous and repeated stimuli

subjective data: information that the patient, his family, or his friends give about the patient's current health care status during the health history; reflects the personal perspective of the patient, family, and friends

synovial joint: type of freely movable joint lined with a synovial membrane that secretes synovial fluid for lubrication

tail of Spence: extension of breast tissue that projects from the upper outer quadrant of the breast toward the axilla

telangiectasis: permanently dilated small blood vessels that form a weblike pattern; may be the result of scleroderma, lupus erythematosus, or cirrhosis or may be normal in healthy, older adults

thrill: palpable vibration felt over the heart or vessel that results from turbulent blood flow

tinnitus: ringing sound in one or both ears

tone: normal degree of vigor and tension; in muscle, the normal degree of tension

tympany: musical, drumlike sound heard during percussion over a hollow organ such as the stomach; a normal sound

vertigo: illusion that one's body or surroundings is moving

vitiligo: areas of complete absence of melanin pigment leading to patchy areas of white or light skin

wheezes: high-pitched breath sounds heard first on exhalation that occur when airflow is blocked

Selected references

Alcenius, M. "Successfully Meet Pain Assessment Standards," *Nursing Management* 35(3):12, March 2004.

Anatomy & Physiology Made Incredibly Easy! 2nd ed. Philadelphia: Lippincott Williams & Wilkins, 2005.

Andrews, M.M., and Boyle, J.S. *Transcultural Concepts in Nursing Care*, 4th ed. Philadelphia: Lippincott Williams & Wilkins, 2003.

Assessment: A 2-in-1 Reference for Nurses. Philadelphia: Lippincott Williams & Wilkins, 2004.

Bickley, L.S. *Bates' Guide to Physical Examination and History Taking*, 8th ed. Philadelphia: Lippincott Williams & Wilkins, 2004.

Bourbonnais, F.F., Perreault, A., and Bouvette, M. "Introduction of a Pain and Symptom Assessment Tool in the Clinical Setting—Lessons Learned," *Journal of Nursing Management* 12(3):194-200, May 2004.

Coviello, J.S. "Cardiac Assessment 101: A New Look at the Guidelines for Cardiac Homecare Patients," *Home Healthcare Nurse* 22(2):116-23, February 2004.

Doughty, D.B. "Wound Assessment: Tips and Techniques," *Home Healthcare Nurse* 22(3):192-95, March 2004.

Elkayam, J., and English, K. "Counseling Adolescents with Hearing Loss with the Use of Self-Assessment/Significant Other Questionnaires," *Journal of the American Academy of Audiology* 14(9):485-99, November 2003.

Giger, J.N., and Davidhizar, R.E. *Transcultural Nursing: Assessment and Intervention*, 4th ed. St. Louis: Mosby–Year Book, Inc., 2004.

McLeod, R.P. "Lumps, Bumps, and Things That Go Itch in Your Office!" *Journal of School Nursing* 20(4):245-46, August 2004.

Middleton, C. "The Assessment and Treatment of Patients with Chronic Pain," *Nursing Times* 100(18):40-44, May 2004.

Montgomery, R.K. "Pain Management in Burn Injury," *Critical Care Nursing Clinics of North America* 16(1):39-49, March 2004.

Potter, P.A., and Perry, A.G. *Fundamentals of Nursing*, 6th ed. St. Louis: Mosby–Year Book, Inc., 2005.

Prabhu, F.R., and Bickley, L.S. *Case Studies to Accompany Bates' Guide to Physical Examination and History Taking*, 8th ed. Philadelphia: Lippincott Williams & Wilkins, 2002.

Professional Guide to Signs and Symptoms, 4th ed. Philadelphia: Lippincott Williams & Wilkins, 2003.

Pullen, R.L., Jr. "Neurologic Assessment for Pronator Drift," *Nursing2004* 34(3):22, March 2004.

Rapid Assessment: A Flowchart Guide to Evaluating Signs & Symptoms. Philadelphia: Lippincott Williams & Wilkins, 2003.

SkillMasters: 3-Minute Assessment. Philadelphia: Lippincott Williams & Wilkins, 2002.

Walsh, S. "Formulation of a Plan of Care for Culturally Diverse Patients," *International Journal of Nursing Terminologies and Classifications* 15(1):17-26, January-March 2004.

Woodrow, P. "Assessing Blood Pressure in Older People," *Nursing Older People* 16(1):29-31, March 2004.

Index

t refers to a table; i refers to an illustration; **boldface** indicates color pages.

t refers to a table; i refers to an illustration; **boldface** indicates color pages.

t refers to a table; i refers to an illustration; **boldface** indicates color pages.

R

S

T

U

V

WXYZ